CANCER BIOLOGY

Books are to be r⊑

We work with leading authors to develop the
strongest educational materials in biology,
bringing cutting-edge thinking and best learning
practice to a global market

Under a range of well-known imprints, including
Prentice Hall, we craft high-quality print and
electronic publications which help readers to
understand and apply their content,
whether studying or at work

To find out more about the complete range of our
publishing, please visit us on the World Wide Web at:
www.pearsoned.co.uk

Cancer Biology

Third Edition

ROGER J B KING
SCHOOL OF BIOLOGICAL SCIENCES,
UNIVERSITY OF SURREY

MIKE W ROBINS
DEPARTMENT OF PHYSIOLOGY,
KING'S COLLEGE LONDON

PEARSON
Prentice
Hall

Harlow, England • London • New York • Boston • San Francisco • Toronto • Sydney • Singapore • Hong Kong
Tokyo • Seoul • Taipei • New Delhi • Cape Town • Madrid • Mexico City • Amsterdam • Munich • Paris • Milan

Pearson Education Limited
Edinburgh Gate
Harlow
Essex CM20 2JE
England

and Associated Companies throughout the world

Visit us on the World Wide Web at:
www.pearsoned.co.uk

First published under the Longman imprint 1996
Second edition 2000
Third edition 2006

ISBN (13): 978-0-13-129454-7
ISBN (10): 0-13-129454-7

British Library Cataloguing-in-Publication Data
A catalogue record for this book is available from the British Library

Library of Congress Cataloging-in-Publication Data
King, R.J.B. (Roger John Benjamin)
    Cancer biology / R.J.B. King, M.W. Robins.—3rd ed.
        p.; cm.
    Includes bibliographical references and index.
    ISBN-13; 978-0-13-129454-7
    ISBN-10: 0-13-129454-7
    1. Cancer. 2. Carcinogenesis. I. Robins, M.W. (Mike W.) II. Title.
    [DNLM: 1. Neoplasms—physiopathology. 2. Neoplasms—etiology.
    3. Neoplasms—therapy. QZ 200 K54c 2006]
    RC254.6.K54 2006
    616.994′4—dc22

                                                    2005056451

10 9 8 7 6 5 4 3 2 1
10 09 08 07 06

Typeset in 10/12pt Bembo by 35
Printed by Ashford Colour Press Ltd., Gosport

The publisher's policy is to use paper manufactured from sustainable forests.

Brief contents

Detailed contents

1. What is cancer?   1

2. Natural history: the life of a cancer   9

3. Pathology: defining a neoplasm   32

8. Familial cancers   128

9. Growth: a balance of cell proliferation, death and differentiation   139

10. Responding to the environment: growth regulation and signal transduction   168

11. Invasion and metastasis   209

12. Principles of cancer treatment 230

13. Approaches to cancer prevention 263

Preface

The basic format of Professor King's successful book has been retained. One small change has been to move the references to the end of each chapter, where hopefully they are more in context. The advances in the field in the four/five years the since the second edition have been considerable, and while I have attempted to cover the area, there will undoubtedly be some gaps. I wish to thank to staff at King's College, especially Dr Rob Brooks, for his help, my students for keeping me on my toes, and those kind enough to offer advice and criticism. Finally thanks to my wife Jackie for her forbearance, without which I would not have completed this work.

Dr Mike Robins

Preface to the second edition

In collecting the information to revise this book, I was impressed by the advances that have been made over the four years since the first edition was written. When one is actively involved in specific areas of cancer research, it is possible to get frustrated at periods of limited progress. However, when one takes a broader perspective, as I have done here, it is clear that substantial progress continues on many fronts: I congratulate the workers involved and I hope they will get 'the cure' before I need it! This will be my last substantial piece of scientific writing, so I would like to conclude with special thanks to four scientists from whose guidance I have benefited enormously: Professor Guy Marrian FRS, Professor Sir Michael Stoker FRS, Professor Sir Walter Bodmer FRS and Dr Veronica King. The first three were successive directors of research at the Imperial Cancer Research Fund and without them I would not have got very far; without the last person, my wife, I would have got nowhere.

Roger JB King

Preface to the first edition

This book is intended to provide information, at undergraduate level, on the biological principles underlying the causes and treatments of cancer. It is structured to illustrate those principles with specific examples taken wherever possible from human cancers. The human emphasis is supplemented with data from other species wherever appropriate.

The basis for the book is a 20-lecture module I give to final-year students in the School of Biological Sciences, University of Surrey. The students are mostly following a biochemistry and molecular biology-based course but include microbiologists with minimal knowledge of mammalian cell function. The microbiologists cope well with the mammalian information and most difficulties arise with the section on how cells communicate with their environment (Chapter 10). There are no medical students at Surrey but the course would be well tailored to their requirements.

The stimulus for preparing the book came from the realisation that a modern affordable book at the appropriate level did not exist. There are good multi-author volumes whose expense precludes widespread student use. The academic level of this book has been pitched somewhat higher than that required for a good degree at this university. The offering of information more detailed than required, particularly in molecular detail, is intentional so as to cater for the wide range of abilities among the students and to lead the more adventurous students to further study.

In addition to the Surrey students, other sources of help in compiling this book should be acknowledged. Veronica King, Tony Avades, Jack Salway, Brian Stace, Ron Hubbard, Maurice Coombes, Ian Hart, Margaret Green and Wynne Aherne contributed greatly to the generation of an understandable text. The Imperial Cancer Research Fund is to be thanked for providing me with a lifetime's working environment in which I learned the basics encompassed by this book and then for giving me the freedom to write it.

Roger JB King

This book is dedicated to
the students of SBS310 in the
School of Biological Sciences,
University of Surrey

Acknowledgements

We are grateful to the following for permission to reproduce copyright material:

Figure 1.1: Adapted from Figure 9.6 in DeVita, V.T., Hellman, S. and Rosenberg, S.A. (eds) (1993) *Cancer: Principles and Practice of Oncology*, Fourth Edition. Philadelphia, PA: Lippincott; Figure 2.3: Graph adapted from Tannock, I.F. (1968) *British Journal of Cancer*, **22**, 258–73. Copyright © 1968. Reprinted with permission of Macmillan Publishers Ltd; Figure 2.4: Based on data in Muller, W.J., *et al.* (1988) *Cell*, **54**, 105–15. Copyright © 1988. Reproduced with permission from Elsevier; Figure 2.8: Based on data in Anderson, M.J. and Stanbridge, E.J. (1993) *FASEB Journal*, **7**, 826–33; Figure 2.9: Reproduced from Figure 24.3 in Alberts, B., Bray, D., Lewis, J., Raff, M., Roberts, K. and Watson J.D. (1994) *Molecular Biology of the Cell*, Third Edition. New York: Garland Publishing. Reproduced by permission of Garland Science / Taylor & Francis LLC; Figure 4.3: Adapted from American Cancer Society (1995) *Cancer Facts and Figures*. Philadelphia, PA: American Cancer Society. Reprinted by permission of the American Cancer Society. All rights reserved; Figure 4.5: Adapted from Crawford, F.G., *et al.* (1994) *Journal of the National Cancer Institute*, **86**, 1398–1402. Reproduced with permission from Oxford University Press; Figure 4.6: Adapted from Greenblatt, M.S., *et al.* (1994) Mutations in the p53 tumor suppressor gene: clues to cancer etiology and molecular pathogenesis. *Cancer Research*, **54**, 4855–78. Reprinted with permission from the American Association for Cancer Research; Figure 4.7: Reproduced from Figure 3 in Greenblatt, M.S., *et al.* (1994) Mutations in the p53 tumor suppressor gene: clues to cancer etiology and molecular pathogenesis. *Cancer Research*, **54**, 4855–78. Reproduced with permission from the American Association for Cancer Research; Figure 4.8: Adapted from Figure 2.8 in Tannock, I.F. and Hill, R.P. (eds) (1992) *The Basic Science of Oncology*, Second Edition. New York: McGraw-Hill. Reprinted with permission of the McGraw-Hill Companies; Figure 4.9: Based on data in World Cancer Research Fund / American Institute for Cancer Research (1997) *Food, Nutrition and the Prevention of Cancer: A Global Perspective*. Washington, DC: American Institute for Cancer Research. Reprinted with permission; Figure 4.10: Adapted from Figure 9 in Hirayama, T.J. (1992) *National Cancer Institute Monograph*, **12**, 65–74; Figure 4.11: Based on data in World Cancer Research Fund / American Institute for Cancer Research (1997) *Food, Nutrition and the Prevention of Cancer: A Global Perspective*. Washington, DC: American Institute for Cancer Research. Reprinted with permission; Table 4.1: Adapted from Table 9.5 in DeVita, V.T., Hellman, S. and Rosenberg, S.A. (eds) (1993) *Cancer: Principles and Practice of Oncology*, Fourth Edition. Philadelphia, PA: Lippincott; Table 4.2: Based on data in Bosch, F.X., *et al.* (1992) *International Journal of Cancer*, **52**, 750–58; Tables 4.4 and 4.5: Adapted from Table 9.5 in DeVita, V.T., Hellman,

S. and Rosenberg, S.A. (eds) (1993) *Cancer: Principles and Practice of Oncology*, Fourth Edition. Philadelphia, PA: Lippincott; Table 4.6: Based on data in World Cancer Research Fund / American Institute for Cancer Research (1997) *Food, Nutrition and the Prevention of Cancer: A Global Perspective*. Washington, DC: American Institute for Cancer Research. Reprinted with permission; Table 4.9: Adapted from Wynder, E.L. (1977) *Nature*, **268**, 284. Copyright © 1977. Reprinted with permission of Macmillan Publishers Ltd; Figure 5.12: Based on data in Kinzler, K.W. and Vogelstein, B. (1996) *Cell*, **87**, 159–70. Copyright © 1996. Reproduced with permission of Elsevier; Figure 6.12: Adapted from Figure 4 in Levine, A.J., *et al.* (1994) *British Journal of Cancer*, **69**, 409–16. Copyright © 1994. Reprinted with permission of Macmillan Publishers Ltd; Table 6.7: Adapted from Table 12.2 in DeVita, V.T., Hellman, S. and Rosenburg, S.A. (eds) (1993) *Cancer: Principles and Practice of Oncology*, Fourth Edition. Philadelphia, PA: Lippincott; Table 6.8: Reproduced from Table 1 in Greenblatt, M.S., *et al.* (1994) Mutations in the p53 tumor suppressor gene: clues to cancer etiology and molecular pathogenesis. *Cancer Research*, **54**, 4855–78. Reproduced with permission from the American Association for Cancer Research; Table 6.9: Reproduced from Table 2 in Greenblatt, M.S., *et al.* (1994) Mutations in the p53 tumor suppressor gene: clues to cancer etiology and molecular pathogenesis. *Cancer Research*, **54**, 4855–78. Reproduced with permission from the American Association for Cancer Research; Table 7.1: Based on data in Simpson, A.J.G. (1997) *Advances in Cancer Research*, **71**, 209–240. Copyright © 1997. Reproduced with permission of Elsevier; Figure 9.5: Adapted from Figure 1 in Peters G. (1994) *Nature*, **371**, 204–5. Copyright © 1977. Reprinted with permission of Macmillan Publishers Ltd; Figure 9.20: Based on data in Sieweke, M.H. and Graff, T. (1998) *Current Opinion in Genetics and Development*, **8**, 545–551. Copyright © 1998. Reproduced with permission of Elsevier; Table 10.3: Based on data in Sawyers, C.L. and Denny, C.T. (1994) Cell, 77, 171–73. Copyright © 1994. Reproduced with permission of Elsevier; Figure 11.4: Adapted from Figure 4 in Maemura, M. and Dickson, R.B. (1994) *Breast Cancer Research and Treatment*, **32**, 239–60; Figure 12.2: Adapted from Figure 1 in Galea, M.H., *et al.* (1992) *Breast Cancer Research and Treatment*, **22**, 207–19; Figure 12.3: From Jordan, V. Craig (ed) (1986) *Estrogen/Antiestrogen Action and Breast Cancer Therapy*. Madison, WI: University of Wisconsin Press. Copyright © 1986. Reprinted with permission of University of Wisconsin Press; Figure 12.4: Läärä, E., Day, N.E., and Hakama, M. (1987) Trends in mortality from cervical cancer in the Nordic countries: association with organised screening programmes. *Lancet* i 1247–9; Figure 12.7: Adapted from Fig. 17.2 in Franks, L.M. and Teich, N.M. (eds) (1991) *Introduction to the Cellular and Molecular Biology of Cancer*, Second Edition. Oxford: Oxford University Press. Reproduced by permission of Oxford University Press; Figure 12.14: Based on data in Lobell, R.B. and Kohl, N.E. (1998) *Cancer and Metastasis Reviews*, **17**, 203–210; Figure 12.15: Based on data in Kohls, W.D., Fry, D.W. and Kraker A.J. (1997) *Current Opinion in Oncology*, **9**, 562–68; Table 12.1: Adapted from Brenner, H. (2002) *The Lancet*, 360, 1131–35. Reproduced with permission of Elsevier; Figure 13.2: Based on data in Stanford, J.L. (1991) *Contraception*, **43**, 543–46. Copyright © 1991. Reproduced with permission of Elsevier; Figure 13.3: Based on data in Thun, M.J., Namboodri, M.M. and Heath, C.W. (1991) *New England Journal of Medicine*, **325**, 1593–96; Table 13.1: Based on data in World Cancer Research Fund / American Institute for Cancer Research (1997) *Food, Nutrition and the Prevention* *of Cancer: A Global Perspective*. Washington, DC: American Institute for Cancer Research. Reprinted with permission.

While every effort has been made to trace the owners of copyright material, in a few cases this has been proved impossible and we take this opportunity to offer our apologies to any copyright holders whose rights we may have unwittingly infringed.

Basic science, terminology and abbreviations

To describe the biology of cancer it is necessary to cover all aspects of cell function. To do this, a decision has to be made on how much basic science is included in a book of this type. We have adopted the approach of providing the pertinent information in boxes and placed each box in the chapter where it is most relevant; the box number refers to the chapter in which it appears. This approach has also been used for molecular biology, genetics and cell biology, which have broad relevance and which may create cross-reference problems. The following chapters contain general details of such topics:

Molecular biology
   Gene regulation: Box 5.1
   DNA structure and synthesis: Box 5.1 and Box 9.1
   Genetic terminology and chromosome structure: Box 8.1, Table 5.1
Cell and animal biology
   Chapter 2
   Transgenic knock-out immunodeficient mice: Box 2.1
   Cytoskeleton, cell adhesion, cell migration: Box 10.1
Classification of tumours
   Box 3.1
Epidemiology
   Box 4.1

Abbreviations can be confusing, especially as illogical names are often used. No one could reasonably expect to know that 'son of sevenless' is a gene involved in signal transduction! To clarify the situation as far as is possible, where an abbreviation is used for the first time, we have put in **bold type** the letters that contribute to the abbreviation, although there are cases where this approach is not possible. Thus, SOS first appears in the text as **s**on **o**f **s**evenless. The literature often uses multiple terminologies for a single entity. As far as possible, we have mentioned the alternatives for the more common abbreviations. Box 5.1 describes abbreviations relevant to oncogenes and tumour suppressor genes.

1 What is cancer?

KEY POINTS

- Cancer is a collection of diseases with the common feature of uncontrolled growth.
- There are multiple causes, but lifestyle factors are a major influence.
- Several cellular changes are required to generate a cancer.
- All cell types are susceptible, but epithelial cells are most prone to change.
- Cell changes continue to occur after a cancer has formed.
- Mutations in tumour suppressor genes and oncogenes are important.
- Invasion and metastasis distinguish cancers from benign growths.
- Cancers are not always lethal.
- It is possible to prevent cancer formation.

Introduction

The most common question asked of cancer specialists is, 'Are you making progress?' This begs the question, 'Progress towards what?' To answer that, one has to know what cancers are. The use of the plural is deliberate because cancer is really a collection of different diseases with three common features: uncontrolled growth is their core property and they are life-threatening, but the third feature is a more philosophical one. It is that generalisations about cancer are invalid because there are always exceptions that disprove the generalisation. Despite this, generalisations are essential in order to convey an understanding of the topic, otherwise one would end up with a jungle of confusing statements. Thus, although cancer has multiple causes, an acceptable clinical definition would be 'a set of diseases characterised by unregulated cell growth leading to invasion of surrounding tissues and spread (metastasis) to other parts of the body'. This definition would be considered too narrow by experimentalists, who would not require evidence of invasion and metastasis. The variable use of definitions sometimes results in confusion, with the terms 'cancer', 'tumour' and 'neoplasm' being used interchangeably. This is not correct, as 'neoplasm' means new growth without qualifying the nature of that growth, and 'tumour' can be applied to both benign and malignant growths.

Carcinogenesis requires several cellular changes

Cancer is an ancient condition and was known to the early Egyptians. Despite this ancient lineage, two modern components, longevity and lifestyle, have major impacts on both the type and the number of cancers encountered. Carcinogenesis, the process by which cancers are generated, is a multistep mechanism resulting from the accumulation of errors in vital regulatory pathways. It is initiated in a single cell, which then multiplies and acquires additional changes that give it a survival advantage over its neighbours. The altered cells must be amplified to generate billions of cells that constitute a cancer. As it takes time to generate these errors and cell numbers, it follows that the longer a person lives, the more likely they are to get cancer. Figure 1.1 shows the age distribution of several cancers, indicating their increase with age. Sadly, the dictum that cancer is a disease of old age has exceptions, in that some cancers are characterised by onset in childhood: cancers of the eye and certain leukaemias fall into this category. This explains the initial high incidence of leukaemia followed by a dip and then a rise in older people (Figure 1.1).

Lifestyle and family influences on cancer

The impact of lifestyle is illustrated by the prevalence of certain cancers in different countries (Figure 1.2): breast and prostate cancer are common in Western countries, while cancers of the cervix and stomach are more prevalent in nations such as China. As lifestyles change, so do the types of cancer; these geographical differences are due to more than just genetic variations between races. Environmental influences are important, even though they exert their effects via the genetic machinery of the cells.

In the majority of situations, the accumulation of errors in the cellular machinery occurs after birth in somatic cells. Important exceptions are those defects inherited

Figure 1.1

Influence of age on cancer incidence (USA).
(Source: Adapted from DeVita, V.T., Hellman, S. and Rosenberg, S.A. (eds) (1993) *Cancer: Principles and Practice of Oncology*, Fourth Edition. Philadelphia, PA: Lippincott.)

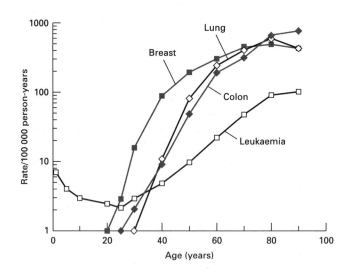

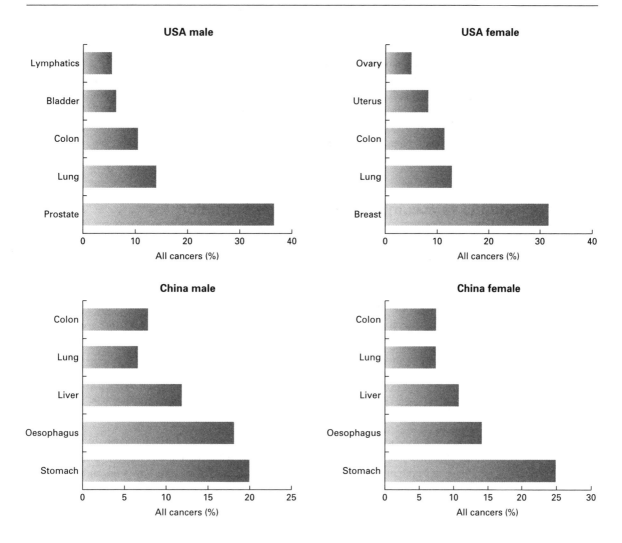

Figure 1.2

Comparison of the five commonest cancers in the USA and China.

via the germ cells (sperm, egg) that contribute to a minority of cancers, such as those of the eye and kidney. Even some of the major cancers include a small proportion of patients who inherit a predisposition for that cancer. Such situations illustrate the diverse nature of cancers even if they have the same name. Thus, the majority of colon cancers have no inherited features but at least three different types of inherited genetic defect have been identified in a minority of cases. This requirement for error generation introduces the linked questions: what agents cause cancer, and how do they generate mutations? Laboratory tests show that an enormous range of products can induce cancers, but the emphasis is on the word 'can' rather than 'do' because such tests are not always relevant to the human situation. The laboratory tests were designed around the idea that cancers were generated by environmental chemicals, a view that was fully justified on the basis of occupational cancers in humans (such as bladder cancers in dye-workers and lung cancers in smokers) and chemical induction of cancers in animals. However, the word 'environmental' conjures up the impression of synthetic, unnatural agents and, with the exception of smoking, these types of reagent have a relatively minor impact on the prevalence of human cancers. Diet and lifestyle changes are of much greater importance, and the feeling is growing that natural events such as generation of free radicals or hormonal stimuli to proliferate may be the driving force for initiators of common human cancers such as those of the colon and breast. This is coupled with the realisation that initial cellular changes accelerate the appearance of subsequent mutations and so carcinogenesis involves the generation of genetic instability.

Changes continue to accumulate after cancer formation

It is not always appreciated that the generation of errors does not stop once a cancer has been formed; cancers continue to change their behaviour as they develop, a fact that creates problems when it comes to treating patients. For example, a breast cancer may initially be sensitive to the same hormones that influence normal breast but then become hormone-insensitive. Such progressive changes in cancers reflect the genetic instability of the cells involved, resulting in more and more of the cells' economy being diverted towards growth.

Cancers are most common in epithelial cells

Figure 1.2 shows that some tissues are more prone to develop cancer than others and that men and women have different cancer patterns. This is emphasised in Table 1.1, which presents data from the UK. Men do not have ovaries or uteri, and women do not have prostate glands, and so the reason for the absence of these cancers in the relevant sexes is clear, but the big sex difference in breast cancer points to sex-related influences. In fact, it is not always realised that men *do* get breast cancer. On the other hand, the percentages of colon cancer are similar in men and women. The three most common cancers in both sexes are of epithelial origin but mesenchymal cells are also affected to a lesser degree (leukaemias/lymphomas in Table 1.1, sarcomas not shown), and thus most cell types are susceptible.

Cancer results from uncontrolled growth

No single explanation accounts for these differences in susceptibility of cells to cancer formation, but proliferation is correctly ascribed to being a core feature of cancer. This is often linked erroneously with faster rather than uncontrolled proliferation. It is true that in experimental systems, such as cell culture and animals, faster proliferation is common, but it is not always so in humans. Mouth and skin cancers, which account for only 5% of all cancers, both contain rapidly proliferating

Table 1.1 Types of cancer in men and women as percentages of all cancers (UK, 2003).

	Men		Women	
	New cancers	Death	New cancers	Death
Breast	–	–	30	17
Prostate	21	13	–	–
Lung	17	25	11	18
Colorectal	14	11	12	10
Bladder	6	4	2	2
Stomach	4	5	2	3
Head and neck	4	–	–	–
Non-Hodgkin's lymphoma	4	3	3	3
Oesophagus	3	6	–	4
Leukaemia	3	3	–	3
Kidney	3	3	–	–
Ovary	–	–	5	6
Uterus	–	–	4	–
Pancreas	–	4	3	5
Melanoma	–	–	3	3
Other	21	24	24	29
All malignancies (total numbers)	80 220		74 327	

Non-melanoma skin cancers are common (in excess of 62 000). However, as they can be diagnosed and treated in general-practice surgeries, and are usually totally cured, they are not included in this table.

cells, whereas breast cancer, the most common female cancer (Table 1.1), proliferates slowly. Many normal cells hyperproliferate on occasions (hyperplasia, see Chapter 3) but otherwise retain their normal appearance and behaviour. The crucial feature of cancer cells is that they are antisocial in that they have a degree of autonomy not experienced by their normal counterparts. Normal cells are subject to internal and external inhibitory signals, which, to varying degrees, are lost during carcinogenesis. Identification of these regulatory signals is, therefore, important to our understanding of how the extracellular environment can influence cell function, how a cancer cell can manipulate its environment and what determines the overall behaviour of a mass of cells (Figure 1.3). A decreased rate of cell death is at least as important as increased proliferation in determining the size of a cancer, and supply of nutrients by the generation of new blood vessels is essential if a tumour mass is to exceed a critical size. As cells differentiate, they divide more slowly. Thus, blocking differentiation (as occurs in some leukaemias) or causing dedifferentiation (as in many advanced cancers) increases growth. Contact with other cells or with the extracellular matrix inhibits growth in cultures of normal cells, but this is not the case for cancer cells.

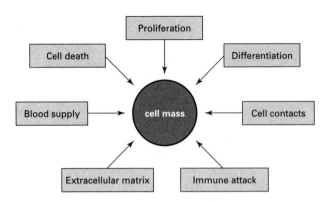

Figure 1.3

Factors influencing a cell mass.

Cancer genes

It is now appreciated that some genes, proto-oncogenes, are concerned specifically with the normal regulation of cell proliferation. These genes can mutate, thus de-regulating cell growth; in this case, the genes are termed oncogenes. Additionally, many cancers are generated by loss of specific genes concerned with the repair of cell damage, cell death or growth inhibition. These are called tumour suppressor genes. It is clear that cancer can develop from changes in either or both of these two regulatory systems.

Invasion and metastasis

Increased cell mass on its own generates what a clinician would consider to be a benign growth and not a cancer. Additional changes are required that enable those cells to invade the surrounding tissue and metastasise to other parts of the body. This ability of cancer cells to overcome the normal containment mechanisms reflects membrane modifications resulting in diminished cell–cell interactions as well as the production of proteases that facilitate movement through the extracellular matrix. Additionally, cancer cells can use chemical messengers to signal normal cells to help them. Thus, they promote the development of new blood vessels, thereby ensuring an adequate supply of essential nutrients. The acquisition of invasive properties is what distinguishes cancer cells from normal cells, while metastasis to other parts of the body is the major cause of clinical problems and death.

Some cancers are curable

Cancer is probably the biggest medical concern of people living in affluent so-cieties. This is understandable, but it is important to put that concern in perspective with other causes of death (Figure 1.4). Death from cancer is second to death from cardiovascular disorders, with other causes lagging quite a way behind. Another way

Figure 1.4

Causes of death in the UK.

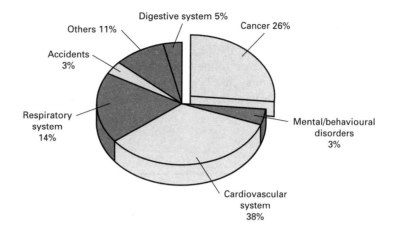

Digestive system 5%

Others 11%

Cancer 26%

Accidents 3%

Respiratory system 14%

Mental/behavioural disorders 3%

Cardiovascular system 38%

of looking at this is to consider the years of life lost through cardiovascular disease and cancer. As cardiovascular disease affects younger people more than cancer does, cancer could be considered less dangerous than heart disease by this criterion. In most people's minds, cancer is linked to death, but this is not the invariable situation: although only 3% of people are alive 5 years after diagnosis of pancreatic cancer, the figure is 91% for testicular cancer and can almost be considered a cure. At present, the major cancers cannot be cured in their entirety, but comparison of the numbers of people developing specific cancers with those dying therefrom indicates that something beneficial is happening with some cancers (Table 1.1). In women, 30% of all cancers arise in the breast, but these account for only 17% of cancer deaths. The same pattern is seen for cancers of the uterus. Unfortunately, the converse pattern of incidence and death occurs with lung cancer. However, some cancers can be cured, e.g. choriocarcinoma in the placenta.

Death is an all too frequent consequence of cancer, but we do not always know how cancer kills. Most frequently, death is due to disruption of vital organs such as the brain or liver, but it is not immediately apparent why bone metastases should be so lethal. The wasting (cachexia) commonly seen in people with cancer may be due to toxins released into the circulation.

Prevention, screening and treatment

As in other diseases, the prevention of cancer is better than its cure. This is understood by governments that endeavour to minimise work-associated cancers by regulation and to recommend good practices such as minimising the smoking habit, discouraging excessive exposure to solar ultraviolet light, and so on. Of course, early detection of the disease is very important; if the number of affected cells is small, then there is a greater probability of a cure. For a few cancers (breast, cervical, colorectal), it is possible to screen susceptible populations for very early signs of the disease and if necessary to initiate treatment, which has a high chance of success.

Treatment of cancer is based on the removal and/or killing of the tumour cells while minimising any unwanted side effects of the therapy on the normal cells. Usually the first option in therapy is surgery or radiotherapy to remove totally or to reduce the mass of the tumour. However, it is often the case that by the time the primary tumour has been detected, secondary tumours have become established, so that chemotherapy and radiotherapy commonly follow surgery.

Further reading

Alberts, B., Johnson, A., Lewis, J., *et al.* (2002) *Molecular Biology of the Cell*, 4th edn. New York: Garland Press.

Hanahan, D. and Weinberg, R.A. (2000) The hallmarks of cancer. *Cell* **100**, 57–70.

Knowles, M. and Selby, P. (eds) (2005) *Introduction to Cellular and Molecular Biology of Cancer*, 4th edn. Oxford: Oxford University Press.

Lodish, H., Berk, A., Matsudaira, P., *et al.* (eds) (2004) *Molecular Cell Biology*, 5th edn. New York: W.H. Freeman.

Pecorino, L. (2005) *Molecular Biology of Cancer*. Oxford: Oxford University Press.

Pollard, T.D. and Earnshaw, W.C. (2002) *Cell Biology*. Philadelphia, PA: Saunders.

Souhami, R.L., Tannock, I., Hohenberger, P. and Horiot, C. (2002) *Oxford Textbook of Oncology*, 2nd edn. Oxford: Oxford University Press.

Stewart, B.W. and Kleihues, P. (eds) (2003) *World Cancer Report*. Lyons: IACR Press.

Tannock, I.F., Hill, R.P., Bristow, R.G. and Harrington, L. (eds) (2005) *The Basic Science of Oncology*, 4th edn. New York: McGraw-Hill.

Websites

The websites of major research organisations are reliable and authoritative.
Cancer Index: www.cancerindex.org
Cancer Research UK: www.cancerresearchuk.org
Cancer Web: http://cancerweb.ncl.ac.uk
National Cancer Institute, US National Institutes of Health: www.cancer.gov

2 Natural history: the life of a cancer

KEY POINTS

- The life history of a cancer can be divided into stages. Carcinogenesis, the process of cancer development from a normal cell, is divided into initiation and promotion stages. Progression describes the additional changes occurring after a cancer has formed.
- Most characteristics identified by laboratory models have counterparts in human cancers, but initiation is difficult to define in some human cancers.
- Altered DNA bases (mutations) are the basis of cellular changes that cause cancer. This can involve chemical alteration of individual bases or the order in which the bases occur.
- Several mutations are required for carcinogenesis. This involves genes that either gain (dominant) or lose (recessive) function as a result of mutation.
- Multiple pathways exist by which a cancer in one cell type is generated.
- Different cancers have different aetiologies, although they may have some common features.
- Cancers arise in single cells (clonal origin).
- Cancers detected by clinical means are at an advanced stage of their natural history.

Introduction

The sequence of events involved in carcinogenesis and the data on which our knowledge of these events is based have been derived from sources ranging from animal studies through cell and molecular biology to clinical experiences. Therefore, it is not surprising that different perspectives and terms exist to describe the various stages in the natural history or pathogenesis of cancer development. Four representations are given in Figure 2.1, which, with varying degrees of overlap, illustrate models derived from animal experiments (1,4), cell biology (2), molecular biology (2,3) and clinical data (4). This chapter will look at the overall process of carcinogenesis and tumour progression from the separate perspectives of the experimental biologist

Figure 2.1

Cancer development: four models. Each connecting arrow represents several events and multiple pathways can exist between each stage.

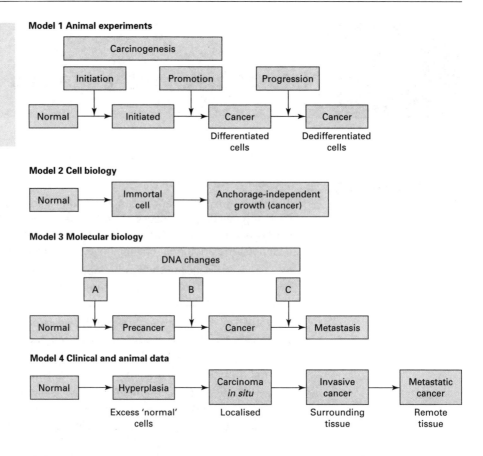

Model 1 Animal experiments

Model 2 Cell biology

Model 3 Molecular biology

Model 4 Clinical and animal data

and the medical practitioner. These two broad categories have been chosen because they provide different insights into the processes involved that reinforce each other in some situations but raise doubts about the relevance of animal data to human cancer in others. By their nature, experimental approaches are capable of providing more clear-cut answers than data derived from clinical experiences, but clinical experiences are more relevant to the human situation. The concluding part of this chapter will bring together the two perspectives with some general comments plus a discussion of their relevance to two human cancers: colorectal cancer and **c**hronic **m**yeloid **l**eukaemia (CML).

Clonal origins of cancer

Evidence favours the concept that all the cells in a cancer arise by proliferation of one abnormal cell; that is, cancers are monoclonal in origin. Several strands of evidence support this idea, but one of the most telling is concerned with the distribution of genetically distinct types of X-linked enzymes such as **g**lucose-**6**-**p**hosphate **d**ehydrogenase (G6PD) in cancers. Genetic variants of such enzymes (say, A and B) can be

Figure 2.2

Cancers arise from single cells: clonal origin.

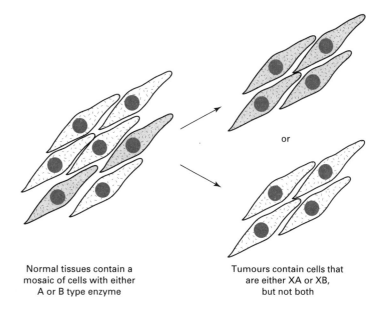

Normal tissues contain a
mosaic of cells with either
A or B type enzyme

or

Tumours contain cells that
are either XA or XB,
but not both

distinguished electrophoretically. In the cells of women, one of the X chromosomes is inactivated, so the tissues are a mosaic of XA and XB cells, as the process of X chromosome inactivation is random (Figure 2.2). In women with CML, the abnormal cells are of one type only, either XA or XB, indicating that all the malignant cells are derived from one cell. Similar evidence is available for leiomyomas (benign tumours of the uterine smooth muscle), melanomas, and cancers of the bladder, pharynx, thyroid, palate and cervix. Although G6PD mutations illustrate the clonal origin of cancers, the enzyme is not the cause of that growth. The tumour suppressor gene p53 fulfils that criterion (see Chapter 5), and mutations of this gene also indicate clonal origins. Ultraviolet-induced skin lesions carry mutation of the p53 gene; all regions of a single lesion contain the same mutation but this is different from mutations elsewhere in the same patient.

Experimental biology

The main feature of models derived from experimental systems is of a discrete, ordered series of changes to which terms such as 'initiation', 'promotion', 'progression' and 'immortality' can be applied. Animal experiments generated terms like 'carcinogenesis', which covers events leading up to the generation of a cancer, whereas 'progression' is the term applied to changes after a tumour has formed (Figure 2.1, model 1). Progression includes invasion and metastasis, but these fundamental features of human cancer occur infrequently in primary animal tumours. Cell culture experiments tend to be described in terms of immortalisation or prolonging the lifespan of cells plus an altered ability to recognise adjacent cells and extracellular components. These properties often result in anchorage-independent growth (ability to proliferate without attachment to the plastic culture dish) (model 2). Molecular biologists think in terms of discrete mutational events (model 3). Progression would be equated to change C in model 3. Model 4 describes the sequence of histological changes observed in human and animal tumours, with progression referring to stages beyond *in situ* carcinoma. Data so derived have emphasised the multifactorial nature of cancer aetiology, the multiple changes required to generate a cancer and the fact that changes continue to occur in established tumours.

Animal studies

Carcinogenesis: initiation and promotion

Percival Potts, an eighteenth-century surgeon, first noted that young male chimneysweeps had a high incidence of scrotal cancer. He assumed that continuous exposure to soot might give rise to this cancer. Later, experimental investigations that involved repeatedly painting the skin of mice with various organic agents, such as coal tar derivatives, showed that these resulted in the development of skin cancer. However, the cancer-producing agents (carcinogens) did not lead to the immediate production of a tumour: cancer developed only after a long period. Several steps are involved in this process (carcinogenesis). The first stage, initiation, was found to involve mutagenic effects of the carcinogen on skin stem cells; there were no outward manifestations at this stage. The second stage, promotion, could be induced by a variety of agents, which need not necessarily be carcinogens. The visible manifestations of promotion were the development of benign skin tumours caused by increased cell proliferation, and a local increase in reddening of the skin. The local development of blood vessels is a reflection of the increased nutritional and respiratory requirements required for rapid proliferation in the adjacent skin (Figure 2.3). The terms 'initiation' and 'promotion' are still used to describe this sequence of steps in the process of carcinogenesis in both humans and experimental animals (Figure 2.1).

Hormones are promoters Carcinogenic polycyclic hydrocarbons were widely used in early experiments because of their availability and the fact that their high potency generated clear-cut results. Two additional features are illustrated in another example of their use – in rat mammary carcinogenesis.

A single oral dose of DMBA generates breast cancers but only under specific conditions. Removal of the ovarian hormone oestradiol immediately after DMBA treatment blocks carcinogenesis, an effect that is reversed by readministration of oestradiol. This is analogous to the skin model but with the hormone rather than TPA acting as the promoter. However, in intact animals, DMBA only works when given at a specific age – when the mammary gland is developing – indicating that cells are only susceptible to initiating agents at certain stages of their development. There is thus a link between carcinogenesis and cell development (differentiation status).

The second feature is that cancers other than breast cancer are rarely caused by DMBA in this model system, indicating different sensitivities of cells to a carcinogen.

Conceptual problems with the term 'initiation'   Important as the concepts of initiation and promotion are, conceptual problems arise if they are applied too widely. Carcinogenicity studies indicate that active agents can be classified into genotoxic and non-genotoxic categories depending on whether or not they damage DNA (Chapter 7). Compounds like DMBA are genotoxi, although they must be metabolised to compounds that react with DNA. The reactive metabolite is referred to as the ultimate carcinogen, which is the actual initiator. Non-genotoxic agents act by diverse mechanisms, some of which raise conceptual problems. Ovarian hormones like oestradiol are non-genotoxic but can generate breast and ovarian cancers in rodents without additional treatments probably by virtue of their mitogenic effect. Ovarian hormones are usually described as tumour promoters, but what is the initiator in this model? A similar situation occurs in humans with cancers generated by a single hormone. This is discussed in the section linking laboratory and clinical results.

On the other hand, the antilipotrophic drug clofibrate acts as a hepatic carcinogen by increasing the number of intracellular organelles, peroxisomes. This increases reactive oxygen, free radical production which, in turn, can damage DNA. It is not certain that clofibrate is an initiating agent.

It is a recurring theme throughout cancer research that definitions resulting from early discoveries are useful but, because of the many aetiologies of cancers, those definitions become too restrictive. The oestradiol and clofibrate problems may be examples where a discrete step under the heading 'initiation' may not always be necessary. This conceptual difficulty does not arise with the term 'promotion' because the molecular changes involved are more diverse and can be accommodated within a multiple change model. These points are also relevant to human carcinogenesis and are further elaborated on p. 23.

Progression

A second set of animal experiments showed that tumours, once formed, underwent further changes (progression) as demonstrated by dedifferentiation, increasingly autonomous growth and aggressive behaviour (Figure 2.1). The original work using spontaneous mouse mammary tumours still serves as a good model for tumour progression. Initially, the tumours grow only when the animals become pregnant, regress at parturition and regrow at the next pregnancy. The hormonal changes accompanying pregnancy stimulate growth of the tumour, which is therefore defined as being hormone-dependent because the cells are completely dependent on the hormones; cessation of hormone production is accompanied by disappearance of the tumour. However, small numbers of tumour cells remain; at the next pregnancy, the tumour regrows at the same place but almost invariably its behaviour changes with time, becoming first hormone-responsive (partial regression at parturition) and then hormone-independent (no regression). Histological examination indicates that loss of hormone sensitivity is accompanied by cellular dedifferentiation and increased mitotic activity. This irreversible sequence of changes does not always occur in the order stated, as hormone-responsive or hormone-independent tumours can arise without prior detection of the dependent stage. This illustrates the variability of the development pathways that can exist even within one tumour type.

Figure 2.3

New blood vessels are required for cancer growth.
(Source: Adapted from Tannock, I.F. (1968) *British Journal of Cancer*, 22, 258–73. Copyright © 1968. Reprinted with permission of Macmillan Publishers Ltd.)

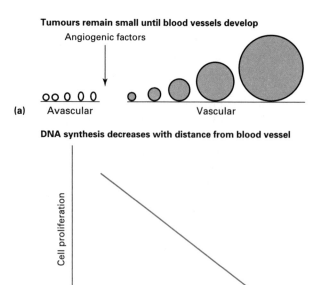

Tumours remain small until blood vessels develop

Angiogenic factors

(a) Avascular   Vascular

DNA synthesis decreases with distance from blood vessel

Cell proliferation

100   200

(b)   Distance from blood vessel (μm)

Progression reflects multiple changes in growth regulatory mechanisms. Promotion can occur by different pathways in different cells, but two common features highlighted by animal studies are altered cell proliferation and the formation of new blood vessels (Figure 2.3). Proliferation rate is discussed later in this chapter, but angiogenesis, the formation of new capillaries, will be considered here. Tumours will grow to a diameter of about 1 mm, but further expansion requires the induction of extra blood vessels by angiogenic growth factors released from the cancer. The role of a well-developed vasculature within the tumour is illustrated by the fact that proliferation is rapid adjacent to the vessels and decreases with increasing distance from the vessels (Figure 2.3b).

Special strains of mice

Mice have provided a valuable means of investigating fundamental aspects of cancer in humans. In spite of species differences, several points favour such an approach: the species have similar organ systems, and there is genetic conservation of the important signalling pathways controlling cell proliferation, apoptosis and so on. Additionally, mice can be genetically manipulated in order to provide many special strains that have experimentally useful features. In particular, two types of mice have facilitated dissection of the steps involved in tumour development (pathogenesis). The first set comprises strains in which specific genes have been altered in all cells within the animal, while the second set comprises animals with defective immune systems.

The availability of engineered mice in which all cells have a specific gene that has been either activated (transgenic mice) or inactivated (knock-out mice) has facilitated analysis of the biological consequences of altered gene function (Box 2.1).

Box 2.1	**Special mice used in cancer research**

Transgenic studies

If a gene, a *transgene*, is injected into a unicellular egg that is then transplanted into a mother, all the cells in the offspring contain that gene and the mice are said to be *transgenic*. Frequently, the gene to be studied is joined to a strong promoter (see Box 5.1) from another gene to ensure adequate expression. This manipulation allows analysis of *potential* function of the gene in question but, in the absence of the normal promoter, quantitative differences in expression do not permit the conclusion that the gene actually generates the observed effects in normal animals. The animal can be monitored to see what biological changes result from having this gene engineered; this technique is used widely to study oncogene function. Alternatively, DNA base changes can be engineered in a gene and the immediate consequences monitored by introduction into cultured cells with a technique called *transfection*. However, cultured cells have different regulatory restraints from those encountered in animals, and so use of transgenic animals overcomes that problem.

Knock-out mice

Repressor genes are important in carcinogenesis when their normal inhibitory function is lost. Somatic cells are diploid, i.e. they contain two copies of each allele. Both copies have to be deleted before the consequences of their loss can be determined, although exceptions do exist (see Chapter 5). This approach requires a complex combination of methodologies. An inactivating mutation is engineered in a tumour suppressor gene such as that coding for the 53 kDa protein p53, and transfected into cultured cells. If recipient cells are from an early stage of egg development (a blastocyst), then they have the ability to develop into any type of adult cell – they are said to be *totipotent* – and so the introduced mutant p53 has the potential to modify all of the adult cells. *Homologous recombination* (see Box 8.1) of chromosomes during mitosis will generate some *heterozygous* cells with one normal allele and one mutant allele. Reintroduction of these cells into the blastocyst followed by implantation into a mother will result in some heterozygous offspring. By cross-breeding two heterozygotes, some of their embryos will be *homozygous* (both alleles the same) for mutant (inactive) p53. These embryos are known as *knock-out*, *null/null* or $^{-/-}$ mice.

Immunodeficient mice

Strains of mice have been developed with immune-system defects. One strain has no thymus gland; the consequent absence of T-cells leads to loss of that cell-mediated immunity, so the mice do not reject foreign cells. Such animals can be hairless and are known as *nude mice*. A different group of mice, known as SCID (**s**evere **c**ombined **i**mmuno**d**eficiency) mice have no B- or

T-lymphocytes of their own. Transplantation of stem cells from human bone marrow repopulates the mouse with human lymphocytes that protect SCID mice from opportunistic infections but will not reject human cells. SCID mice can be used to analyse the effects of drugs and growth factors on human samples whose cellular architecture is maintained. Additionally, many normal tissues will not survive in immunodeficient mice, whereas cancers will survive; changes related to carcinogenesis can thus be monitored. It is not known why normal cells have difficulty in surviving this environment, but presumably it is related to their more complex growth requirements.

Inbred strains

Inbred strains derived from brother–sister matings over many generations become genetically homogenous. Different strains have marked differences, such as variation in the incidence of specific cancers. The strains A, BALB/c, C3H, DBA, GR and RIII have a high incidence of mammary tumours, while BALB/c show a susceptibility to pristan-induced plasmacytomas. Additionally, as mice within a strain are genetically very homogenous, it is possible to transplant tumours between individuals of that strain without graft rejection.

Transgenic mice Genes in which mutations activate function (oncogenes, see Chapter 5) can be analysed by inserting that gene (a transgene) into mouse cells. Thus, *ras*, *myc* and *neu* oncogenes code for proteins involved in signal transduction, gene transcription and cell membrane receptor, respectively. The transgenic approach showed that the *ras* gene generated breast tumours in some but not all mice and that other cell types did not become cancerous (Figure 2.4). In the context of tumour pathogenesis, this indicates that single gene changes can inefficiently generate cancers and that cell-specific influences exist that determine which cells can be transformed into cancers. The *myc* gene had a similar effect to that of *ras*, but together the two were synergistic. This cooperation between oncogenes fits well with multistage models of carcinogenesis. The third oncogene, *neu*, generated breast cancers in all the female offspring. This example illustrates the multiple ways in which a cancer type can be generated.

Figure 2.4

Transgenic mice are used to analyse oncogene effects. (Source: Based on data from Muller, W.J., *et al.* (1988) *Cell*, 54, 105–15, Copyright © 1988. Reproduced with permission from Elsevier.)

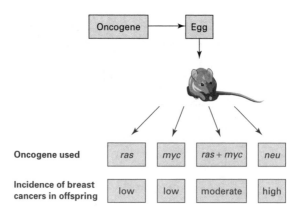

Knock-out mice   To define effects of genes whose normal function is inhibitory, it is more informative to delete the inhibitory factor. Tumour suppressor genes are studied in this way; inactivation of both alleles is usually necessary because of their recessive characteristics (see Chapter 5). Thus, p53$^{-/-}$ mice appear normal at first, indicating that p53 is not required for early development, but in later life about three-quarters develop cancers such as lymphomas and sarcomas. This indicates that normal p53 is not required for early development, but in its absence errors accumulate that lead to cancers. This is compatible with its normal role in inhibiting cell proliferation when damaged DNA is present (see Chapter 7). It also highlights the existence of cell-specific factors, because only certain cells develop into cancers. Another example is found in the *MIN* mouse, which has both alleles of the **a**denatomous **p**olyposis **c**oli gene knocked out (Apc$^{-/-}$). This results in a high incidence of intestinal and mammary tumours. PTEN$^{+/-}$ p27$^{KIP+/-}$ mice are prostate-tumour-prone, while PTEN$^{-/-}$p27$^{KIP+/-}$ mice all develop prostate cancer.

Immunodeficient mice   The response of solid human tissues or cultured human cells to growth manipulation *in vivo* can be studied in such mice as the host immune mechanisms are lost (Box 2.1). The *in vitro* carcinogenesis example described in the next section provides an illustration of their use.

Cell and molecular biology

When methods became available to culture cell lines, less complex and therefore more readily interpretable experiments were possible. It was noted that in the media available, cancer cells grew more readily than their normal counterparts, which gave rise to the notion that carcinogenesis was accompanied by the need for less stringent growth conditions. This has developed into the autocrine/paracrine model of growth regulation, whereby cancer cells produce or respond, via altered receptors, to locally synthesised growth factors (see Figure 10.3). It was further noted that cultured cancer cells often lose a normal property called density or contact inhibition (Figure 2.5). As the name implies, when normal cells become crowded and contact

Figure 2.5

Proliferation characteristics of cultured cells.

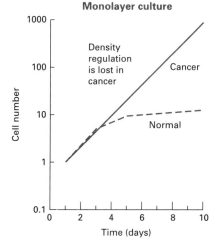

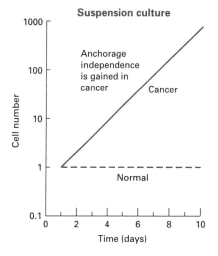

adjacent cells, they stop and will not overgrow their neighbours, whereas many cancer cells continue to proliferate. This 'antisocial' behaviour is a reflection of altered interactions between the cell membranes in contact with other cells and with the plastic substrates on which they were growing. Normal cells must attach to plastic in order to grow (monolayer culture); free-floating normal cells do not proliferate. However, some cancer cells grow without attachment, a phenomenon known as suspension culture or anchorage independence. Cultured cells are said to be transformed if they exhibit these behavioural changes, which are often accompanied by morphological alterations.

Carcinogenesis can be mimicked in culture

Comparison of various cell biological properties with ability to grow as tumours in immunodeficient animals indicated that anchorage independence was the best, but not invariate, indication that the cell in question was cancerous. This was demonstrated by an *in vitro* carcinogenesis experiment in which cultured normal fibroblasts were briefly treated with the carcinogen benzopyrene and the subsequent behaviour of the cells in culture was monitored. The cultured cells were periodically injected into immunodeficient mice to see whether the mice formed tumours (Figure 2.6). By analogy with *in vivo* animal studies, carcinogen treatment was equivalent to initiation and additional changes in culture to promotion. Several post-initiation events were observed, such as changed morphology and secretion of proteases like plasminogen activator, but it was not until the cells acquired the ability to grow in suspension culture that they also behaved as cancer cells when injected into mice. As these promotional events did not occur without prior benzopyrene exposure, the benzopyrene must have set in train a series of changes leading to cells capable of an autonomous existence. Several inheritable changes are required before cultured cells can grow as tumours in mice, and so, in this respect, the experimental model mimics the situation seen in patients and animals. However, differences also exist. In culture, benzopyrene acts as both initiator and promoter, whereas in animals it often requires a promoter as well. The different pattern of behaviour probably reflects the strong proliferative environment in culture. Culture conditions have been deliberately established in order to maximise proliferation and minimise inhibitory influences, whereas in animals there exists an equilibrium between positive and negative controls. The culture medium with its plentiful supply of growth factors may be equivalent to the promotional agent needed *in vivo*.

Figure 2.6

Carcinogenesis in cell culture: changes over time.

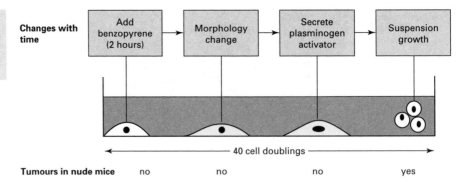

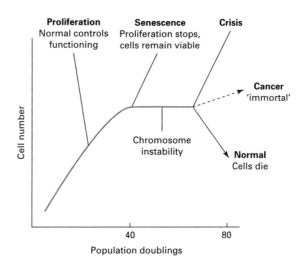

Figure 2.7

The life cycle of normal cultured cells.

Are cancer cells immortal?

When normal cells are cultured, they have a lifespan of about 40 generations (cell doublings) by which time the build-up of errors results in senescence and death (Figure 2.7). A component of the carcinogenic process is disruption of these events, so that cells live longer and there is greater probability of error accumulation. The term 'immortal' (see Figure 2.1, model 2) is sometimes used, but it is inappropriate because cancer cells do die, even in fast-growing tumours. It is better to think in terms of extended life rather than immortality. Senescent cells are viable but have lost the ability to replicate. Increasing numbers of abnormal chromosomes accumulate, and eventually 'crisis' occurs, a loosely defined set of events during which most cells undergo programmed cell death (see Chapter 9). A few cells may restart proliferating during the crisis period and become immortal cell lines. Cancer cells *in vivo* may have acquired some of the properties of these post-crisis cultured cells. Little is known about causative events linked to senescence and crisis, except that chromosome instability and the enzyme telomerase are involved (Chapter 9).

Genes involved in carcinogenesis are sometimes classified into those that influence the lifespan of cells and those that have other effects, such as altering sensitivity to external stimuli. The former group tend to code for nuclear tumour suppressor proteins, such as p53 and Rb, whereas the latter category code for extranuclear oncogene proteins such as ras and erbB2. The functions of these gene products are described in Chapter 5. This generalisation should not be taken too far; one exception is the mitochondrial protein Bcl2. Loss of Bcl2 effectively extends lifespan by decreasing cell death (see Chapter 9). Immortalisation of cultured cells has been equated with initiation.

Any discussion on build-up of errors in cell DNA (see above) must involve mutation rates. Mutation rates for normal cells increase with age. In culture, this means the number of cell doublings; the same phenomenon occurs with normal human cells *in vivo*. Biological age of cells is related to the number of divisions they have undergone; the higher the number of divisions, the 'older' the cell. This behaviour in culture equates with the clinical picture of cancer being more common in older people (see Figure 1.1). Mechanisms must exist in normal cells in order to generate and accelerate mutations with age. The same applies in cancer cells, but there is unresolved debate as to whether the normal picture is adequate to explain the mutator phenotype ascribed to cancer cells (see Chapter 7). The mutation rate varies according to cell type, and it may be that the rate in embryonic cells determines the rate in normal adult cells, which in turn influences cancer risk for that cell type. This is only a hypothesis, but the inference would be that high-incidence sites such as the breast would have higher mutation rates than low-incidence sites such as the brain.

Genes can be carcinogenic: oncogenes

Cell culture provides a means of growing cells whose genetic complement has been manipulated by molecular techniques and analysing the biological effects of those manipulations. The technique of transfection (introducing foreign DNA into intact cultured cells) was initially used to compare DNA fragments from normal and cancer cells. The carcinogenic potential of the *ras* gene from bladder cancer was identified in this way (see Chapter 5). This experiment indicated that a single gene, *ras*, was capable of generating cancers, whereas animal biologists (see above), epidemiologists and clinical geneticists (see below) had shown a requirement for multi-hit mechanisms. This was resolved when it was realised that the host cells were not truly normal but had already undergone genetic changes before transfection. Similar experiments with different oncogenes showed that although a few, such as *Rb* and *neu*, could generate cancers on their own, in the majority of cases at least two were required.

Transfection experiments are also used to test the effects of specific mutations on gene function. For example, mutations engineered in codon 12 of the *ras* oncogene increased its transforming potential and decreased its guanosine triphosphatase (GTPase) activity, thus providing a cause-and-effect link between these two functions.

Loss of gene function can be carcinogenic

The above results indicate that cancers can result from acquisition of genetic information, but loss of such information is at least as important. If a normal fibroblast is fused with a cancer cell in culture, then the hybrid behaves not as a cancer but as a normal cell when transplanted into nude mice (Figure 2.8). Thus, the normal phenotype is dominant as it generates a product capable of inhibiting the cancer phenotype. Several such inhibitory genes have been identified, many of which are involved in regulating cell proliferation and death. Terms such as 'tumour suppressor', 'anti-oncogene', 'recessive' and 'loss of function' have been used to describe this phenomenon (see Chapter 5). When these 'normal' hybrids are cultured further, they lose chromosomes and revert to a cancer-like behaviour because a tumour suppressor gene on a normal chromosome is lost.

This type of experiment also demonstrates the inverse link between differentiation and carcinogenesis. Normal fibroblasts synthesise collagen (an index of differentiation). This property is retained by the hybrid but is lost when cells become tumorigenic.

DNA sequences that do not code for proteins are important

The above discussion about DNA changes conveys the impression that only coding sequences or their immediate regulatory regions are altered during carcinogenesis. This is not correct, as mutations in microsatellite DNA may also participate. This type of DNA is made up of multiple two- to four-oligonucleotide repeats of C : A/G : T,

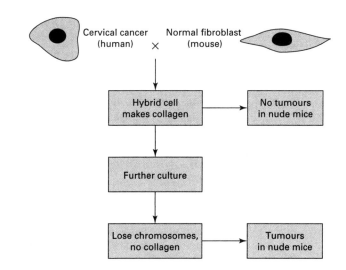

Figure 2.8

Cell-fusion experiments show that inhibitory factors are lost in cancers. (Source: Based on data in Anderson, M.J. and Stanbridge, E.J. (1993) *FASEB Journal*, **7**, 826–33.)

whose functions are unknown. Currently, the important relevance of microsatellite DNA is that an increased size is a marker for one type of DNA repair defect (mismatch repair). Such defects contribute to accelerated accumulation of mutations (see Chapter 7). A second situation where non-coding sequences are relevant to carcinogenesis is in the replication of telomeric termini of chromosomes. These are composed of tandem TTAGGG repeats, which require a special replication process. Chromosome instability occurs if telomere replication is disrupted (see Chapter 9).

Clinical data

Data relevant to pathogenesis of cancers can be obtained from several sources.

Epidemiology

Age at which cancers occur indicates the number of changes required for carcinogenesis

Cancers most commonly arise in older people (see Figure 1.1) because time is needed to accumulate the multiple changes required. It follows that the more changes (hits, errors) required, the greater the age at which that cancer is likely to occur. Most cancers show a linear relationship between log (age) and log (incidence):

$$\text{probability of getting cancer} = \text{age}^n$$

where n = number of changes. For colon cancer (see Figure 1.1), $n = 3 - 6$, which is gratifyingly close to the number of genetic changes actually identified thus far in this cancer (see below).

A limited number of cancers arise at an earlier age because fewer changes are required. Retinoblastoma (eye cancer) is one such example that results from the loss of both alleles of the **retino**blastoma (*Rb*) gene. In the familial form of this cancer, one hit is inherited through the germ cells and one hit is acquired after birth. The early age of onset of retinoblastoma (before age 2 years) is due to only two hits being required, one for each *Rb* allele (see Chapter 8). The *Rb* gene codes for a protein that normally blocks cell division (see Chapters 5 and 9).

The changes identified by the above mean values represent the number of rate-limiting mutations required and do not imply that additional mutations cannot contribute to the overall process of carcinogenesis.

Rate of error accumulation accelerates: genetic instability

In the retinoblastoma example, acquisition of the first hit invariably leads to the second one, which would be unexpected if it were a random event. Something about the first hit increases the probability of the second one occurring. Similarly, the mutation rates measured in young normal cells are too low to explain the observed age–incidence data for many common cancers (see Chapter 7); something happens to accelerate change. This genetic instability, also called mutator phenotype or **r**epli-cation **e**rror **r**epair (RER) phenotype, occurs in many cancers.

Risk factors characterise carcinogenic events

The changes identified by the above methods do not indicate their relationship to the stages of carcinogenesis identified by experimental biologists. Other types of epidemiological study can provide such data. The causes of occupational cancers associated with certain industries have been identified through epidemiological studies and the causative agents equated with initiation. Thus, the genotoxic chemical β-naphthylamine (2-naphthylamine) previously used in the rubber industry caused bladder cancer, whereas ionising radiation from atomic bombs had widespread carcinogenic effects because of the DNA damage it caused (see Chapter 7). Clear-cut as these examples are, it is difficult to prove an initiation and promotion requirement for common cancers like those of colon, prostate and breast. In these situations, the strength of epidemiological data is in identifying risk factors that influence human carcinogenesis without necessarily showing the stage at which those factors work. For example, people who have a diet high in saturated fats have an elevated probability of developing one of several types of cancer, but why this should be is unclear (see Table 4.7). The increasing linkage of molecular and epidemiological studies will help us to resolve this type of problem. With cervical cancer, comparison of specific types of human papilloma virus by **p**olymerase **c**hain **r**eaction (PCR) in normal and abnormal cervical tissues implicates this virus as an early and possible initiating influence in this cancer (see Chapter 5).

Pathology

The judgements made by pathologists as to the nature, malignant or otherwise, of tissue samples are based largely on the divergence from normal appearance of the material being examined. It is, therefore, logical that the more abnormal a sample, the more likely it is to have progressed towards malignancy. This conclusion is substantiated by clinical observation of the behaviour of such abnormalities, such that simple hyperproliferation (hyperplasia) is less dangerous than more complex types of hyperproliferation accompanied by additional cellular changes. This equates with model 4 in Figure 2.1. Thus, in one series of endometrial (lining of the uterus) analyses, untreated patients with simple (cystic) hyperplasia had a less than 1% chance of developing cancer, compared with 27% and 82% for those with the more complex histologies of adenomatous and atypical hyperplasia, respectively; carcinoma *in situ* invariably became invasive if treatment was withheld.

For glandular epithelial cancers such as those of breast and endometrium, the sequence shown in model 4 in Figure 2.1 would be a typical description of their natural history, but variations do occur, e.g. colorectal and thyroid adenocarcinomas progress through stages known as adenomas.

Progression is monitored histologically according to the degree of differentiation and of tumour spread. Various grading protocols are used to assess differentiation. Increasingly, immunohistochemical, biochemical or molecular markers are used to better define this feature. Thus, good morphological data have been crucial in generating information on where specific pathological changes are sited within the carcinogenic sequence and have provided the material that biologists can use to identify molecular changes. This is compatible with models 3 and 4 in Figure 2.1. Molecular data from colon cancers indicate that the sequence in which changes occur is less important than the number accumulated, which is difficult to reconcile with model 1 in Figure 2.1, in which initiation must precede progression (see below).

Clinical evidence

Clinicians come into contact with a cancer at a relatively late stage in its development. The first diagnosis of cancer commonly involves the physical detection of a lump. By this stage, the number of cancer cells is large and the cancer has already passed the halfway stage in its life (Figure 2.9). Special early-detection methods, such

Figure 2.9

Clinical symptoms related to cancer size. (Source: From Figure 24.3 in Alberts, B., Bray, D., Lewis, J., Raff, M., Roberts, K. and Watson J.D. (1994) *Molecular Biology of the Cell*, Third Edition. New York: Garland Publishing. Reproduced with permission of Garland Science/Taylor & Francis LLC.)

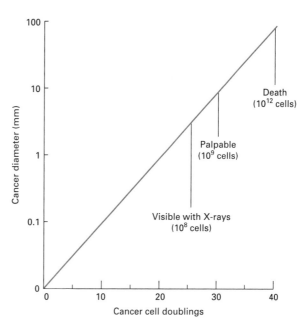

as those used in screening, can detect smaller cancers, but even this is late in the development of cancer. In either case, the clinician is dealing with progression rather than carcinogenesis and must plan a treatment that will cater best for the situation as it is (see Chapter 11).

Linking laboratory and clinic

Initiation and promotion

The various mechanisms described above all refer to the same entity, a specific cancer, and so it is necessary to relate the various terms and descriptions used in laboratory experiments to human conditions. The initiation and promotion model is especially relevant as it has been so influential. This is more than an exercise in semantics because the concept of initiation has generated an industry devoted to the identification of agents that cause it. This is valid if it results in better health but questionable if natural processes such as metabolic free-radical generation, diet and endogenous hormone changes account for the majority of human cancers. There are clear examples with lung cancer (tobacco smoke), bladder cancer (β-naphthylamine) and leukaemia (ionising radiation), where initiating agents have been identified. However, with the exception of smoking and lung cancer, these are not of the first importance. Of greater relevance are the common cancers. It is difficult to define initiating events in colon cancer, leukaemias unrelated to radiation, or hormone-related breast and prostate cancers. The main feature of hormones, which are usually defined as promotional agents, is that they are mitogenic for the cells whose risk they increase, and proliferation alone might generate sufficient errors to cause a breast or prostate cancer. This idea has attractions for other cancers – brain cells (slow growth) rarely develop into cancers, whereas colon epithelium (fast growth) frequently becomes neoplastic. However, the inevitable exceptions exist, such as the mucosal epithelium of the mouth (fast growth), which is not a major cancer. It might be explained by the continual loss (exfoliation) of both normal and damaged cells during eating. If the 'proliferation alone' model has merit, then a discrete early step under the heading 'initiation' may not be necessary. It might clarify conceptual problems about the word 'initiation' (see Animal studies, p. 12) if it were dropped in favour of 'DNA damage' or 'mutation'. It may be that for some human tumours, the clear-cut distinction between an initiating event followed by promotion (see Figure 2.1, model 1) should be modified (Figure 2.10). Continual

Figure 2.10

Initiation and promotion: modified model.

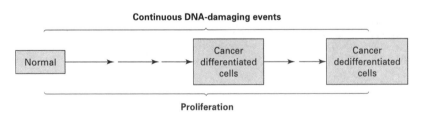

exposure of cells to mutational events (DNA damage) linked with proliferative pressure (promotion) could generate the cellular changes required for carcinogenesis. Cancer progression to a more dedifferentiated state would be a continuation of these events.

Mutation rate increases with cell age (see Chapter 7) in both normal and cancer cells, and so it is not clear whether there is anything special about cancer cells in this respect. Based on the data from normal cells, it has been hypothesised that carcinogenesis is a natural consequence of getting old. Acceleration in the mutation rate can be caused by defective DNA repair, increased proliferation, decreased apoptosis or combinations of these processes (see Chapter 9).

As depicted in Figure 2.10, both damaging and proliferative influences are continuous. This would be correct for damaging events of endogenous origin, such as free-radical formation or incomplete repair of misaligned bases, but it does not preclude additional exposures to exogenous carcinogens, such as ultraviolet light and drugs (see Chapter 7). Proliferative signals could derive from exogenous factors such as diet, viral infection and hormones (contraceptive pills, hormone replacement therapy) or endogenous sources such as hormonal changes. In the case of hormones, they fluctuate on a monthly basis (menstrual cycle) and at different stages of development (puberty, menopause).

No single model will explain the pathogenesis of all human cancers, but it is important to have appropriate models against which data can be tested.

Angiogenesis

Animal studies identified angiogenesis as a crucial event in cancer growth; the same is true in humans, both in the transition from *in situ* to invasive growth and for metastasis. It has been shown that there is a marked quantitative increase in vascular supply at the transition between early non-invasive and the later invasive stages.

Summary

At the molecular level, animal and cell biological experiments have identified DNA sequences and proteins directly relevant to human cancers. The *ras* oncogene and tumour suppressor genes were first identified by combinations of molecular and cell biological techniques, and numerous other examples are provided throughout this book. Molecular analysis is also helping us to identify causative agents for specific human cancers (see Chapter 4). Knowledge is accumulating about types of mutation generated by different carcinogens (mutational spectral analysis), so that it is becoming possible to predict the type of agent causing a mutation (see Chapter 7).

No single model will explain the pathogenesis of all human cancers. Two specific examples – a solid tumour (colon cancer) and a blood cancer (chronic myeloid leukaemia) – will be used to illustrate the relevance of the terms and features derived from experimental systems to these very different human cancers. More detailed molecular descriptions of the events to be described will be found in subsequent chapters.

Colorectal cancer

Clinical picture

Adenocarcinoma of the colon is a common cancer accounting for about 15% of all cancers in Western countries and occurring equally in men and women, mainly between the ages of 55 and 70 years. Appendix A gives more clinical details. About half of all patients survive for 5 years after first detection, but this depends on the degree of spread (stage) when the cancer is first detected. A commonly used staging system (Dukes') divides degree of spread into three categories depending on whether the cancer is localised (A), has invaded through the colon wall (B) or has spread outside the colon (C). The cancer metastasises by several routes. Direct invasion through the colonic mucosa results in peritoneal outgrowths, whereas liver is the major site of blood-borne spread. Lymph nodes become involved via the lymphatic vessels.

Presenting symptoms include irregular and problematic bowel movements and the appearance of blood in the faeces. Blood in the faeces has been developed as a method for early detection of abnormal changes based on the detection of faecal iron derived from haemoglobin. Surgery is the main treatment, together with chemotherapy and radiotherapy.

Several types of colorectal cancer can be identified according to the degree and type of familial involvement. About 80% are sporadic, but the remaining 20% exist in two hereditary forms: **f**amilial **a**denomatous **p**olyposis coli (FAP) and **h**ereditary **n**on-**p**olyposis **c**olon **c**ancer (HNPCC) or Lynch's sydrome. As the names imply, FAP is characterised by thousands of benign adenomatous polyps at an early age (about 20 years), which if untreated progress to invasive cancer. Cancers appear in HNPCC without passing through this intermediate stage. Both familial types occur before age 50 years, earlier than the sporadic cancers.

Cellular changes

Colorectal cancers have clonal origins in the epithelial stem cells at the base of the crypt (see Figure A.4). The subsequent sequence of events defined from pathology samples is analogous to model 4 in Figure 2.1, although some of the names are different (Figure 2.11). Benign adenomas are classified largely by size and degree of cellular abnormality, while 'carcinoma *in situ*' is not a term that is applied to colorectal cancer. The availability of tissue from each of these stages has allowed analysis of DNA alterations at each stage, and a picture has been built up to describe

Figure 2.11

Major gene changes during colorectal carcinogenesis.

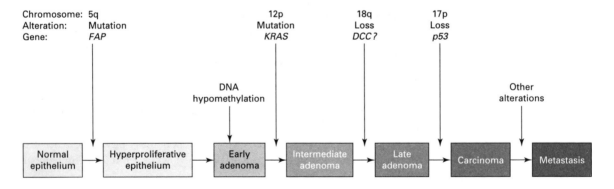

Table 2.1 Major gene changes involved in colorectal cancers.

Gene	Type of change	Chromosome	Function	Cancers showing that change (%)
APC	Loss	5	Cell adhesion	> 70
K-ras	Gain	11	Signal transduction	50
SMAD				
(*DCC*)	Loss	18	Proliferation, differentiation	> 70
p53	Loss	17	DNA repair, apoptosis	> 70
MSH2	Loss	2	DNA repair	5
MLH1	Loss	3	DNA repair	35
TGFβ2			Growth factor receptor	
IGF2R			Growth factor receptor	
PMS				
MLH				
GTBP				
DCC	Loss	18	Tumour suppressor	
CMYC			Transcription factor (regulates p53 acTERT, the main compound of telomerase complex)	

which DNA changes contribute to different stages of development. The mutations identified in familial cancers also occur in sporadic cases, but to different extents. **A**denomatous **p**olyposis **c**oli (*APC*) mutations occur in most sporadic colorectal cancers (Table 2.1), and alteration of this gene is the rate-limiting step in colorectal carcinogenesis. Because of its importance, the gene has been called a gatekeeper gene. The difference between FAP familial cancers and sporadic forms is that the sporadic forms result from somatic cell mutations whereas germline mutations contribute to the familial connection. This difference in source of mutational events is compatible with the earlier appearance of the familial cancers as fewer errors have to be generated. In contrast to FAP, HNPCC mutations have been identified in only a minority of sporadic cancers (Table 2.1).

Additional DNA alterations have been identified by their loss of heterozygosity (see Chapter 8), whereas more general defects occur during progression that increase the DNA content per nucleus (ploidy).

DNA mutations can result in loss or gain in function of the base sequences affected. Both loss and gain are required for colorectal carcinogenesis (Table 2.1), with the loss predominating. Loss of function is characteristic of tumour suppressor genes, whereas gain of function occurs with oncogenes (see Chapter 6).

Mechanisms

The functions of the genes listed in Table 2.1 can be related to general behavioural changes discussed earlier. The normal *APC* gene codes for a protein that mediates signal transduction from a cell-membrane adhesion molecule (a cadherin) to the cytoskeleton and nucleus (see Chapter 10). Loss of this function disrupts the tight linkage of epithelial cells in normal colon and represents an early step in the process of invasion. Its gatekeeper role might suggest that it functions as an initiator, but this creates conceptual problems for the classical model (Figure 2.1, model 1) in that it is not always the first gene to be altered (see below) in sporadic cancers. However, it is compatible with a promotional or proliferative role in either that model or its modified form (see Figure 2.10).

The original model of gene changes associated with colorectal carcinogenesis included one gene called **d**eleted in **c**olon **c**ancer (*DCC*). This was initially described as coding for a cell-adhesion molecule (N-CAM) and then for a membrane receptor for polypeptides (netrins) responsible for directional movement of cells (see Chapter 11). It now appears that due to an error in the mapping of the chromosomal location of *DCC*, the real culprit is a nearby gene, *SMAD4*, involved in the signalling pathway for **t**ransforming **g**rowth **f**actor β (TGF-β). TGF-β is a growth-inhibitory differentiation-inducing cytokine (see Chapters 9 and 10) and so loss of signal transduction from this factor could mediate tumour promotion. In mice containing an *APC* deletion on one allele, knocking out *SMAD4* increased the size and invasiveness of adenomas, whereas *DCC* deletions had no effect. The relevance of these mice experiments to human colon remains to be established, but in this book the original *DCC* terminology has been changed to *SMAD*.

The *K-ras* mutation activates signal transduction from membrane to nucleus by virtue of the loss of its GTPase activity (see Chapter 10), while DNA repair defects (MSH2 and MLH1) increase the probability of accumulating further errors in the DNA (see Chapter 7). The p53 protein links three cellular functions: proliferation, death and DNA repair (see Chapter 9). In normal cells, p53 blocks proliferation and enables completion of DNA repair before DNA synthesis takes place. If repair is incomplete, then the cell dies. Loss of p53 function therefore contributes to propagation of damaged DNA to daughter cells. A minority of cancers exhibit gene changes not listed in Table 2.1. These include various cyclins (4% of cancers), *myc* (2%) and *erbB2* (2%).

The functions listed in Table 2.1 embrace many cell functions and indicate the varied nature and chromosomal involvement of the multiple changes required for carcinogenesis and progression. The sequence of the changes shown in Figure 2.11 is highly simplified. Not all colorectal cancers pass through all stages (Table 2.1), the order in which changes occur can vary, and any one gene can have mutations in different bases.

One signalling pathway not shown in Figure 2.11 is the pathway for prostaglandins. Clinical trials on the beneficial effects of aspirin, a **n**on-**s**teroidal **a**nti-**i**nflammatory **d**rug (NSAID), in patients with heart and rheumatism problems also indicated a marked protective effect against colorectal carcinogenesis; aspirin markedly decreased the risk of getting both cancer and polyps (see Chapter 13). Aspirin inhibits **c**yclo**o**xygenase (COX) enzymes responsible for prostaglandin synthesis, although the mechanisms by which COX enzymes influence colorectal carcinogenesis are unclear (see Chapter 10).

The multiple pathways are most clearly seen by comparing FAP and HNPCC; FAP involves polyp formation whereas HBPCC does not. Variation in sequence or requirement for specific events is demonstrated by the fact that, of colorectal cancers exhibiting changes in four of the genes in Table 2.1 (*K-ras*, *APC*, *p53*, *SMAD*), 10% had all four, 40% three and 80% only two alterations. The overall accumulation of errors rather than their sequence may be important. The late involvement of *p53* in this cancer contrasts with that seen in other tumours and accentuates the point about variable routes of carcinogenesis. This diversity is seen even at the single-gene level. Most germline mutations of the *APC* gene generate stop codons, and a truncated protein is therefore produced. However, amino-acid substitutions and frameshifts have also been identified. Somatic cell mutations in the *APC* gene show a lower proportion of stop codons with a more localised distribution than seen with germline mutations (see Chapter 10).

Relevance to models of carcinogenesis

The histological picture fits with model 4 in Figure 2.1, with the caveats that colon adenoma and polyps should be considered as stages between hyperplasia and carcinoma. Also, the term 'carcinoma *in situ*' is not used with colorectal cancer. The sequence of gene changes is compatible with model 3. Initiation (model 1) is usually shown as the first event in carcinogenesis; thus, if the *APC* gene is that event, then it is difficult to reconcile changes in cell–cell contact with initiation, and the modified model in Figure 2.10 might be more appropriate. On the other hand, DNA repair defects resulting from *MSH2* and *MLH1* mutations by generating a mutator phenotype would be prime candidates as an initiating event, but they occur in only a minority of sporadic cancers.

It is important to identify the causes of the genetic alterations. Chemical carcinogens can generate colorectal cancers in rodents but, in humans, one is largely confined to talking about environmental or dietary carcinogens with minimal definition of what that means. There is a 19-fold difference between countries with the highest incidence (USA) and lowest incidence (India) of colorectal cancer; this indicates a lifestyle effect, probably dietary. Diets high in meat and animal fat and low in fibre increase the risk, but the mechanism remains to be established. Production of carcinogens during cooking of meat is one possibility; animal and cell-culture experiments indicate that fat can be a promoter (see Chapter 4). Activated *ras* would increase cell proliferation and play a promotional role.

Chronic myeloid leukaemia

Clinical picture

CML is characterised by the progressive replacement of normal bone marrow cells by mature myeloid cells that have altered sensitivity to normal regulatory mechanisms (Figure 2.12). The ratio of leukaemic to normal cells increases gradually to a critical level, when a 'blast crisis' occurs. If uncorrected, this leads to blast-cell invasion of vital organs such as the brain. These abnormal blast cells have variable phenotypes; myeloblasts are commonly seen in about two-thirds of cases and lymphoblasts in one-third, although the phenotypes can change with time or can be a mixture (Figure 2.12). The acute phase results rapidly in death due to haemorrhage in the invaded organ. It takes about 4 years from first detection to death.

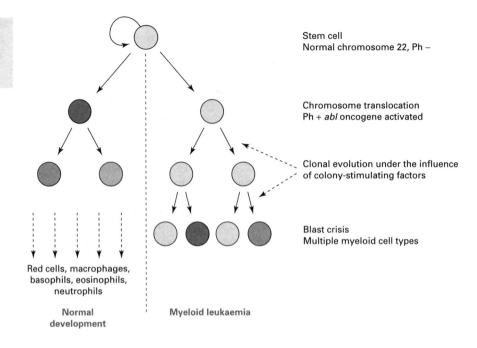

Figure 2.12

Development of chronic myeloid leukaemia.

Stem cell
Normal chromosome 22, Ph –

Chromosome translocation
Ph + *abl* oncogene activated

Clonal evolution under the influence
of colony-stimulating factors

Blast crisis
Multiple myeloid cell types

Red cells, macrophages,
basophils, eosinophils,
neutrophils

**Normal
development**

Myeloid leukaemia

Cellular changes

CML is characterised by the possession of an abnormally small chromosome 22, the **Ph**iladelphia chromosome (Ph), caused by the translocation of part of its genetic material to chromosome 9. This brings the *abl* oncogene from chromosome 9 under the regulatory influence of oncogene *bcr* on chromosome 22, increasing the tyrosine kinase activity of *abl* (see Chapter 5). Different breakpoints occur in the *bcr* gene in different patients, although the biochemical end result is the same – elevated tyrosine kinase activity in the myeloid cells, which renders them hyperresponsive to growth factors. This variability in breakpoints with the same end result illustrates the multiple pathways to cancer evident from experimental models. The importance of the ABL tyrosine kinase in the progress of this disease is illustrated by the fact that the disease is treated with an inhibitor specific for this tyrosine kinase (see Chapter 12).

When CML progresses to the terminal acute phase, additional chromosome abnormalities can be detected such that the chromosome number changes from the normal 46 (diploid) to a modal number of 47–50. Cell-proliferation rates of CML do not increase in the acute phase, and so progression involves more than simply increasing growth rate.

Analysis of chromosomes and of isoenzymes such as G6PD indicates that clonal selection occurs at least twice: the original generation of Ph and during events leading up to blast crisis.

Mechanisms

CML results from blocked differentiation and continued proliferation of immature myelocytes (see Figure A.5). The chromosome translocation resulting in increased tyrosine kinase activity is a crucial event, as transfection of the *abl* cDNA into normal cells generates leukaemias. This is probably not equivalent to initiation because although the protein product of the translocation has the properties of an initiating agent as defined in experimental models, it begs the question of what causes the translocation. Whatever causes the chromosome change would have a better claim to be the initiator. Candidates identified through animal experiments include viruses, radiation, immune deficiency and carcinogenic chemicals. Of these, only radiation has been identified as a causal influence in humans.

Little is known about promotional events other than the increased activity of growth factors such as **c**olony-**s**timulating **f**actor (CSF). Animal experiments show that continuous exogenous or autocrine production of CSF will produce hyperplasia in normal cells but not leukaemias. On the other hand, if the cells are first immortalised with a virus, overproduction of CSF will generate leukaemias. Similar changes may occur with human CML, but as none of the observed chromosome changes involves CSF genes, more subtle changes must be happening.

Transition to the acute phase, characterised by the blast crisis, is equivalent to progression. Multiple events are required for each stage, much as in the experimental models, but apart from the chromosome changes, the nature of these events is obscure. The only other identified agent is a family of growth factors, CSFs. As their name implies, these glycoproteins are required for proliferation of CML colonies, analogous to anchorage-independent growth. CML cells will survive but not grow if suspended in agar, but addition of CSF stimulates this anchorage-independent growth; they are, therefore, CSF-dependent for growth, a property that is retained by most but not all blast cells. As in the experimental models, human CML can progress by more than one pathway.

Further reading

Fearon, E.R. and Vogelstein, B. (1990) A genetic model for colorectal tumorigenesis. *Cell* **61**, 759–767.

Fialko, P.J. (1972) Use of genetic markers to study cellular origin and development of tumours in human females. *Adv Cancer Res* **15**, 191–226.

Goldman, J.M. and Melo, J.V. (2003) Chronic myeloid leukaemia: advances in biology and new approaches to treatment. *N Engl J Med* **349**, 1451–1464.

Hann, B. and Balmain, A. (2001) Building 'validated' mouse models of human cancer. *Curr Opin Cell Biol* **13**, 778–784.

Kemp, Z., Thirlwell, C., Sieber, O., Silver, A. and Tomlinson, I. (2004) An update on the genetics of colorectal cancer. *Hum Mol Genet* **13**, R177–R185.

Kinzler, K.W. and Vogelstein, B. (1997) Cancer-susceptibility genes: gatekeepers and caretakers. *Nature* **386**, 761–762.

Weidner, N., Semple, J.P., Welch, W.R. and Folkman, J. (1991) Tumour angiogenesis and metastasis: correlation in invasive breast carcinoma. *N Engl J Med* **324**, 1–8.

3 Pathology: defining a neoplasm

KEY POINTS

- Tissue and cell architecture are used to decide whether a growth is malignant.
- Pathology can distinguish between benign and malignant growths.
- Pathology defines the type of cancer.
- Pathology helps to determine prognosis and treatment.

Introduction

An understanding of pathology is essential to any description of cancer biology because it plays important roles in diagnosis and prognosis as well as helping to elucidate the steps in carcinogenesis. The steps in carcinogenesis were described in the previous chapter and so more general aspects of pathology will be dealt with here. Three types of pathology can be defined depending on whether intact tissues, individual cells or chemical analysis of body fluids or tissues are involved (Table 3.1). Cancer is the growth of one or, occasionally, a few cell types at the expense of others, and this differential growth disrupts the normal interrelationships between the different cell types and their extracellular matrix. These features can be visualised by microscopic examination of stained tissue sections (histopathology). Cytology, on the other hand, deals with single or small clumps of cells removed from a suspect site. Chemical pathology, which will be described more fully in Chapter 12, involves chemical analysis of tissue, blood or urine.

The term 'cancer' tends to be used differently in experimental and clinical settings; experimentalists adopt a more general usage than clinicians. Experimentalists use the term to include abnormal growth regardless of whether invasion and metastasis occur. This is understandable, as most chemically induced growths in animals tend not to metastasise and cultured cells have no opportunity to exhibit this property. The terms 'neoplasm' (new growth) and 'tumour' cover this broader definition of abnormal growth. Clinically, a cancer is defined more precisely as being invasive and able to metastasise (malignant) in contrast to benign growths, which remain localised. Use of the term 'cancer' should be confined to invasive growths. Other distinctions between benign and malignant growths are listed in Table 3.2 and further described below. Benign growths are sometimes, but not always, precursors of malignant growths. Colorectal cancer and thyroid cancer are examples where benign

Table 3.1 The objectives of pathology in oncology.

Pathology
Histopathology: tissues
Cytology: individual cells
Chemical pathology: analysis of tissue, blood and urine

Diagnosis
Is it cancer?
What type of cancer?

Histogenesis
Has the surgeon removed it all?

Prognosis
What is the clinical outlook?

Identifying features
Cell and tissue architecture
Differentiation: degree to which it resembles normal
Cell structure: nucleus, mitoses, nuclear/cytoplasmic ratio
Localised or invasive (stroma, blood vessels)

Methods
Staining
Immunohistochemistry: protein
In situ hybridisation: mRNA
DNA characterisation

Table 3.2 Comparison of benign and malignant growths.

Feature	Benign	Malignant
Edges	Encapsulated	Irregular
Metastasis	No	Yes
Invasion	No	Yes
Comparison with normal	Good	Variable, often none
Growth rate	Low	High
Nuclei	Normal	Variable, irregular
Life-threatening	Unusual	Usual

growths turn malignant, whereas benign prostate and breast growths are not precursors of malignant growths.

One role of pathology is to distinguish between benign and malignant cells, because benign cells are not usually life-threatening and therefore treatments of the two types of growth are different. A second function is to determine the cellular origin of a cancer (histogenesis), as a cancer in an organ can have several origins. Thus, in lung, smoking generates epithelial cancers, whereas mesothelial cancers result from asbestos exposure. As treatments are different, the importance of determining histogenesis is clear. Likewise, it is not axiomatic that a liver growth originated in the liver, as it may have metastasised from elsewhere. There are even tumours whose cellular origins cannot be determined (cancers of unknown origin).

Carcinogenesis involves a series of changes that are reflected in an increasing departure from normal morphology. Pathology helps to define boundaries in this sequence of events, but as changes continue to occur after a cancer has formed, cell characterisation also has a role to play as a predictive (prognostic) tool in determining the likely course of the disease. Another function of pathology is in monitoring completeness of surgery. Because cancers have ill-defined margins, it is sometimes difficult for a surgeon to decide what should be removed; microscopic analysis of an excised lump can inform whether cancer cells occur at its edges and thereby provide evidence as to efficiency of removal.

Box 3.1 Classifying cancers

Neoplasms are classified as being benign or malignant; malignant neoplasms are equivalent to cancer. Cancers are described according to their cell of origin and the tissue in which they arise (Table 3.3). Most common cancers arise in

Table 3.3 Terminology.

General
 Growth: vague term that covers any collection of hyperproliferative cells
 Neoplasm: general term used to identify a new growth without defining the characteristics of that growth
 Tumour: general term used to describe any abnormal growth
 Cancer: invasive growth with abnormal cellular and architectural features.

Epithelium (carcinoma)
 Glandular, e.g. prostate: adenocarcinoma
 Squamous, e.g. cervix: carcinoma

Mesenchyme (sarcoma)
 Smooth muscle: leiomyosarcoma; benign hyperproliferation is called a leiomyoma (fibroid)
 Bone: osteosarcoma
 Fat cells: liposarcoma; benign hyperproliferation is called a lipoma

Nervous system
 Eye: retinoblastoma
 Astrocytes: astrocytoma

White blood cells (leukaemia)★
 Myeloid cells: myelocytic leukaemia
 Lymphocytes: lymphocytic leukaemia
 Lymphoma: solid tumour derived from B- or T-lymphocytes

★ Can be subdivided into chronic and acute forms.

epithelial cells; these carry the suffix 'carcinoma' preceded by the name of the cell type involved. Frequently, the type of epithelium is additionally identified, so that a glandular epithelium generates an adenocarcinoma (e.g. prostatic adenocarcinoma) whereas a cancer of squamous epithelium would be a squamous cell carcinoma (e.g. cervical squamous cell carcinoma). Mesenchymal cells give rise to 'sarcomas' prefixed by the cell of origin, a format followed for other cancers. White-blood-cell cancers, leukaemias, are typical in this respect but are defined further according to the speed with which they develop. Thus **a**cute **m**yelocytic **l**eukaemia (AML) and **c**hronic **m**yelocytic **l**eukaemia (CML) exhibit rapid and slow onset of symptoms, respectively, and are different diseases with different causes. In contrast to leukaemic cells that circulate in the bloodstream, lymphomas of either B-cell or T-cell origin remain as solid-cell aggregates. For historical reasons, confusingly some cancers are named after their discoverers: Burkitt's lymphoma is a B-lymphocyte cancer, Wilms' tumour is a renal carcinoma in young children and Kaposi's sarcoma arises from endothelial cells of blood vessels.

Histopathology

Histopathology is the routine method for characterising an excised lump. Diagnosis relies not only on the appearance of the cells but also on the tissue architecture, reflecting neoplastic cell relationships to the extracellular matrix and other cells (Figure 3.1). The main features that distinguish an epithelial cancer from its normal progenitor cells are shown in cartoon format in Figure 3.1, and a real example is given in Figure 3.2. The comparison of normal and cancerous colon in Figure 3.2 conveys the partial change in epithelial characteristics associated with a moderately differentiated cancer. The regular arrangement of crypt cells is retained in places but lost elsewhere in the section; invasive cancer cells are present in the stroma. The normal cells have regularly shaped nuclei in contrast to the heterogeneous sizes in the cancer; mitotic (proliferating) cells are evident in the cancer but not the normal colon. No secretory vacuoles are present in the cancer, indicating some loss of differentiated function. Such examples do not convey the remarkable heterogeneity of structures contained within a cancerous growth. Figure 3.3 shows a section of a breast cancer that indicates this heterogeneity with normal ducts, *in situ* carcinoma, invasive carcinoma and infiltrating lymphocytes all present in one area of a cancer excised by surgery. This section provides a snapshot in time of what happens during carcinogenesis. The normal mammary epithelium surrounds a duct; during carcinogenesis, the epithelium proliferates into and fills the duct but does not penetrate the basement membrane. The cells have the abnormalities represented in Figure 3.1 but they have not become invasive; this stage is known as *in situ* carcinoma. Cancer cells that have become invasive are dispersed throughout the stroma (extracellular matrix proteins such as collagen plus mesenchymal cells). Blood vessels supplying nutrients and as potential routes for metastasis are also present in the

Figure 3.1

Glandular epithelium.

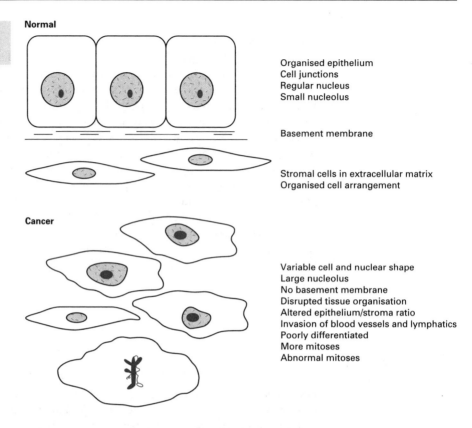

Normal

Organised epithelium
Cell junctions
Regular nucleus
Small nucleolus

Basement membrane

Stromal cells in extracellular matrix
Organised cell arrangement

Cancer

Variable cell and nuclear shape
Large nucleolus
No basement membrane
Disrupted tissue organisation
Altered epithelium/stroma ratio
Invasion of blood vessels and lymphatics
Poorly differentiated
More mitoses
Abnormal mitoses

stroma. The section in Figure 3.3 has been immunohistochemically stained with an antibody against a **h**eat-**s**hock **p**rotein (HSP27) to illustrate another aspect of heterogeneity within the cells that make up a cancer. Expression of specific proteins alters during carcinogenesis and can be used for diagnostic purposes (see Chapter 12). In this example, expression is low in normal epithelium, is slightly raised in *in situ carcinoma* but is greatly enhanced in the invasive cancer.

Benign growths such as lipomas (fat cells) and leiomyomas (muscle cells) caused by overproliferation of specific cell types that resemble the cell of origin are encapsulated and do not invade surrounding areas. Malignant lesions, on the other hand, can profoundly damage their surroundings. Epithelial cancers destroy the basement membrane and invade the stroma, thus increasing the ratio of epithelial cells to stromal cells. Leukaemic cells take over the bone marrow and disrupt the balance of haemopoietic cells; sarcomas also disrupt normal architecture.

The cells themselves are also informative (see Table 3.1). Benign cells closely resemble their normal antecedents, and their nuclei have a regular shape with a small nucleolus. Malignant cells have a more varied appearance, with convoluted cell membranes, irregularly shaped and large nuclei, pronounced nucleoli and little heterochromatin; the latter two features reflect an active transcription machinery. If the cancer arose from cells with specialist functions, such as a glandular epithelium involved in production of a secretion, then cytoplasmic changes are evident, such as disorganisation of the endoplasmic reticulum and absence of secretions (see Figure 3.2).

Cellular stroma below a single layer of epithelial cells

Disorganised structure with few stormal cells.
Some residual crypt organisation

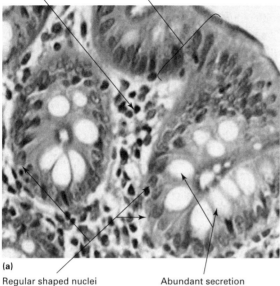

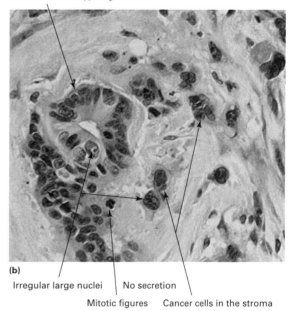

(a)

Regular shaped nuclei
No mitoses

Abundant secretion

Well-organised tissue with distinct glands and stroma

(b)

Irregular large nuclei   No secretion

Mitotic figures   Cancer cells in the stroma

Figure 3.2

Colon epithelium:
(a) normal and
(b) moderately
differentiated cancer.

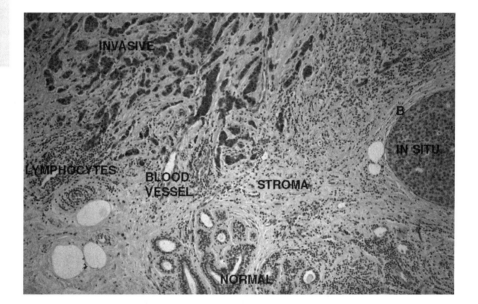

Figure 3.3

Histological sections of a breast cancer. NORMAL: mammary duct lined by
epithelium. IN SITU: carcinoma that has not invaded the basement membrane (B).
INVASIVE: carcinoma cells in the stroma; the stroma also contains infiltrating
lymphocytes and blood vessels. The section has been stained with an antibody against a
heat-shock protein (HSP27) to highlight differential expression of this protein in breast
cells at different stages of cancer development.

This loss of differentiation (dedifferentiation) is a common accompaniment of carcinogenesis. Many cancers are graded on the above features to give an index of their degree of malignancy, which in turn can be used to predict subsequent behaviour of the cancer. Several grading systems exist (see Chapter 12); some use all features of the cells and tissues, including number of mitotic figures, while others rely only on nuclear characteristics.

Cytology

This increasingly useful diagnostic technique relies on the characteristics of isolated exfoliated cells alone, but because it loses the benefit of tissue architecture, it provides less precise information than histopathology. It has the advantage over histopathology of requiring a less invasive procedure. Its most widespread use is in screening women for early signs of cervical cancer and with fine needle aspirates of suspicious breast lumps.

Immunohistochemistry

This technique enables workers to detect the location of specific proteins within tissues and cells. Tissue sections or smears are treated with antibodies tagged with a coloured or fluorescent dye, a heavy metal or an enzyme. Sites of antibody–antigen reaction can be visualised either directly (dye, fluorescent dye, heavy metal) or following a subsequent reaction (enzyme). This technique is useful in determining the presence of tumour suppressor genes such as *p53* and *Rb* in tumours. In colorectal cancer, the cells are often *p53*-positive, while benign (adenoma) and normal epithelium are not.

Molecular techniques

This section is intended only as a brief introduction to a rapidly developing area.

In situ hybridisation
This is used to determine where a particular mRNA is expressed. Tissue sections are reacted with probes, which are single-stranded RNA molecules synthesised from a suitable DNA. Such a probe must be 'antisense', that is, an RNA version of the non-coding strand. This can be used to detect viral RNA in sections of cancer; an example here would be EBV in nasopharyngeal cancer.

Tissue microdissection
This involves isolation of pure populations of cells from tissue sections viewed under the microscope. For example, microdissected DNA can be used as a template for

other techniques such as **p**olymerase **c**hain **r**eaction (PCR, see below) and loss of heterozygosity.

Polymerase chain reaction

This is repeated copying of target sequences of DNA by use of oligonucleotide primers unique to the sequence of interest.

Gene expression profiling

RNA is extracted from the sample and tagged with a fluorescent dye. This is hybridised with a microarray, which consists of a systematic array of specific cDNAs or oligonucleotides of known sequence that have been robotically spotted on to a glass surface. This allows determination of the expression of thousands of genes simultaneously. Analysis of such displays is complex, but essentially it involves computer-based filtering and arranging data into significant groups. This technique can be used, for example, to identify prognostic subclasses of adult myeloid leukaemia.

Further reading

Crnogorac-Jurcevic, T., Pulson, R., Banks, R.E. (2005) The molecular pathology of cancer. In *Introduction to the Cellular and Molecular Biology of Cancer*, ed. M. Knowles and P. Selby. Oxford: Oxford University Press.

Fletcher, C.D.M., Unni, K.K. and Mertens, F. (2002) *Pathology and Genetics of Tumours of Soft Tissue and Bone*. Lyons: IACR Press.

Notterman, D.A., Alon, U., Sierk, A.J. and Levine, A.J. (2001) Transcriptional gene expression profiles of colorectal adenoma, adenocarcinoma, and normal tissues by oligonucleotide arrays. *Cancer Res* **61**, 3124–3130.

Stevens, A., Lowe, J.S. and Young, B. (2002) *Wheater's Basic Histopathology*, 4th edn. Edinburgh: Churchill Livingstone.

4 Epidemiology: identifying causes for human cancers

KEY POINTS

- Incidence of cancers in different populations provides clues about the causes.
- Risk factors can be identified that indicate causative events in cancer development.
- Geographical differences in cancer incidence indicate the importance of diet and solar radiation.
- The influence of diet on cancer is a complex one in which fat, vitamins, fibre and other agents are involved.
- Smoking, diet, sex hormones, increasing age and family history of cancer alter the risk of developing cancer.
- Most cancers could be prevented.
- Biochemical analyses provide additional information for epidemiological studies by identifying people at risk.
- Molecular epidemiology can be used to identify causative agents.

Introduction

Epidemiology, the study of disease distributions in human populations, is probably the single most important discipline that generates clues about factors that influence specific types of human cancers. Although laboratory experiments with animals and cell cultures can dissect molecular mechanisms and indicate the potential of chemicals or conditions to influence carcinogenesis, their applicability to real life can only be tested in humans. Epidemiological analysis is a major way of achieving that objective. This discipline involves comparisons of groups of people. Its methodology has progressed markedly from the eighteenth-century observations that nuns get more breast cancer than other women and that scrotal cancer was common in chimneysweeps. The methods by which groups of people are compared are critical to decisions as to whether observed differences reflect a causal or artefactual link. Therefore, those methods must be understood as well as the information generated therefrom.

Epidemiology is divided conveniently into two categories, descriptive and analytical, based on the type of data being used. A third category, molecular epidemiology, has entered the lexicon; here, molecular analyses such as DNA and protein profiles are included as variables in the epidemiological studies.

Descriptive epidemiology

Descriptive epidemiology uses data from large populations. It draws general conclusions on which more specific analyses can be based. Figure 4.1 shows deaths from three cancers in the USA, indicating lung cancer to have been an increasing problem that has now reached a plateau, cancer of the stomach to be declining and colorectal cancer to be static. Such data indicate that a problem exists with lung cancer whereas something beneficial is happening for stomach cancer. However, the data tell us nothing about what causes those changes or what should be done in order to increase the benefits and decrease the adverse effects. Geographical distributions and influences of lifestyle, such as diet and environment, also provide important clues as to what might cause cancers.

Descriptive epidemiology is good at highlighting trends or differences, but more rigorous analytical epidemiology is needed in order to reveal aetiological relationships. Both methods are also useful for defining biological hypotheses that can be tested by other means.

Figure 4.1

Age-corrected male cancer deaths in the USA.

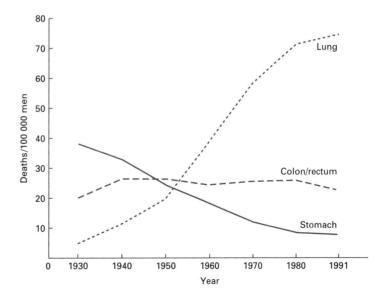

| Box 4.1 | **Epidemiological methods and terminology** |

Descriptive epidemiology

Records of people's health and causes of death are used to correlate events such as the first detection of (*incidence*) or death from (*mortality*) a specific cancer with personal details like age, sex and race. Death certificates are an important source of information on mortality, but incidence data are better obtained from population-based registries maintained by national and international organisations. From these data, *incidence rates* can be calculated as follows:

$$\frac{\text{Number of people developing a cancer in a specific time period}}{\text{Total population at that time}}$$

A similar calculation is used to obtain *mortality rates*, but the number of people dying replaces those developing cancer. The time period can be one year or several years. If the period is extended to encompass people of all ages throughout their life, it is called the *cumulative* or *lifetime rate*. This gives an index of the probability of getting (incidence) or dying from (mortality) a specific cancer at some time during a person's life.

Population numbers are usually corrected per 100 000 people. According to Figure 4.1, the mortality rate from lung cancer in US men during the period 1989–91 was 75 per 100 000 population. The equivalent incidence rate for that population was 80 per 100 000 (not shown in Figure 4.1). US men born in 1940 have a one in ten likelihood of getting lung cancer at some time in their life. These numbers are known as *crude incidence* or *mortality rates* because the data have not been corrected in any way. As many cancers occur in older people, it follows that an older population will have higher rates than a younger population, so uncorrected data can result in erroneous conclusions. For example, if we wish to know how a Japanese lifestyle, based on a high-fish, low-fat diet, compares with a low-fish, high-fat Western diet, then it is important not to let the different age profiles of the two populations confuse the results. This is remedied by correcting the crude data for age, so that we can compare rates for populations of equivalent ages, a process that yields *age-corrected incidence* or *mortality rates*. *Prevalence* is analogous to incidence, except that it represents the *number of cancer cases in a defined population at the time of data collection*, not just the new cases over a given period.

Age-corrected data are useful for comparing populations to get an idea of whether incidence of certain cancers is changing with time or whether a particular lifestyle correlates with specific cancers, but it gives little information on whether there is a cause-and-effect relationship. In the Japanese–Western comparison, it turns out that stomach cancer is high in Japan whereas breast cancer shows the opposite pattern. However, it would be wrong to immediately conclude that differences were due to diet, because breast cancer also correlates with many other factors. This highlights an important principle relevant to all epidemiological methods: any explanation for differences observed must be biologically plausible.

Analytical epidemiology

The essence of analytical work is the comparison of two or more groups of people with different characteristics. This generates a number called *relative risk*, which indicates the risk associated with a given factor, e.g. smoking, compared with an identical group not influenced by that factor. The term *odds ratio* approximates to the same thing. Because the range of values in a study can be large, it is important to obtain an estimate as to the limits within which the real risk lies. A commonly used method to achieve this is the *95% confidence limit*. This gives the range of values between which the real value has a 95% probability of lying. If the value exceeds 1.0, then there is a strong probability that the exposure in question has a real effect.

There are two approaches for analytical analyses, case–control studies and cohort comparisons. In *case–control studies*, two groups of people are compared, one having cancer and the other not. Because they rely on past events, these are sometimes called *retrospective analyses*. In *cohort studies*, a healthy, well-defined population (a cohort) is followed for many years in order to identify the characteristics that distinguish people who subsequently get cancer from those who do not. Because cohort studies monitor events following the start of analysis, these are known as *prospective studies*. Cohort studies provide more reliable information than case–control studies but are more complex and more expensive to conduct.

To avoid drawing false conclusions, it is important that the groups being compared are identical apart from the specific factor being analysed. This can be difficult to achieve and errors arise through *bias* and *confounding factors*. *Selection bias* occurs through inappropriate selection of people for comparison; *recall bias* occurs through inadequate measures of exposure. For example, in case–control studies, it is common to ask both groups to recall past events. Compared with the controls, people with cancer have more reason to think about events that might have led to their disease, so the recall may be different in the two groups. In case–control studies, controls are often selected from people attending hospital for non-cancerous conditions. This tends to underestimate real differences (selection bias).

Because several factors may be indices of the same underlying influence, if we want to identify causative agents it is important to identify the real agent rather than a *confounding factor*. For example, eating red meat is a risk factor for several cancers, but this may be due to its fat content rather than the meat protein component. There are often difficulties in recruiting sufficient numbers of individuals for one study in order to provide the statistical power needed to detect small effects on risk. This problem can be overcome by using mathematical models to combine data from several different studies (*meta-analysis*).

Types of information obtained from descriptive data

Changes with time

If incidence or mortality changes with time, then this indicates that something is happening for which an explanation must be sought. Figure 4.1 illustrates examples of male cancer deaths that are increasing (lung), decreasing (stomach) or showing little change (colorectal) over recent years. Analytical data (see below) indicate that the increase in lung cancer is due to smoking, as the amount of tobacco smoked mirrors this increase and a decline in smoking lessens the rate of increase. Biological plausibility is provided by the identification of carcinogens in cigarette smoke. The decrease in stomach cancer is intriguing, but conclusions about cause are elusive, although diet is a prime candidate. Analytical epidemiological data have shown that high intake of fruit, vegetable, fibre and vitamins A and C and low intake of salted meat and fish all correlate with a low incidence of stomach cancer (see below). Laboratory data provide biological plausibility for such concepts. Highly salted foods contain nitrates capable of conversion to oxidising agents that damage cells; vitamins such as A (converted to retinoic acid) and C (ascorbic acid) are antioxidants that prevent these adverse effects.

Geography

There are enormous geographical differences in cancer incidence, and their study has provided important insights into cancer causation. It has also given cause for optimism that a high proportion of common cancers may be preventable. These points are illustrated in Table 4.1, which compares incidence rates for selected cancers in high- and low-risk countries. Japan has high levels of stomach cancer but low numbers of melanomas, whereas China has low rates of prostate cancer but high rates of liver cancer.

From these types of data, we can generate testable hypotheses as to what might be the causes of such large intercountry differences. Perhaps they could be explained by genetic differences between races, but according to studies of Chinese people migrating to Hawaii or the USA (Figure 4.2), this does not seem to be the case. Both prostate and breast cancer incidence rates increase, although not to the levels

Table 4.1 Incidence of cancers in different countries.

Cancer	High	Low	Relative risk (high/low)	Cause?
Skin	Australia	Japan	155	Sunlight (UV)
Prostate	USA	China	70	?
Colorectal	USA	India	19	Diet
Stomach	Japan	Kuwait	22	Diet
Cervix	Brazil	Israel	28	Sexual practices
Liver	China	Canada	49	Viruses/toxins

(Source: Adapted from Table 9.5 in DeVita, V.T., Hellman, S. and Rosenberg, S.A. (eds) (1993) *Cancer: Principles and Practice of Oncology*, Fourth Edition. Philadelphia, PA: Lippincott.)

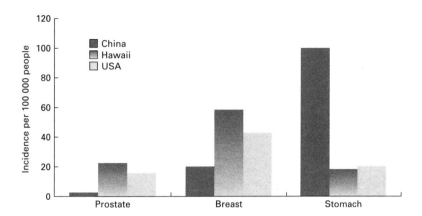

Figure 4.2

Cancer incidence for Chinese people according to place of residence.

in the indigenous white population. Conversely, stomach cancer decreases in the migrating population. If the migrants maintain an Eastern diet, then they retain an Eastern pattern of high rates of stomach cancer and low rates of breast cancer; if they adopt a Western diet, then the incidence of these two cancers reverses to mimic that seen in the white US population. Analytical epidemiological studies indicate that fat is one culprit, and laboratory studies are attempting to identify how this might work at a cellular level.

The large high : low cancer ratios illustrated in Table 4.1 plus the link between smoking and lung cancer indicate that many cancers are potentially preventable (see below). Identification of the reasons for the high : low risk ratios in various populations should facilitate corrective measures, although major problems exist for their implementation. The incidence of skin cancer in pale-skinned races varies with latitude, being highest near the Equator, where solar radiation is highest. Preventive measures such as the use of sun-block, wearing suitable protective clothing and avoiding the midday sun are known to be effective in reducing the incidence of skin cancer.

Age

The older people get, the more likely they are to develop the common cancers. Carcinogenesis requires multiple cellular changes that take time to accumulate. Using data on cancer incidence at different ages, it is possible to obtain a minimal estimate of how many changes are required (see Chapter 2).

Effects of treatment

Descriptive studies can also be used to generate information on effectiveness of treatment, although not as efficiently as with clinical trials. Alterations in 5-year survival rates with time can provide clues as to whether changing clinical practices are beneficial (Figure 4.3). Success rates with ovarian cancer have changed little, whereas for testicular cancer the increased survival is such that one can begin to talk of a cure. Figure 4.3 also illustrates the markedly different life expectancies associated with various cancers, such that the majority of breast cancer patients survive 5 years whereas hepatoma patients do not. The latter reflects the essential functions performed by the liver, disruption of which has dire consequences.

Figure 4.3

Five-year survival rates for consecutive three-year periods (US data). (Source: Adapted from American Cancer Society (1995) *Cancer Facts and Figures*. Philadelphia, PA: American Cancer Society. Reprinted by Permission of American Cancer Society.)

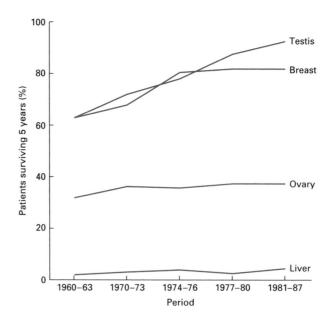

Analytical epidemiology

Factors that influence the probability of getting cancer, such as where one lives or what one eats, are referred to as risk factors. They can be identified by comparing populations of people who have a given cancer with healthy people, or comparing people exposed to a certain environment with people who are unexposed. An example would be a comparison of lung cancers in smokers and non-smokers, which defines smoking as a bad risk factor; an example of the other kind would be relating the number of breast cancers in women who have had children (parous) with those who have not (nulliparous), which shows that having children reduces the risk. Thus, the term 'risk factor' can be used in both positive and negative ways.

Analytical information is obtained from questionnaires on lifestyles and past events, but molecular data are increasingly being built into such analyses, a practice known as molecular epidemiology (see below).

Case–control studies

This method compares the characteristics of cases, either patients who have a cancer or healthy individuals with specific characteristics, with controls who do not have cancer or the characteristic in question. Details are compared in order to identify factors that are different between the two groups. Case–control studies have the advantage of providing quick answers because a relatively small number of people can be used and data are already available on both cases and controls. Major disadvantages are deciding on the appropriate controls and the fidelity of recall for past events. It is essential that the characteristics of cases and controls should be matched carefully so as not to confound the factors that do influence cancer.

Table 4.2 Case–control analysis of cervical cancer in Colombia.

Factor	Relative risk	95% Confidence limits
A. All women		
HPV DNA positive	16	7–35★
More than six sexual partners	7	2–24★
First intercourse before age 16 years	3	1–9★
Lack of schooling	3	1–8★
Oral contraceptive use	1.5	0.8–3
B. HPV-positive women only		
Oral contraceptive use	6	1.3–31★
Lack of schooling	3	0.6–12
More than six sexual partners	1	0.2–6
First intercourse before age 16 years	2	0.5–6

★ Statistically significant differences.
HPV, human papilloma virus.
(Source: Based on data in Bosch, F.X., *et al.* (1992) *International Journal of Cancer*, 52, 750–58.)

A study designed to identify risk factors for cervical cancer (Table 4.2) illustrates the general features of a case–control study. In panel A of Table 4.2, all of the factors except oral contraceptive use fall into this category.

Women with cervical cancer were 16 times more likely than controls to be **h**uman **p**apilloma **v**irus (HPV)-positive, with indices of sexual activity (number of partners, age at first intercourse) also indicating increased risk. If all women were included in the analysis, then lack of schooling was a risk factor but oral contraceptive use was not. If the sexually transmitted virus HPV is a causative agent, then other indices of sexual activity that increase the likelihood of viral infection would also show up as risk factors. Lack of schooling would be an indirect index of promiscuity (a confounding factor) in Colombia for economic reasons or due to poor social environment. This is the case because if the analyses are undertaken only on HPV-positive women, then schooling and indices of sexual activity are no longer risk factors (panel B). Interestingly, use of oral contraceptives becomes a risk factor in this subgroup, which indicates a synergism between the virus and hormones in the contraceptive.

Cohort studies

These require a well-defined healthy population (a cohort). The principle is to compare those of the cohort who get cancer in the ensuing years with those who do not. These prospective studies provide more reliable data by circumventing many of the defects of case–control studies. There are none of the problems of finding a control group, although confounding factors still occur. The reasons cohort studies are not used more widely are expense and time. Carcinogenesis is a long process, so cohorts must be followed for many years and must contain large numbers of people to ensure there are enough cancers to analyse. There is also the problem of

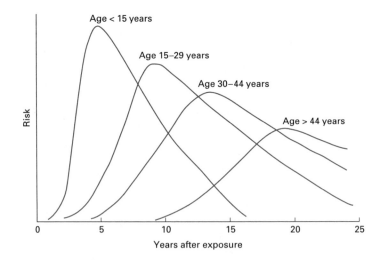

Figure 4.4

Prospective cohort analysis of relative risk of developing leukaemia in people of various ages at the time of exposure to atomic radiation in Hiroshima/Nagasaki.

maintaining contact with those people over a long period. When atom bombs were dropped on Japan in 1945, the radiation they released was a powerful carcinogen and people living at different distances from the epicentres were subjected to quantifiable levels of exposure. Those cohorts have been followed up with inform-ative results. All age groups subsequently had an increased likelihood of developing leukaemia, but it occurred more rapidly in younger people than in older people (Figure 4.4). This was a common feature with all types of cancer induced by atomic radiation, and it may reflect the increased sensitivity of cells to carcinogenic agents before reaching their fully differentiated state (see Chapter 6).

Criteria required to establish causality

With the exception of rare inherited cancers, everything to do with human cancers concerns probabilities of events rather than clear-cut distinctions. This is also true for epidemiological conclusions about establishing causal links between risk factors and cancers. Conclusions can be drawn only from repeatable studies designed to minimise bias and identify confounding factors. There should be a dose–response relationship between 'factor' and cancer risk, the time course of events should be logical and a plausible biological link should be established.

Biomarkers

Inclusion of molecular data can greatly strengthen the power of epidemiological research. Recall bias is a problem in many studies in which exposure to an agent has to be quantitated: independent ways of assessing exposure help to determine that exposure. The HPV/cervical cancer study discussed above monitored viral

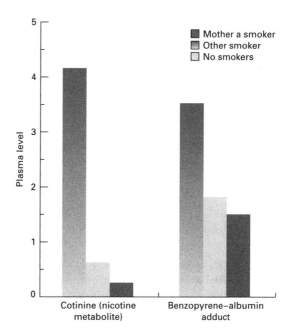

Figure 4.5

Families and smoking. Cigarette smoke metabolites were measured in the plasma of non-smoking children. (Source: Adapted from Crawford, F.G., *et al.* (1994) *Journal of the National Cancer Institute,* 86, 1398–1402.)

infection by PCR methods. Another study on liver cancer in China used a urinary metabolite of the fungal hepatocarcinogen aflatoxin to indicate people who had been exposed. The results indicated a synergism between aflatoxin and hepatitis B virus, such that a marginally increased risk with either agent alone was amplified 50-fold when both agents were involved.

Biochemical markers are also useful when carcinogen exposure cannot otherwise be determined. Passive smoking is known to increase lung cancer risk in non-smokers. The extent of carcinogen exposure in this group is difficult to quantify using questionnaires, but plasma analysis of cotinine and polycyclic aromatic hydrocarbon–albumin adducts can be so used. Cotinine is a metabolite of nicotine, while the albumin adduct of benzopyrene indicates exposure to this tobacco carcinogen. Figure 4.5 shows the levels of the two metabolites in plasma of children in three family categories: no smokers, mother a smoker and a member other than the mother who smokes. The children of smoking mothers are clearly exposed to elevated levels of noxious chemicals, and the levels are related to the number of cigarettes smoked by the mother.

Molecular epidemiology

Molecular epidemiology combines epidemiological methods with molecular analysis to help determine carcinogenic events. The molecular dissection of colorectal carcinogenesis (see Figure 2.11) was a forerunner of the approach, but a better idea of the information obtainable involves p53 mutations. This tumour

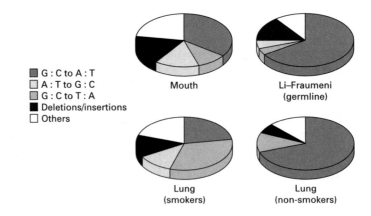

Figure 4.6

Types of *p53* mutation in different cancers. Each segment represents the percentage of all mutations in the stated category. (Source: Adapted from Greenblatt, M.S., *et al.* (1994) Mutations in the p53 tumor suppressor gene: clues to cancer etiology and molecular pathogenesis. *Cancer Research*, 54, 4855–78. Reprinted with permission from the American Association for Cancer Research.)

suppressor gene plays a pivotal role in the genesis of many cancers (see Chapter 5) and so changes in its structure are relevant to carcinogenesis. Over 2000 mutations have been identified, which has enabled correlations of mutation types with different cancers. This may point to causative agents (Figure 4.6). The Li–Fraumeni syndrome is due to a germline mutation in the *p53* gene, resulting in an inherited risk of breast, bone or brain cancers (Chapter 8). The pattern of *p53* mutations is different in this syndrome from the pattern of somatic mutations in mouth and lung cancers, and variable patterns are seen in the various cancers generated by somatic cell mutations. This dissimilar mutational spectrum is even seen in comparisons of lung cancers from smokers and non-smokers. As different carcinogens generate different mutations (see Chapter 6), molecular epidemiology may provide evidence as to the identity of causative agents independent of the evidence obtained by conventional epidemiology. Thus, the pattern of *p53* mutations seen in lung cancers from smokers is consistent with exposure to a spectrum of carcinogen types, each having a major influence, whereas the different pattern seen in non-smokers (Figure 4.6) suggests that one type of carcinogen is predominantly responsible. Another example of this approach is the spectrum of *p53* mutations seen in liver cancers in China, Japan and Taiwan (Figure 4.7). Hepatitis B virus infection is a risk factor in all three countries, but the Qidong province of China has an additional exposure to a fungal toxin, aflatoxin, from poorly stored peanuts. Most *p53* mutations in liver cancers from that region are of one type (G : C → T : A) characteristic of an adduct between a guanine and a bulky carcinogen like aflatoxin. The other regions of Japan and Taiwan have more variable mutational spectra. Analysis of *p53* mutational spectra to identify human carcinogens is discussed further in Chapter 6.

Factors that influence human carcinogenesis

If we look at the five major cancers in men and women, four factors occur most frequently – smoking, diet, sex hormones and family history (Table 4.3) – each of which will be described separately here.

Figure 4.7

Liver cancers in Southeast Asia: *p53* mutations. (Source: From Figure 3 in Greenblatt, M.S., *et al.* (1994) Mutations in the p53 tumor suppressor gene: clues to cancer etiology and molecular pathogenesis. *Cancer Research*, 54, 4855–78, Reproduced with permission from the American Association for Cancer Research.)

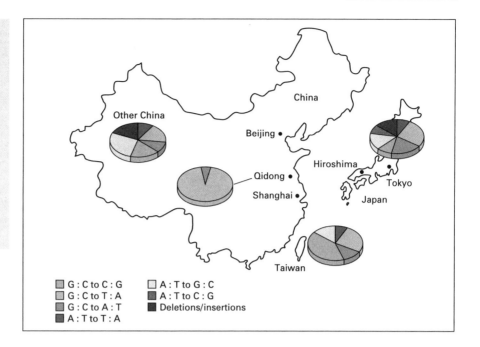

G : C to C : G
G : C to T : A
G : C to A : T
A : T to T : A
A : T to G : C
A : T to C : G
Deletions/insertions

Table 4.3 Incidence of the five main cancers in the USA and their risk factors.

Cancer	Percentage of all cancers	Risk factors	Possible mechanisms
Men			
Prostate	36	Sex hormones	Proliferation
		Diet	Hormones
Lung	13	Smoking	DNA damage
Colorectal	12	Diet	Antioxidants/toxic chemicals
		Family history	Gene defects
Urinary tract	9	Smoking	DNA damage
		Industrial★	DNA damage★
Leukaemia/lymphoma	7	?	?
Women			
Breast	33	Sex hormones	Proliferation
		Family history	Gene defects
		Diet	Hormones
Lung	13	Smoking	DNA damage
Colorectal	12	Family history	Gene defects
		Diet	Antioxidants/toxic chemicals
Leukaemia/lymphoma	6	?	?
Ovary	5	Ovulation	Tissue damage
		Family history	Gene defects

★ No longer significant.

Table 4.4 Statistics associated with cigarette smoking in the USA.

	Annual number of smoking-related deaths
All deaths	400 000★
Lung cancer	150 000
Other cancers	30 000
Passive smoking	
All deaths	40 000
Lung	3 000

Smoking is responsible for 30% of all cancer deaths and 17% of all deaths.

Less than 10% of people with lung cancer are alive 5 years after first diagnosis.

★ Worldwide, this figure is estimated to be 3 million.
(Source: Adapted from Table 9.5 in DeVita, V.T., Hellman, S. and Rosenberg, S.A. (eds)
(1993) *Cancer: Principles and Practice of Oncology*, Fourth Edition. Philadelphia, PA: Lippincott.)

Smoking

The statistics related to smoking as a cause of premature death are frightening. In the USA, 17% of deaths and 30% of all cancer deaths are due to smoking; the figures are similar in other countries. These figures translate into 3 million people worldwide each year dying uneccessarily (Table 4.4). The outlook for people contracting lung cancer is poor, with less than 10% being alive 5 years after diagnosis. What is worse is that non-smokers (passive smokers) are also affected due to inhalation of tobacco-related products in the air. A non-smoker who lives with a smoker has a 30% higher risk of dying from lung cancer compared with their risk when living with a non-smoker.

Although most attention is directed at lung cancer, there are also increases in mouth, pharynx, oesophageal, bladder and kidney cancer (Table 4.5). Smoking is the main cause of lung and mouth cancers and accounts for half of bladder and kidney growths. Most of the affected sites are those that come into contact with the carcinogens in the smoke, but inhaled carcinogens enter the bloodstream through the lungs and

Table 4.5 Increased risk of cancers at different sites due to smoking.

Cancer	Relative risk smoker/non-smoker	Attributable to smoking (%)
Lung	22	90
Mouth	28	92
Bladder	3	47
Kidney	3	48

(Source: Adapted from Table 9.5 in DeVita, V.T., Hellman, S. and Rosenberg, S.A. (eds)
(1993) *Cancer: Principles and Practice of Oncology*, Fourth Edition. Philadelphia, PA: Lippincott.)

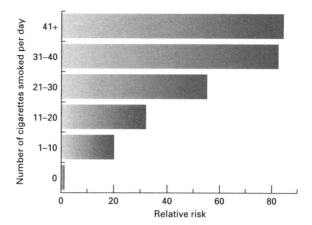

Figure 4.8

Lung cancer risk increases with the number of cigarettes smoked.
(Source: Adapted from Figure 2.8 in Tannock, I.F. and Hill, R.P. (eds) (1992) *The Basic Science of Oncology*, Second Edition. New York: McGraw-Hill. Reprinted with permission of the McGraw-Hill Companies.)

are excreted via the kidneys and bladder. Both these sites are affected, and it is interesting that inactivating mutations in the tumour suppressor gene *p53* are different in bladder and lung cancers (see Chapter 6). This suggests that carcinogens in the smoke reaching the bladder are different from those acting on lung epithelium.

Causation has been established by all of the criteria mentioned in the previous section. Over 40 potent carcinogens have been isolated from tobacco, including hydrocarbons such as benzopyrene and nitrosamines such as dimethylnitrosamine. There is a dose–response relationship between the number of cigarettes smoked and the increased lung cancer risk (Figure 4.8). Maximal increased risk of contracting lung cancer occurs with the smoking of more than 30 cigarettes per day, but even smoking fewer than 10 cigarettes per day increases the risk 20-fold. There is a 20-year gap between increased tobacco consumption and lung cancer changes, and although stopping smoking decreases the risk, the risk remains higher than in people who have never smoked for about the same period. There is a synergistic effect between smoking and alcohol consumption in mouth cancer, for example.

Diet

The evidence linking diet with several types of cancer is strong, but the basis of that link is obscure, as both beneficial and detrimental components have been identified. Fruit and vegetables are protective against several types of cancer analysed, whereas bad factors are more discriminating (Table 4.6). Not surprisingly, the biggest effects tend to be seen in the gastrointestinal tract, but sites such as breast and lung, which do not come into direct contact with food, are also affected. Good factors identified in fruit and vegetables include fibre (non-starch polysaccharides), complex phenols and micronutrients such as carotenoids, and vitamins A, C and E.

The current conclusion about the influence of diet on carcinogenesis is that it is important, multifaceted and confusing. Part of this confusion arises from the fact that altering diet changes several components, so that it is difficult to decide whether a beneficial effect is due to addition of a 'good' factor or removal of a 'bad' factor; both types exist. An Eastern diet rich in plant products contains many beneficial

Table 4.6 Association between diet and major cancers.

Site	Dietary factor	
	Good	**Bad**
Lung	Fruit and vegetables	
Stomach	Fruit and vegetables	Salt, salty foods
Breast	Fruit and vegetables	Fat, alcohol
Prostate	Fruit and vegetables	–
Colon	Fruit and vegetables	Meat, alcohol
Mouth, pharynx, nasopharynx	Fruit and vegetables	Alcohol, salty fish

(Source: Based on data in World Cancer Research Fund/American Institute for Cancer Research (1997) *Food, Nutrition and the Prevention of Cancer: A Global Perspective*. Washington, DC: American Institute for Cancer Research. Reprinted with permission.)

ingredients, whereas fat-rich Western diets have the opposite effect. The so-called Mediterranean diet is thought to be beneficial because it has a high content of fruit and vegetable, red wine (phenols) and complex carbohydrate and a low content of saturated fat. The major dietary components that influence carcinogenesis will now be considered.

Fruit and vegetables

High fruit and vegetable consumption is associated with a decreased risk of many cancers and may have a general inhibitory effect (Table 4.6). This conclusion is based on epidemiological analysis of food-consumption patterns in different communities at an international level (different countries) and within specific countries (vegetarian and non-vegetarian groups). Biologically plausible mechanisms exist to explain the beneficial effects via components such as antioxidants, vitamins, fibre and phyto-oestrogens (see below). However, in many cases, the effect of these individual factors is less than is seen for the food as a whole; additional dietary components have yet to be identified. For simplicity, fruit and vegetables will be discussed as a single entity because common components are involved, but beneficial effects have been noted with each on their own and with individual items within each group (green vegetables and lung cancer, citrus fruits and stomach cancer). The effect of vegetable intake on risk of lung cancer is shown in Figure 4.9. There is a 50% difference between the lowest- and highest-intake groups. A beneficial effect occurs in both smokers and non-smokers.

Fruit and vegetable consumption linked with low fat intake (see below) goes a long way towards explaining geographical differences in incidence of cancers such as breast, prostate and colon (see Table 4.1), but additional components have yet to be identified. Carotenoids are present in many plants; they are especially abundant in carrots. In theory, carotenoids could have a two-fold beneficial effect, both as antioxidants and as precursors of vitamin A, which promotes cellular differentiation and blocks proliferation (see Chapter 9). However, trials of β-carotene to prevent lung cancer in smokers have shown it to have a detrimental effect (see Chapter 13). The plant-derived vitamins A (retinol), C (ascorbic acid) and E (tocopherol) have antioxidant properties

Figure 4.9

Association between lung cancer and vegetable consumption. (Source: Based on data in World Cancer Research Fund/American Institute for Cancer Research (1997) *Food, Nutrition and the Prevention of Cancer: A Global Perspective.* Washington, DC: American Institute for Cancer Research. Reprinted with permission.)

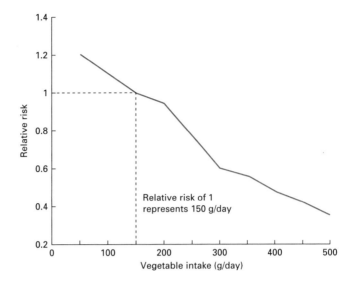

that contribute to their protective effect. Reactive oxygen species such as superoxides or OH⋅ radicals are carcinogenic through their ability to damage DNA (see Chapter 6); antioxidants counteract this effect. Two classes of plant phenols, lignans (metabolised by gut microflora to phenols) and isoflavones, have specific beneficial effects on cancers requiring sex hormones for their genesis. The phenols antagonise the mitogenic effects of the natural sex hormone oestradiol (see Chapter 13).

Dietary fibre such as cellulose from plant cell walls has little nutritional value, and its mode of action in decreasing cancer risk is unclear. The major protective effects are seen in the gastrointestinal tract, where the dietary agents are in close contact with the cells involved, although small effects are noted elsewhere. A protective effect of fibre was first suggested from the observation that elephants have bulky faeces because of the fibre they eat but they do not get colon cancer. It is unclear why fibre is protective, but there are several suggestions. Fibre accelerates the rate of gut emptying and this might reduce the contact time between dietary carcinogens and nearby cells; fibre might help to bind or inactivate carcinogens in the gut; and fibre might alter the profile of microflora within the intestine. A high-fibre diet is often accompanied by low fat consumption, but low fat consumption is unlikely to account for all of fibre's protective effect. Comparisons of groups with the same high fat intake but low (New York) or high (Finland) fibre indicate a lower incidence of colorectal cancers in the Finnish group. The same is true for breast cancer (Figure 4.10).

Fat and meat

A high meat consumption is linked with an elevated risk of colorectal cancers and possibly breast, prostate, pancreatic and kidney cancers. As meat is a major source of animal fat in Western diets (in the USA, one-third of saturated fat intake comes from red meat), meat will be assumed to be a surrogate measure of saturated fat intake. This may be an oversimplification of meat's true role, as high-temperature roasting may generate carcinogens from non-fat components.

Figure 4.10

Deaths from breast cancer may be linked to fat consumption. (Source: Adapted from Figure 9 in Hirayama, T.J. (1992) *National Cancer Institute Monograph*, 12, 65–74.)

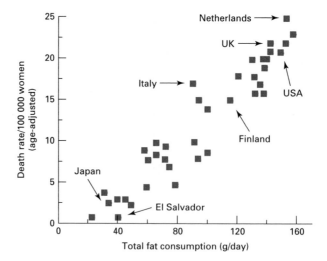

Breast cancer incidence in different countries correlates with the total per-capita fat consumption in that country (Figure 4.10). The same type of relationship exists if different ethnic groups within one country (Hawaii) are compared. A similar link exists between total fat intake and cancers of the colon, pancreas, prostate, kidney and endometrium. The potential importance of these data is illustrated by the theoretical calculation that if total fat consumption in the USA was halved, then the incidence of common cancers, such as those of the breast, endometrium and colon (women) or prostate and colon (men), would be reduced by up to two-thirds. Unfortunately, this calculation is unrealistic because this degree of fat reduction is impossible to achieve and because we do not know why these international correlations between fat and cancer exist (the fat hypothesis). Sorting out the contribution of fat rather than the potential confounding factors has not been achieved for any cancer type. It is not clear whether reduced fat intake is beneficial because fat contributes a 'bad' factor or whether the switch to fruit and vegetables (see below) increases a 'good' factor. Probably both are important.

Animal feeding experiments support a causal relationship between fat intake and cancer production, but besides the international comparisons just mentioned epidemiological studies in humans are equivocal. Retrospective case–control analyses in which fat consumption by people with cancer was compared with fat consumption in controls suggest a weak association; prospective cohort studies addressing the same question indicate little association (see Chapter 13).

One factor that may help to clarify this confusion is the heterogeneous nature of the fat. There are animal and vegetable fats to consider, along with saturated and unsaturated fats, cholesterol and total calories provided by the fat. In the Western world, fat of mainly animal origin provides about one-third of the energy intake, whereas fat consumption in developing countries derives primarily from plants and constitutes only about one-fifth of energy intake. There is also a qualitative difference between the two populations in that animal fat contains mainly saturated fatty acids whereas unsaturated fatty acids predominate in plants. The story is complicated further by the fact that the number and position of double bonds in unsaturated fatty

Table 4.7 Association between fat consumption and cancer.

The following fats are correlated with increased risk of cancer:
- Total fat: lung, colon, breast, prostate
- Saturated/animal fat: lung, colon, breast, uterus, prostate
- Cholesterol: lung, pancreas

Breast cancer shows no relationship to levels of cholesterol, monounsaturated fats or polyunsaturated fats

Absence of other sites from the above indicates lack of data rather than no effect

No protective effect of fat has been identified for any site

acids influences their biological effects. Animal fat is also a rich source of cholesterol but plant fat does not contain this lipid. It is difficult to reach any firm conclusions about the relative contributions of individual components of fat except to say that a high total fat consumption, especially of animal origin, increases cancer risk at many sites (Table 4.7).

The uncertainty about the role of fat in carcinogenesis extends to ideas about its biological role in the process. Animal experiments indicate fat to be involved in promotion rather than initiation, but, beyond that, ideas become speculative. High fat intake increases obesity, and obesity has been identified conclusively as a risk factor for breast and uterine cancers in women because of its effect on the production of female sex hormone (oestradiol). Fat cells can synthesise the mitogenic steroid oestradiol: increased fat equates to increased oestradiol and hyperproliferation (see Table 10.5 and Figure 12.12).

Micronutrients

Micronutrients are constituents that are small in quantitative terms but not necessarily in terms of their biological effect. Vitamins and carotenoids were described above, but minerals can also be important. A high salt (sodium nitrate) intake increases the risk of stomach cancer. The breast/fat data illustrated in Figure 4.10 can be mimicked by a graph of deaths from stomach cancer against the salt content of preserved soya beans in different rural prefectures in Japan. This practice of food preservation has now declined, such that per-capita intake has fallen in Japan by 16% and deaths from stomach cancer have fallen by 50% since 1970.

High selenium or calcium consumption may also be protective, but the mechanism of this is obscure. Some proteins need these ions for their biological effect, e.g. glutathione peroxidase needs selenium to destroy mutagenic free radicals (see Figure 6.8).

Alcohol

Alcohol is an important constituent of many diets (including students!). It has adverse effects on cancers of the breast, colon, liver and upper digestive tract (Table 4.6). For cancers of the oesophagus and larynx, the carcinogenic effect is seen in both smokers and non-smokers, but smoking and alcohol consumption have a synergistic effect rather

Figure 4.11

Association between oesophageal cancer and alcohol consumption. (Source: Based on data in World Cancer Research Fund/American Institute for Cancer Research (1997) *Food, Nutrition and the Prevention of Cancer: A Global Perspective.* Washington, DC: American Institute for Cancer Research. Reprinted with permission.)

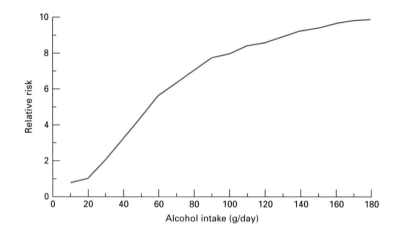

than an additive effect. There is a 20-fold difference in relative risk between a daily consumption of 10 g alcohol or less (10 g is half a pint of beer) and a daily consumption of more than 160 g (8 pints of beer or 500 ml of spirits) (Figure 4.11).

Sex hormones

Sex hormones are crucially involved in the most frequent non-smoking-related cancers in men (prostate) and women (breast) as well as others, including those of the ovary and uterus (Table 4.3). The hormones are produced mainly in the testis (androgens, men) or ovary (oestrogens and progestins, women); people who have had these organs removed have a dramatically reduced incidence of the disease. Both male and female hormones influence proliferation of their respective target cells, and this contributes to their promotional effects. Actions of these hormones are discussed elsewhere (see Chapters 10 and 12), but note that they interrelate with other risk factors in a complex way. Diet influences both endogenous hormone levels and their bioavailability as well as provides plant compounds that antagonise the actions of endogenous hormones. Thus, a low-fat diet reduces androgen (testosterone) levels in men and is associated with a low risk of prostate cancer, while obesity in women increases the incidence of breast cancer due to oestrogen synthesis in fat tissue. Stages in a woman's reproductive history (age at first birth, age at start and end of ovulation) are hormone-mediated features that influence the likelihood of breast cancer. Interestingly, the contraceptive pill, whose active ingredients are the two types of female sex steroid, oestrogen and progesterone, has little influence on breast cancer, although it can reduce the risk of both uterine and ovarian cancers by half. In a slightly different context, hormone replacement therapy causes a small but significant increase in the risk of breast cancer, though when combined with progesterone may decrease the risk of endometrial cancer. Ovarian cancer is listed in Table 4.3 as possibly being due to tissue damage resulting from ovulation, in which release of the egg requires disruption of the surrounding tissue. Hence, there is decreased risk when ovulation is suppressed, as occurs with oral contraceptives containing oestrogen and progestin, but there is increased risk when ovulation is increased during fertility treatment.

Family history

Inherited genetic factors make a minor contribution to most types of cancer. Nevertheless, studies in the incidence of cancer in twins have implied that genetic factors play a distinct role in three major cancers: prostate (42% of total risk), colorectal (35% of total risk) and breast (27% of total risk). There are also rare childhood cancers such as retinoblastoma (eye) and Wilms' tumour (kidney) where the majority of children carrying a genetic trait are affected. Familial cancers are discussed in Chapter 8.

Other factors

Tables of carcinogenic agents are available. Most agents relate to animal data but some have been proved to cause cancer in humans through epidemiological studies (Table 4.8). With improvements in occupational health regulations, many carcinogens have been eliminated, as in the case of bladder cancer. Original observations showed that people working in the rubber and dyestuff industries had a high incidence of bladder cancer. A metabolite of 2-naphthylamine, one of the culprits, forms adducts with DNA (see Chapter 6).

Exposure still occurs to some forms of radiation that carry a degree of risk, mostly due to their DNA-damaging properties (see Chapter 6). Ultraviolet (UV) light is a major determinant of skin cancer in pale-skinned people and debate continues over the nuclear industry's contribution to leukaemia. Accumulation of radon-222 gas (an alpha-particle emitter) in homes can increase lung cancers (see Chapter 6).

Table 4.8 Agents known to cause human cancer.

Agent	Source	Cancer
Current		
Radon-222	Geological seepage	Lung
X-rays	Radiotherapy	Breast, thyroid, bone
UV radiation	Sunlight	Skin
Cytotoxic drugs	Chemotherapy	Leukaemia/lymphoma
Immunosuppression	Organ transplants	Leukaemia/lymphoma
Asbestos	Industry	Lung
Aflatoxin	Diet	Liver
Human papilloma virus	Prostitutes	Cervix
Historical		
Soot	Chimneysweeps	Scrotum
2-Naphthylamine	Rubber, dye industry	Bladder
Chromium/nickel compound	Industry	Lung

Table 4.9 Potential for cancer prevention.

Factor	Percentage of deaths that could be avoided	
	Potential	Achievable now
Diet	35	2
Tobacco	30	30
Reproductive factors	7	?
Alcohol	3	3
Food additives	< 1	< 1
Industrial products	< 1	< 1
Total	76	34

(Source: Adapted from Wynder, E.L. (1997) *Nature*, **268**, 284. Copyright © 1977. Reprinted by permission of Macmillan Publishers Ltd.)

Cancer prevention

Many of the risk factors identified by epidemiological means reflect elements of lifestyle that can be changed and therefore have the potential of altering cancer risk (Table 4.9). However, potential and reality do not equate, so although tobacco-related cancers could be prevented now by banning tobacco use, getting people to change their diets to include more fruit and vegetables and less fat is more problematic. This is even more true for reproductive factors such as when a woman has her first child or whether a barrier method of contraception is used to minimise HPV transmission.

Routes to preventing cancer formation in humans based on many of the factors described in this section are discussed in Chapter 13.

Further reading

Adami, C.D.M., Hunter, D. and Trichopoulos, D. (2002) *Textbook of Cancer Epidemiology*. Oxford: Oxford University Press.

Collaborative Group on Hormonal Factors in Breast Cancer (1997) Breast cancer and hormone replacement therapy: collaborative reanalysis of data from 51 epidemiological studies of 52 705 women with breast cancer and 108 411 women without breast cancer. *Lancet* **350**, 1047–1059.

Darby, S., Whitley, E., Silcocks, P., *et al.* (1998) Risk of lung cancer associated with residential radon exposure in south-west England: a case–control study. *Br J Cancer* **78**, 394–408.

Doll, R., Peto, R., Boreham, J. and Sutherland, I. (2005) Mortality in relationship to smoking: 50 years observation on male British doctors. *Br J Cancer* **92**, 426–429.

Lichtenstein, P., Holm, N.V., Verkasalo, P.K., *et al.* (2000) Environmental and heritable factors in the causation of cancer: analyses of cohorts of twins from Sweden, Denmark, and Finland. *N Engl J Med* **343**, 78–85.

Million Women Study Collaborators (2003) Breast cancer and hormone replacement therapy in the Million Women Study. *Lancet* **362**, 419–27.

Norat, T., Lukanova, A., Ferrari, P. and Riboli, E. (2002) Meat consumption and colorectal cancer risk: dose response meta-analysis of epidemiological studies. *Int J Cancer* **98**, 241–256.

Office for National Statistics (2002) *Cancer Statistics Registrations: Registrations of Cancer Diagnosed in 1999, England.* London: HMSO.

Peto, J. (2001) Cancer epidemiology in the last century and the next decade. *Nature* **411**, 390–395.

Riboli, E. and Lambert, R. (2002) *Nutrition and Lifestyle: Opportunities for Cancer Prevention.* Lyons: IARC Press.

Woodman, C.B.J., Collins, S., Winter, H. *et al.* (2001) Natural history of cervical human papillomavirus infection in young women: a longitudinal cohort study. *Lancet* **357**, 1831–1836.

5 Oncogenes, tumour suppressor genes and viruses

KEY POINTS

- Oncogenes and tumour suppressor genes play major roles in carcinogenesis.
- Oncogenes are normal regulatory genes whose activity is increased as a consequence of genetic alteration. This gain of function can be due to qualitative or quantitative change in the protein product.
- Only one allele of an oncogene needs to be changed for a biological effect to occur. The effect is dominant.
- Oncogenes can be activated by mutation in a coding sequence that generates an altered product. Alternatively, chromosome rearrangement can result in increased production of a normal protein or a fusion protein with altered biological activity. Gene amplification commonly occurs during progression.
- The function of many metabolic pathways can be altered as a result of oncogene activation. These include membrane receptors, signal transduction and gene transcription.
- Tumour suppressor genes code for inhibitory proteins whose function is lost in cancers.
- Both gene copies of a diploid cell usually must be lost before a biological effect is seen. This type of gene is recessive; *p53* is an exception in that mutation in one allele generates an abnormal p53 that inactivates the normal product of the other allele. The first mutation is dominant-negative.
- Tumour suppressor proteins can be inactivated by protein phosphorylation, mutation or binding to other proteins.
- Some carcinogenic RNA viruses carry an oncogene. Others cause cancers by influencing host genes through viral regulatory sequences (insertional mutagenesis).
- Carcinogenic DNA viruses code for tumour-suppressor-binding proteins or may act by indirect methods.
- Many pathways are influenced by tumour suppressor genes, including those regulating cell proliferation and death.
- Inactivating mutations can occur at many loci within a tumour suppressor gene.
- Oncogenes and tumour suppressor genes cooperate in the genesis of cancers.

Introduction

Oncogenes and tumour suppressor genes, and the proteins for which they code, describe the functional features that drive carcinogenesis at a molecular level. The two terms have historical origins. Oncogene, or cancer gene, was so named to account for the properties of a viral gene that caused cancers in animal cells. Tumour suppressor genes were identified later when it became clear that normal cells contained inhibitory functions (suppressors) whose loss resulted in uncontrolled growth. Tumour suppressor genes are sometimes referred to as anti-oncogenes, which is not a good term, as it implies erroneously that they always act by counteracting the function of oncogenes. In fact, the two functions synergise in carcinogenesis. Oncogenes can be described as genes whose protein products gain a function as a result of mutation, whereas tumour suppressor genes lose a function.

This chapter is concerned mainly with molecular changes in the genes and their products; the biological consequences of these changes are discussed in Chapters 8–11. Terminology and molecular detail can create problems for those not immersed in the topic, so some general points are explained in Box 5.1.

Box 5.1

Molecular terms relevant to genes and their regulation

Abbreviations

Oncogenes are described by a three-letter code usually derived from their first discovery. Thus, the *ras* oncogene refers to a gene originally identified in **ra**t **s**arcomas and the name *abl* derives from its first discovery in the **Abl**eson virus. Sometimes, the three-letter code is followed by a letter or number. This became necessary when a function allocated to one 'gene' was subsequently found to have multiple activities. The *erb* gene, identified in the **er**ythro**b**lastosis virus, is now divided into *erbA* and *erbB* categories. The functions of the genes were originally unknown but, even when rectified, the original nomenclature is retained. Thus, *erbA* is the viral homologue of the thyroid hormone receptor and *erbB* is homologous to the epidermal growth factor receptor. Allocation of a number conveys the fact that many of these genes are members of closely related families. The number refers to its place in the family.

Tumour suppressor genes have a more varied terminology; two- and three-letter codes are used in some situations, and the size of the protein product is used in others. Thus, *Rb* refers to the **r**etino**b**lastoma gene and *Bcl2* describes a gene first identified in a **B-c**ell lymphoma. The '2' was added to distinguish it from another gene in the same tumour type. The *p53* gene is so named because the protein synthesised from its coding sequence has a molecular mass of 53 000 daltons (53 kDa). Some clarity is beginning to emerge with regard to the situation in humans, where the abbreviations for human genes are

▶

written in upper-case italics (e.g. *MYC*), while those for the respective proteins use upper-case non-italics (e.g. MYC).

The protein products from these genes are named using the molecular mass in kDa, preceded by a 'p' or by the same code as the gene. Thus, the *ras* gene produces the ras protein or p21. Little can be done about these multiple nomenclatures, and common sense has to be used in deciding whether a term refers to a gene or its protein product. The confusion is confounded by the fact that different genes can produce proteins of the same size. The ras p21 GTP-binding protein (see Chapter 10) has different functions from the p21 cyclin-dependent kinase inhibitor (see Chapter 9); once again, all that can be done is to translate the abbreviations in the context of their use.

Genetic terminology

Most cancers arise in somatic rather than germ cells. Somatic *mutations* are therefore said to underlie most types of cancer. As somatic cells are diploid, they carry two copies (alleles) of each autosomal gene and, as both alleles can be transcribed, it follows that a mutation in one allele will influence cell activity only if the change results in a gain of function that is *dominant* over that of the unaffected allele (Table 5.1). This gain of function is characteristic of oncogene mutations such as *ras* that generate a constitutively active protein. Where a mutation in one allele has no effect, that mutation is said to be *recessive* and biological consequences result only when the second normal or **wild-t**ype (wt) allele is lost. When the second allele is lost, the cell changes from being *heterozygous* to being *homozygous* (loss of heterozygosity, LOH),

Table 5.1 Terminology used to describe effects of gene changes.

Diploid alleles

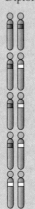

Normal: both alleles active

Dominant: gain of function in one allele overrides activity of normal allele

Dominant-negative: mutation results in loss of usual function but will block normal activity

Recessive: loss of function of one allele has no effect; must change both alleles to generate change

Loss of heterozygosity (LOH): change from heterozygous to homozygous state due to mutations in second normal allele

which is characteristic of repressors such as Rb, whose normal function is inhibitory. Functional loss of each of the two alleles can be via different mechanisms. Thus, inactivation of the first *p53* allele is often by a point mutation whereas a deletion/insertion destroys the second allele. However, the function of one suppressor, *p53*, is altered after a single allelic mutation. This protein is a transcription factor and two *p53* molecules must interact (homodimer) as part of the activation process. If mutant *p53* is formed from one allele, then the normal and mutant products form an inactive dimer (heterodimer). Oligomer is the general term used for these protein interactions. The single mutation in the first allele is *dominant* but *negative*.

Oncogenes and tumour suppressor genes produce key regulatory proteins, so there is a tendency for homologies, at both nucleic acid and protein levels, to be conserved throughout evolution, such that similarities are seen in genes from yeast, fruit flies, frogs and humans. This has helped us to elucidate functions, as information is available from lower organisms that has relevance to humans. However, it has confused the terminology as non-mammalian names become adopted for functions of human cells.

DNA structure   In mammalian nuclei, DNA exists as two strands twisted into a double helix. This forms part of a higher structure, the chromosome, described in Box 8.1. Each DNA strand has a backbone of deoxyribose units joined to each other by phosphate groups. One end of the chain has free 3′-hydroxyl group, known as the *3′ end*, and there is a terminal 5′-hydroxyl at the other end, the *5′ end*. This polarity is such that the two chains of the double helix are of opposing polarity (Figure 5.1). The polarity determines the direction in which the genetic code is read because the enzyme RNA polymerase, which reads (transcribes) the code into messenger RNA (mRNA), will do so only in a 5′ to 3′ direction. Local regions within the helix have to be separated (melted) so that the code can be read into mRNA; the strand being read is called the *sense strand* in contrast to the complementary *antisense strand*. The genetic code is formed by the sequence of four bases attached to the deoxyribose phosphate backbone. The two pyrimidine bases, thymine (T) and cytosine (C), and the two purines, adenine (A) and guanine (G), can pair with complementary bases on the other strand of the DNA double helix in the format G : C and A : T (Figure 5.1). The cytosines can sometimes be methylated (see Figure 7.2). Each amino acid is coded by three bases (a codon) specific to that amino acid.

Gene regulation

The DNA bases code for the sequence of amino acids in a protein, with each amino acid being specified by a three-base sequence known as a *codon* (Figure 5.1). Mutations in the bases can result in their being misread, so that a

▶

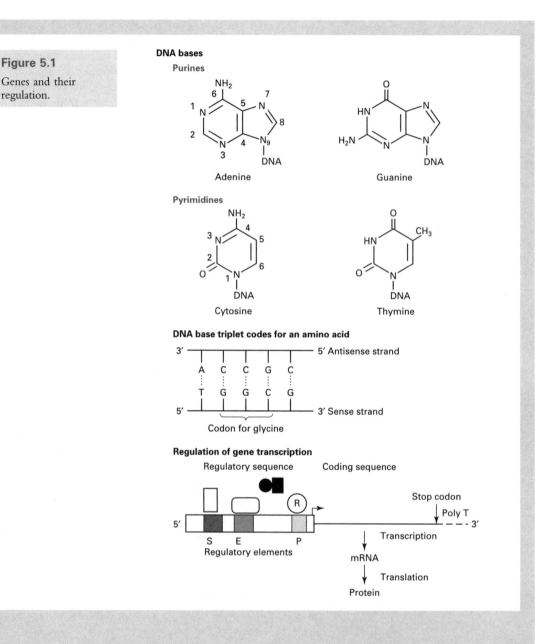

Figure 5.1

Genes and their regulation.

different base is inserted at the next round of DNA synthesis. In colon cancers, the middle base of -GGC- (codon 12) in the *ras* oncogene is often mutated to an adenine, which results in aspartate rather than glycine being incorporated into the protein. Other types of mutation result in complete loss of protein, a truncated protein or fusion proteins derived from two genes; these are described in Box 8.1.

A gene is composed of a *coding sequence* that codes for a protein and *regulatory regions*. The regulatory regions can occur at several places within a gene, but they are usually depicted at each end (Figure 5.1). The 5′ end contains base sequences that are recognised by DNA-binding proteins. These include RNA polymerase (R), which transcribes the DNA sequence into messenger RNA (mRNA), and *transcription factors*, which regulate transcription. Several types of transcription factor are required, but some features are especially relevant to carcinogenesis. Many of the metabolic pathways by which the cancer cell responds to extracellular signals are focused into altering the function of transcription factors that either enhance (E) or silence (S) gene transcription. Both of these functions are mediated by proteins called *enhancers* or *silencers* binding to DNA base sequences (regulatory elements). Proteins that act in this way have the ability to recognise specific DNA bases and other proteins that must be recruited into the transcription complex (*coactivators*). Many DNA-binding proteins of this type bind not as single molecules but as dimers. Dimers can consist of two similar proteins (homodimer) or two dissimilar proteins (heterodimer).

At the 3′ end of the gene are triplet bases that stop transcription, often followed by polythymine tails. The coding sequence is transcribed into RNA but some of them are removed (*spliced out*) to give mature mRNA that will be translated into protein. The DNA sequences that are eventually transcribed and translated into protein are called *exons*; those that are transcribed and then spliced out are called *introns*.

Protein structure   The first amino acid translated from the 5′ end of the mRNA has a free amino group (N-terminus) whereas the last amino acid has a free carboxyl group (C-terminus). Regulatory proteins are composed of different regions (domains), each with a specific function. Thus, the DNA-binding transcription factors have a DNA-binding domain and a transactivation domain. The transactivation domain is responsible for binding other proteins, thereby forming the transcription complex. Other proteins are described later with domains responsible for ligand binding (e.g. hormones, growth factors), GTP binding (e.g. ras) and tyrosine kinase activity (e.g. growth factor receptors). There can be complex interactions between domains, and so the function of the full protein does not simply reflect the sum of the individual domains. The domain function of regulatory proteins is often altered by phosphorylation of protein hydroxyl groups. One class of protein kinase phosphorylates serine and threonine residues, while another group phosphorylates tyrosines.

Proteins are destroyed by proteolysis, either in lysosomes or by macromolecular complexes called *proteasomes*. The lysosomal pathway is relatively non-specific, whereas proteasomes can selectively inactivate proteins. They do this by attaching the polypeptide ubiquitin to the protein; this marks the protein for proteolysis within the proteasome. As proteolysis destroys function, it represents an off-switch for biochemical reactions.

67

Oncogenes

Oncogenes are genes that gain oncogenic or transforming potential as a result of genetic changes in either their coding region or regulatory sequences. The gene present in normal cells is called a *proto-oncogene* to distinguish it from the altered gene in the cancer cell. The term 'proto-oncogene' can be misleading as it implies a latency in normal cells that is unwarranted, since the normal genes have important functions. The normal gene is sometimes referred to as a cellular oncogene (*c-onc*) to distinguish it from its viral homologues (*v-onc*). This arose for historical reasons as the original oncogene, *v-src*, was first identified as a viral gene responsible for the sarcoma-producing properties of the Rous sarcoma virus; a cellular homologue, *c-src*, was subsequently identified in normal cells. Virus-induced cancers are not as important in humans as in animals, so the term 'v-onc' has minimal application to humans. The term 'proto-oncogene' can be synonymous with 'c-onc', which becomes an oncogene after its expression is altered. However, additional clarification is necessary about the use of the term 'c-onc'. Figure 5.2 depicts the oncogene model of carcinogenesis in which gene modification results in either qualitative or quantitative changes in gene expression. Altered regulation can bring about quantitative change in a normal product. As shown in Figure 5.2, the 5′ upstream regulatory sequences are changed, thereby altering transcription. However, post-transcriptional effects can occur, as in the *fos* gene, where mutations in the 3′ non-coding region increase the half-life of *fos* mRNA. Overproduction of a normal product is also achieved by gene amplification, as in the case of the growth factor receptor erbB2.

Qualitative changes due to the generation of an abnormal product can occur either by mutation in the coding region or by gene rearrangement resulting in production of a fusion protein made up of parts of each participating gene. In the latter case, there may be confusion as to which of the two genes is the proto-oncogene. The confusion is circumvented if one considers the gene to include both coding and regulatory sequences.

Examples of each type of change are described later.

Viral carcinogenesis

Analysis of mechanisms whereby viruses cause cancer was fundamental to the understanding of molecular carcinogenesis, the original concept being that the virus

Figure 5.2

Models of oncogene activation.

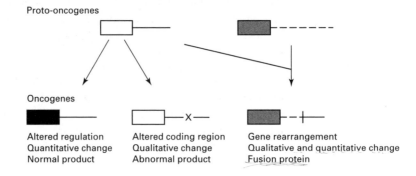

Table 5.2 Viral carcinogenesis.

Virus	Gene	Function	Compartment
RNA			
Rous sarcoma	*pp60^{src}*	Tyrosine kinase ⎫	Cytoplasm, membranes
Rat sarcoma	*ras*	GTPase ⎭	
Erythroblastosis	*erbA*	Thyroid hormone receptor	Nucleus
Feline osteosarcoma	*fos*	Transcription factor	Nucleus
Simian sarcoma	*sis*	Platelet-derived growth factor	Secreted
Mouse mammary tumour	None	Insertional mutagenesis	–
DNA			
Human papilloma 16, 18	*E6, E7*	Bind suppressors (p53, Rb)	Nucleus
Adenovirus	*E1A, E1B*	Bind suppressors (p53, Rb)	Nucleus
Simian virus 40	*Large T antigen*	Binds suppressors (p53, Rb)	Nucleus
Epstein–Barr	*BZLFI, EBNA5*	Binds p53; rearranges *myc* genes?	Nucleus
Hepatitis B	*HBX*	Binds p53	Nucleus

carried a gene capable of disrupting cell regulation. This has since been modified to include viruses that do not carry such genes but that alter cell function in other ways. Table 5.2 gives examples of viruses that contribute to carcinogenesis; it is evident that they influence many different host functions. The RNA viruses shown all relate to animal cancers and have little impact on human carcinogenesis, except for human immunodeficiency virus (HIV, sarcomas) and human T-cell lymphotropic virus (HTLV, leukaemia). This is less true of the DNA viruses mentioned in Table 5.2, as only adenovirus and simian virus 40 (SV40) are not human-related.

RNA viruses

RNA viruses infect competent cells. By reverse transcription, their RNA is converted into DNA and incorporated into the host genome, hence their classification as retroviruses. The DNA generated from the virus is called the provirus. Carcinogenesis is influenced in one of two general ways (Figure 5.3): by provision of an oncogene, or insertional mutagenesis in which regulatory viral sequences alter host gene activity. The former acutely transforming group has a short latent period, as oncogene insertion does not have to be at a specific locus. The latter group shows a prolonged induction period because of the low probability of being inserted in the right place next to a relevant host gene. In humans, insertional mutagenesis is unknown, although it is a common cause of animal cancers.

Provision of an oncogene　Many oncogenic RNA viruses contain an oncogene additional to the sequences needed for viral replication (Figure 5.3). The case illustrated is Rous sarcoma virus, in which the oncogene *v-src* codes for a 60 kDa phosphoprotein (pp60^{src}) that has tyrosine kinase activity. In its active form it is bound to the inner face of the cell membrane, but it can also be found in the cytoplasm and other membranes. It is attached to the membrane by a 14-carbon side chain, myristic

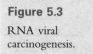

Figure 5.3

RNA viral carcinogenesis.

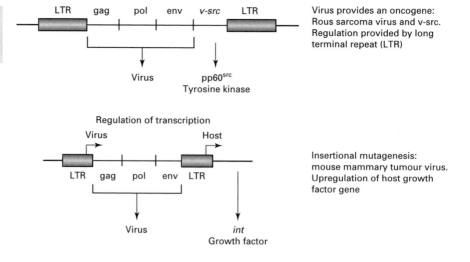

acid. Viral oncogenes differ from cellular oncogenes in both specific and general ways: *c-oncs* are typical eukaryotic genes in possessing both introns and exons, the introns being spliced out in the mRNA; *v-oncs* have lost their introns during the evolutionary time since the virus acquired the gene from the host cell. In the *src* example, specific differences include a longer C-terminal region in *c-src* and the last 12 codons of *v-src* differ from their *c-src* counterparts.

Insertional mutagenesis **M**ouse **m**ammary **t**umour **v**irus (MMTV) does not contain a v-onc but its regulatory sequences can stimulate adjacent host genes (Figure 5.3). The regulatory sequences are repeated at each end of the viral genome (**l**ong **t**erminal **r**epeats, LTRs) and so either end of the virus has the potential to influence host genes. LTRs contain enhancer sequences capable of increasing transcription from nearby genes. The DNA base sequences that make up the enhancer are effective in either 5′–3′ or 3′–5′ orientations, and so the orientation of the virus relative to host genes does not matter. Mapping MMTV in mouse mammary tumours indicated that although the insert locus could vary, it was always near a gene (*int*) that codes for a fibroblast growth factor (Figure 5.3).

The modes of action of the two human retroviruses HIV and HTLV are indirect but obscure. Neither carries an oncogene and no meaningful pattern of tumour insertions has been identified. HIV may work by suppressing immune attack on early cancers, but this is not a complete answer. HTLV can code for transcription factors that regulate host genes such as *fos*, but the link with carcinogenesis is tenuous.

DNA viruses

DNA viruses can act directly by virtue of one of their protein products binding to and inactivating host protein (Table 5.2). The suppressor protein p53 was first identified by its interaction with large T antigen of the SV40 virus, whereas the E7 oncoprotein of **h**uman **p**apilloma **v**irus (HPV) binds to and inactivates the Rb suppressor protein. The consequence of either of these interactions is altered cell proliferation. Note that there is frequently viral production of proteins capable of binding p53 and Rb suppressors; this may represent a common pathway for the carcinogenic effects of directly acting DNA viruses. In some cases (HPV, adenovirus) the virus codes for two separate proteins, one inactivating p53 the other Rb; by contrast, SV40 codes for a single protein, large T (tumour) antigen with separate domains for recognising p53 and Rb.

Several DNA viruses are important in specific human cancers: human papilloma virus (HPV) in cervical cancer, **h**epatitis **B** **v**irus (HBV) in liver cancer, the **E**pstein–**B**arr **v**irus (EBV) in Burkitt's lymphoma and nasopharyngeal cancer, and the **K**aposi **s**arcoma **v**irus (KSV) in Kaposi's sarcoma. There are many HPVs, and about 30 of them cause infections of the genital tract. Infection with some members of this group (HPV 16, 18, 45, 56) greatly increase the risk of development of cervical cancer. The cellular responses to these viruses derive from the component proteins E6 and E7. These oncoproteins together can transform cultured cells, while those from low-risk papilloma viruses do not. The synergy of actions of these two proteins is helped by the fact that both genes are transcribed as a single mRNA regulated by one promoter; the individual E6 and E7 mRNAs are generated by cleavage of the larger RNA.

In HPV, the viral DNA initially exists as individual elements (episomes) within the host cell nucleus (Figure 5.4), but as part of the carcinogenic process specific segments become inserted in a random way into host chromosomes. For cervical cancer to occur, the viral E6 and E7 sequences have to be present. Given the randomness in the choice of viral segments and their positions of insertion in the host DNA, it is not surprising that increasing the viral exposure of cervical epithelium raises the risk of developing cancer. This is not a single-hit process as transient HPV infections are not carcinogenic: prolonged exposure is required. This may be related to the fact that carcinogenesis is a time-dependent, multistage process (Chapter 2); inactivation of Rb and p53 by viral E7 and E6 proteins, respectively, is required at several stages.

Figure 5.4

Association between cervical cancer and human papilloma virus (HPV). See Chapter 9 for consequences of E6 and E7 production.

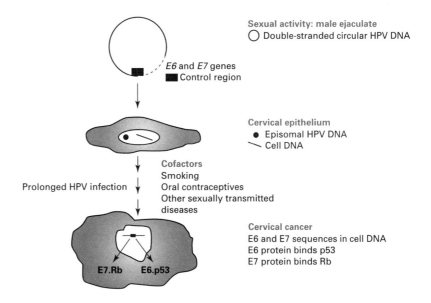

Infection with the dangerous forms of HPV does not necessarily result in cervical cancer; there is normally a relatively long time between infection and the development of cervical cancer. During this latent period, it is assumed that the progress of the disease is favoured by various cofactors such as tobacco smoke and oral contraceptives. In the former case, it is easy to appreciate that genotoxic carcinogens in tobacco smoke favour progression. Oral contraceptives on the other hand contain progestins, which, in combination with receptor proteins (see Chapter 10), can bind to and activate HPV promoter sequences. It is also possible that the infection could be overcome by the immune system.

The geographical distribution of hepatocellular cancer coincides with that of chronic hepatitis B virus (HBV) infection. Chronic hepatitis causes cirrhosis of the liver, essentially a form of chronic inflammation. It is this condition that is vulnerable to successive action by cofactors such as alcohol and aflatoxin. Progression commonly follows the sequence: inflammation, increased proliferative activity (dysplasia), dysplastic nodules, carcinoma and metastasis. Upregulation of the pro-inflammatory cytokine **t**umour **n**ecrosis **f**actor **a**lpha (TNF-α) in adjacent endothelial and inflammatory cells activates the transcription factor **n**uclear **f**actor **k**appa **B** (NF-κB), which results in enhanced cell proliferation and reduced cell death. The development of this cancer is slow (up to 20 years), which implies that cofactors are necessary for progression.

Most people have been infected with the Epstein–Barr virus (EBV), the causal agent of glandular fever. However, only in tropical Africa and New Guinea can this infection give rise to Burkitt's lymphoma. EBV infects and immortalises B-cells. Normally this cell population is held in check by the immune system. However, when additionally chronic malarial infections occur, the immune system cannot cope with the dual challenge and the immortalised B-cell population develops to form the lymphoma. Inactivation of p53 and Rb by viral proteins is also involved (Table 5.2). EBV is also less commonly associated with other malignancies such as Hodgkin's lymphoma, post-transplantation lymphomas, and nasopharyngeal and gastric carcinomas, and so several other cofactors may be concerned with the progression of these cancers.

Kaposi sarcoma virus (KSV) is a herpes virus that opportunistically infects immune suppressed/incompetent patients, such as people with acquired immuno-deficiency syndrome (AIDS) and recipients of grafted organs. Here, a G-protein-coupled receptor (KSV-GPCR) encoded by KSV induces an angiogenic switch to cause the angioma.

People infected with DNA viruses do not inevitably develop cancer. This implies that the immune system may overcome the infection. Nevertheless, the risk of acquiring the cancer is considerably increased (200-fold in the case of HBV). The long latent period between infection and the emergence of cancer indicates that cofactors are necessary for progression.

Specific examples of oncogene changes

More than 60 oncogenes have been identified. An oncogene is contained in each of the diverse regulatory pathways that govern cell behaviour. Selected examples

Table 5.3 Characteristics of eurkaryotic oncogenes.

Oncogene product	Chromosome	Function
Extracellular		
sis	22	Platelet-derived growth factor
Membrane		
ras	11	GTPase
erbB2	7	Growth factor receptor
fms	5	Growth factor receptor
Cytoplasm★		
src	20	Tyrosine kinase
raf	3	Serine/threonine kinase
Nucleus		
myc	8	Transcription factor
fos	14	Transcription factor

★ Can be transferred to membranes.

are shown in Table 5.3 and are referred to in later chapters dealing with biological functions. This section presents specific examples from human tumours to illustrate the main features of oncogene involvement in carcinogenesis.

Increased normal product

Increased normal product is achieved either by amplifying the gene or by altering its regulation. Amplification is common in advanced cancers but is infrequently a causative event in early stages of carcinogenesis. Altered regulation is encountered at both early and late stages of tumour development.

Altered regulation   In some cancers, chromosome rearrangement results in the coding sequence of an oncogene coming under the influence of the strong regulatory (promoter) sequences of another gene (promoter insertion). Little is known about mutations in regulatory regions of oncogenes in the absence of chromosome rearrangements.

Increased c-myc due to promoter insertion is found in Burkitt's lymphoma, a B-cell cancer common in Africa where malaria and Epstein–Barr virus infection are cofactors of unknown function (see Appendix A). In the majority of such tumours, the *c-myc* gene on chromosome 8 is translocated next to an **i**mmuno**g**lobulin (*Ig*) gene on chromosome 14 (Figure 5.5). The *Ig* remains silent, so the body's defence mechanisms are not compromised, but normal c-myc is overproduced because the strong Ig promoter can upregulate the adjacent *myc* gene. The c-myc protein heterodimerises with another protein, Max, to generate a transcription factor that regulates genes involved in both proliferation and apoptosis (see Chapter 9).

Different lymphomas have different chromosome breakpoints, and the orientation of the two genes can be head-to-head (5′ of *c-myc* to 5′ of *Ig*) or head-to-tail

Figure 5.5

Increase in a normal protein: c-myc and Burkitt's lymphoma translocation between chromosomes 8 and 14.

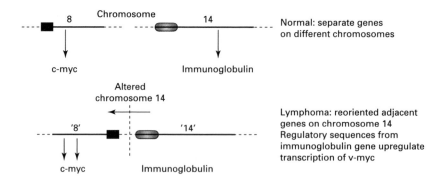

(5′ of *c-myc* to 3′ of *Ig*), although head-to-head is more common. As depicted in Figure 5.5, the c-myc promoter is unaffected by the translocation, but this is not always the case. Whatever happens to the myc promoter, the coding region is always retained and is upregulated by the strong Ig promoter.

Gene amplification This common feature of advanced cancers often accompanies the acquisition of increased aggressiveness, a good example being the *c-erbB2* oncogene. This is a transmembrane growth factor receptor whose cytoplasmic domain has tyrosine kinase activity capable of upregulating growth-promoting signal transduction pathways (see Chapter 10). Cancers of the breast and cervix overexpress normal protein due to gene amplification. The chromosome instability associated with cancer progression is accompanied by multiple duplications of specific regions of DNA due to defective start signals at DNA replication forks (see Chapter 7). In rat neuroblastomas, the *erbB* homologue *neu* has a T → A mutation that changes a glutamate to a valine in the transmembrane region. This may facilitate ligand-independent dimerisation of the receptor and therefore it is constitutively active. Hence, increased receptor activity is achieved by increased normal protein in humans and an abnormal constitutively active product in rats.

Altered product

Two commonly used ways of achieving this result are mutation and production of a fusion protein made up of incomplete parts of two separate genes.

Normal-sized product with altered activity The *ras* oncogene is commonly mutated in tumours such as colon and pancreas. The term 'ras' is a generic one covering different members of a family that includes *H-ras*, *K-ras*, and *N-ras*, the prefixes referring to the condition in which they were first identified: H and K refer to **H**arvey and **K**iersten murine sarcoma viruses, respectively and N indicates **n**euroblastoma. The proto-oncogene codes for a key intermediary in signal transduction between cell membrane and nucleus (see Chapter 10) – it is a GTP-binding protein with latent GTPase activity that is active when bound to GTP and inactive when the GTP is hydrolysed to GDP (Figure 5.6). The 21 kDa ras protein (p21) has intrinsic GTPase activity that is regulated by other proteins (see Chapter 10).

Figure 5.6

Functional change in oncogene product. Ras: mutation in a coding sequence.

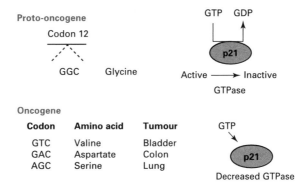

Proto-oncogene

Codon 12

GGC   Glycine

GTP   GDP

p21

Active ———→ Inactive

GTPase

Oncogene

Codon	Amino acid	Tumour
GTC	Valine	Bladder
GAC	Aspartate	Colon
AGC	Serine	Lung

GTP

p21

Decreased GTPase

Table 5.4 Domain functions of the *ras* oncogene.

Function	Codons
GTP phosphates	12, 13, 59–69
GTP guanine	116–119, 147
Bind other proteins	32–40
Prenylation of CAAX motif	C-terminal end
Carcinogenesis, decreased GTPase	12 (frequent)
	13, 1 (infrequent)

CAAX, cysteine.alanine.alanine.any amino acid.

The GTP-binding region (domain) is diffuse, involving five codons between 12 and 69 and four between 116 and 147 (Table 5.4), although all the carcinogenic mutations occur in the first group. Ras is bound to the cytoplasmic face of the cell membrane via a 15-carbon isoprenyl (farnesyl) group linked to a C-terminal cysteine. Experimentally engineered loss of this isoprenylation site inactivates the protein.

Ras protein is a focal point in the signal-transduction pathways for several input signals, and it relays those signals to a number of effector pathways. This requires ras to interact with other proteins (see Chapter 9). The codons responsible for these interactions are located between positions 32 and 40.

Point mutations in *ras* have been identified in several codons, notably 12, 13 and 61, the first being most commonly affected. Whatever the codon, the result is decreased GTPase activity, leading to constitutive *ras* activity. This heterogeneity in affected codons is also seen when individual base changes within codon 12 are identified; different tumours exhibit different point mutations such that the glycine in the proto-oncogene can be substituted with one of valine, aspartate or serine (Figure 5.6). In humans, we know neither the mechanism behind these mutations nor the carcinogens involved, but more complete information is available in the rat. Chemically-induced tumours have codon 12 mutations due to covalent interaction between the carcinogen (*N*-methylnitrosourea) and the O-6 of guanine (see Chapter 6).

Figure 5.7

An abnormal fusion protein. Acute promyelocytic leukaemia: translocation between chromosomes 15 and 17.

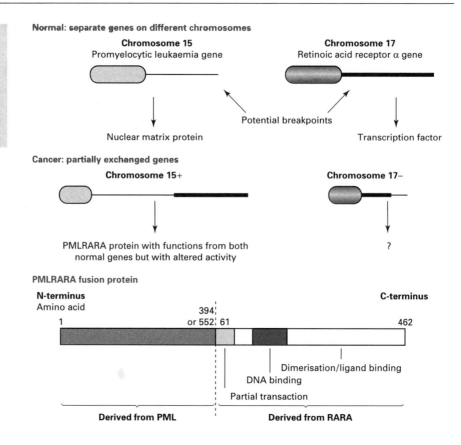

Normal: separate genes on different chromosomes

Chromosome 15
Promyelocytic leukaemia gene

Chromosome 17
Retinoic acid receptor α gene

Potential breakpoints

Nuclear matrix protein

Transcription factor

Cancer: partially exchanged genes

Chromosome 15+

Chromosome 17–

PMLRARA protein with functions from both normal genes but with altered activity

?

PMLRARA fusion protein

N-terminus
Amino acid

C-terminus

1

394
or 552 61

462

Dimerisation/ligand binding

DNA binding

Partial transaction

Derived from PML

Derived from RARA

Abnormal-sized product: retinoic acid receptor α/acute promyelocytic leukaemia
Acute **p**romyelocytic **l**eukaemia (APL) is a form of leukaemia in which differentiation is blocked at the promyeloid cell stage (see Appendix A). It is characterised by a reciprocal chromosome translocation such that the **r**etinoic **a**cid **r**eceptor **α** (*RARA*) gene from chromosome 17 is translocated next to the **p**romyelocytic **l**eukaemia gene (*PML*) on chromosome 15 (Figure 5.7). The altered chromosome 15 is said to be 15+ and the altered chromosome 17 is referred to as 17–; the translocation is designated t(15;17) (see Box 8.1). There are two classes of breakpoints that result in the production of two different PMLRARA fusion proteins (Figure 5.7). Both have a common *RARA* segment that has lost the N-terminal region including part of the transactivation domain (see Figure 10.21), but the *PML* contribution differs in the two sets of patients. A subtype of acute promyelocytic leukaemia is characterised by a different t(11;17) chromosome translocation; the *RARA* gene is involved but the fusion protein (PLZFRARA) has a different N-terminal sequence. The presenting symptoms of the two types of APL patient are similar; this suggests that those symptoms are a consequence of the altered *RARA* gene but it does not rule out a contribution from the other partner of the fusion protein, as treatment responses differ between the two types of patient.

In normal cells, RARA is a transcription factor whose DNA-binding activity relies on the presence of the ligand *trans*-retinoic acid. The RARA receptor plus the *trans*-retinoic acid forms a functional transcription factor by heterodimerising with the **r**etinoic acid **X** receptor (RXR) plus its ligand *cis*-retinoic acid. RXR also heterodimerises with receptors for vitamin D and thyroid hormone; heterodimerisation is essential for the biological function of all these ligands (see Chapter 10). Hence, anything that disrupts RXR availability interferes with the actions of these other agents. Retinoic acid isomers, vitamin D and thyroid hormone all promote cell differentiation so their blockade inhibits differentiation; this is a hallmark of leukaemias (see Chapter 2 and Appendix A). The normal function of *PML* is less clear, but it is expressed in the nuclei of most cells and the protein is a component of the nuclear matrix, possibly involved in regulating gene function. Its predicted structure indicates the presence of DNA-binding and dimerisation domains characteristic of some transcription factors. PML protein can form homodimers with itself and heterodimers with another member of the RARA family, RXR.

The protein produced from the chromosome rearrangement is a fusion of partial products from each participating gene (Figure 5.7). The PMLRARA fusion protein contains most of the functional domains of both *PML* and *RARA* but the *RARA* is the major contributor to the genesis of leukaemia. Nevertheless, RNA transcripts from the 17− fusion gene are detected in some people with APL and so additional effects may derive from this product. The PMLRARA product is under the regulation of the *PML* promoter and the fusion protein made therefrom is mainly cytoplasmic. The RARA part of the fusion protein retains its DNA-binding, dimerisation and ligand-binding domains but loses part of the transactivating mechanism. The protein can bind *trans*-retinoic acid and dimerise and interact with DNA, but it inefficiently recruits other transcription factors. At least two features of this fusion protein contribute to blocked promyelocyte differentiation and their resultant accumulation in the blood. PMLRARA fusion protein will heterodimerise with RXR and interfere with RXR function. This also has the potential to disrupt vitamin D and thyroid hormone effects on differentiation; vitamin D can induce promyelocyte differentiation. Also, loss of part of the *RARA* transactivation domain interferes with *trans*-retinoic acid function. Nevertheless, high concentrations of *trans*-retinoic acid induce remission in most people with APL, and so some elements of normal RARA function are retained. Whatever the mechanisms involved, they are lost in the t(11;17) type of APL as these patients are unresponsive to *trans*-retinoic acid.

In this example and others, such as chronic myeloid leukaemia (see Chapters 2 and 10), components from both the normal genes contribute to the oncogenic potential of the fusion protein, so the terminology becomes problematic about whether one or both of the normal genes are proto-oncogenes.

Tumour suppressor genes

Tumour suppressor genes have proved to be of critical importance in human carcinogenesis and their limited number indicates a more general role than that of the more diverse oncogenes. The basis of their importance is that in normal cells, growth and other functions are restricted by inhibitory (suppressor) proteins that must be reversibly inactivated for growth to occur.

The relevance of such suppressor proteins and their genes to human cancer is apparent from two data sets, one clinical and the other experimental. Familial retinoblastoma is caused by loss of both alleles of a gene, *Rb*, encoding a suppressor protein; loss of functional protein results in uncontrolled growth (see Chapter 8). The experimental data come from studies in which normal and cancer cells are fused, the hybrids having a normal phenotype. The normal cells express suppressor proteins that inhibit the cancerous properties (see Chapter 2).

The involvement of a tumour suppressor gene is advertised by the requirement for inactivation of both alleles, so that neither can make an inhibitor. However, the converse is not always true: biological change resulting from inactivation of only one allele does not exclude a suppressor mechanism. This is exemplified by *p53*, which can act in a dominant–negative manner. When first identified, *p53* was described as an oncogene on the basis of its ability to transform cultured cells. When the original *p53* was shown to be mutant and not the wild-type product, it was reclassified as a tumour suppressor gene. The original experiment worked because the mutation was dominant-negative, so that heterocomplexes with wild-type protein from the other allele produced an inactive complex. Hence, the presence of one mutant allele was sufficient in this situation to generate an inactive product.

Tumour suppressor gene inactivation

Tumour suppressor proteins inhibit cell functions by complexing with other effector proteins and blocking their action. Inactivation of the tumour suppressor gene product and therefore the lifting of its blocking effect is achieved by preventing its binding to the effector protein, a process that can be achieved in several ways (Figure 5.8). In quiescent normal cells, proliferation is blocked because Rb protein binds and inactivates a transcription factor. Serine/threonine phosphorylation of Rb protein disrupts this interaction, thereby releasing the cell-cycle block characteristic of this protein.

Figure 5.8

Methods of tumour suppressor inactivation.

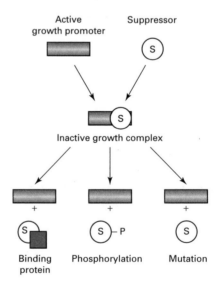

Table 5.5 Tumour suppressor genes.

Gene	Chromosome	Location	Function
Rb	13	Nucleus	Cell cycle
p53	17	Nucleus	DNA repair, apoptosis
INK4A	9	Nucleus	Cell cycle/p53 function
Bcl2	18	Mitochondria	Apoptosis
nm23	17	Mitochondria	Metastasis
BRCA2	17	Nucleus	DNA repair
APC	5	Cytoskeleton	Cell–cell recognition

Mutation resulting in altered product or loss of product is another way of escaping from this inhibition. Alternatively, a tumour suppressor gene need not be changed but the normal product can be inactivated by other proteins. Rb and p53 adopt both mechanisms depending on the cancer concerned (see below).

Examples of tumour suppressor genes inactivated in human cancers are given in Table 5.5; many more are known by virtue of their loss of heterozygosity in various tumours but their functions are unknown. Repressors are found in various cell compartments and influence varied functions. Because Rb and p53 have such a wide and interrelated involvement in carcinogenesis, molecular aspects of their actions will be considered here; biological implications are discussed in Chapters 8–11. Biological features of the other repressors listed in Table 5.5 can be found in Chapters 2 (APC), 8 (BRCA2), 9 (Bcl2) and 11 (nm23).

Retinoblastoma

The *retinoblastoma* gene codes for a 110 kDa nuclear protein of the same name. It was so identified because its loss of function is a causal event in retinoblastoma development (see Chapter 8), but loss has also been noted in a proportion of common cancers such as those of lung, prostate and breast. *Rb* is a large gene (300 kb), although most mutations are in the 3 kb coding region and mostly involve gross chromosomal changes. However, about one-third of the cases are point mutations. Several retinoblastomas can arise in one eye, each with a different *Rb* mutation. This illustrates both the clonal origin of these tumours and the varied ways in which one gene can be inactivated. The gene is crucial for normal development, so homozygous $Rb^{-/-}$ mice die as embryos while heterozygous animals develop pituitary and thyroid cancers. The normal protein inhibits proliferation. In these events, it synergises with p53, so that in many tumours there is loss of both suppressors (see Chapter 9).

The Rb protein has more than ten phosphorylation (ser/thr) sites mainly in the C and N terminal regions. Conversion from hypo- to hyperphosphorylated states alters the ability of Rb to interact with other proteins. Over 25 Rb-binding proteins have been identified, with functions relating to nucleosome structure (Brm), tyrosine phosphorylation (abl), protein dephosphorylation (phosphatases, pp-1a2), oncogenes (Mdm2) and transcription (E2F, DP) of genes involved in proliferation. Thus,

Figure 5.9

Actions of the retinoblastoma suppressor protein (Rb).

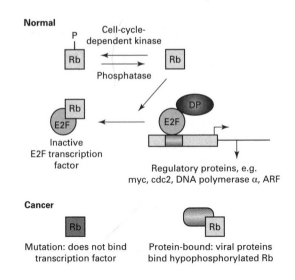

Rb can influence many cell functions but most attention has been directed at its influence on gene transcription. Hypophosphorylated Rb binds and inactivates the transcription factor E2F, whereas the hyperphosphorylated (se/thr) form will not (Figure 5.9). The proliferation cycle of the cell, the cell cycle, is regulated by a series of protein kinases that are activated by another set of proteins, the cyclins. These **c**yclin-**d**ependent **k**inases (CDKs) phosphorylate and inactivate Rb, thereby relieving the cycle block (see Chapter 9). Little is known about dephosphorylation mechanisms except that they involve a protein phosphatase. The released E2F stimulates transcription of genes that regulate growth, such as *cdc2*, *myc* and *DNA polymerase* α. The active transcription complex is a heterodimer of E2F with DP protein. Rb also inhibits transcription from ribosomal and transfer RNA genes by binding with transcription factors UBF (**u**pstream **b**inding **f**actor) and TF-IIIB (**transcription factor IIIB**) respectively (Figure 5.10; see also Chapter 9). Rb thus influences the mass of a cell (protein content) as well as its replicative ability.

Relief of *Rb* suppression occurs normally by hyperphosphorylation and abnormally by *Rb* mutation or binding to other proteins. Binding occurs with hypophosphorylated Rb and human papilloma virus E7 or adenovirus E1B proteins (Figure 5.9). Thus, Rb is inactivated by mutation in retinoblastoma, by E7 protein in cervical cancer and by phosphorylation in the normal cell cycle.

p53

The *p53* gene, which produces the p53 tumour suppressor protein, is the gene most frequently altered in human cancers. If we had to nominate one protein to illustrate the multiplicity of molecular mechanisms involved in carcinogenesis, then p53 would be that protein. There are other members of the p53 family (p41, p51, p73), but information on their functions is sparse. In normal cells, p53 has been well described as the 'guardian of the genome' because it protects DNA from insults as varied as radiation and drugs. It achieves this protection by coordinately blocking cell proliferation, stimulating DNA repair and promoting apoptotic cell death (see Chapters 8

Figure 5.10

Rb inhibits several types of RNA synthesis by binding to different proteins.

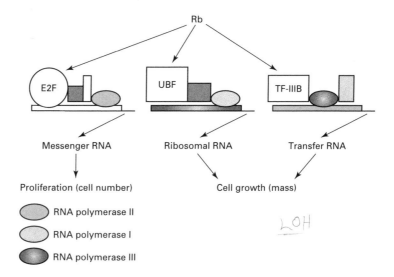

and 9). Given the importance of *p53* in cell function, it is surprising that mice in which both alleles have been deleted or humans who have a germline mutation in one allele (Li–Fraumeni syndrome) develop at all, although they do have a propensity to develop multiple tumours in adulthood. This suggests that knocking out *p53* destabilises the genome in a general way so that deleterious agents such as mutagens are more likely to be effective and errors are more likely to accumulate.

The *p53* gene can be inactivated by mutation or the normal p53 protein can be rendered non-functional by binding to other proteins.

Normal **p53**   Over 10 000 inactivating *p53* mutations have been identified in human tumours. To understand how such diverse and numerous changes achieve the same end result, it is essential to understand the domain structure of *p53* (Figure 5.11). It has four functional domains involved in regulation of transcription (*transactivation*),

Figure 5.11

Domain structure of p53 protein and how its function may be altered.

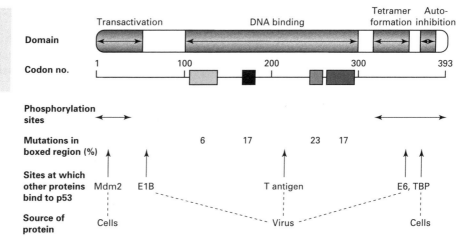

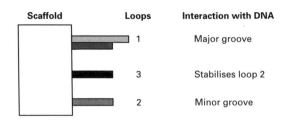

Figure 5.12

Regions of the DNA-binding domain of p53 that interact with DNA. The loop symbols compare directly with those shown in Figure 5.9 to indicate the regions in which most inactivating mutations occur.

(Source: Based on data from Kinzler, K.W. and Vogelstein, B. (1996) *Cell*, 87, 159–70. Copyright © 1996. Reproduced with permission of Elsevier.)

binding to specific DNA sequences, reacting with other p53 molecules (*oligomerisation*), and a C-terminal 30-amino-acid tail capable of inhibiting functions relating to DNA binding (autoinhibitory domain). The transactivation domain stimulates transcription indirectly by binding other nuclear proteins and recruiting them into the transcription complex. Normal cells can produce a protein, Mdm2, capable of inactivating wild-type p53 by binding to the transactivating domain as well as increasing p53 degradation. The functional p53 unit that interacts with DNA is a tetramer made up of two dimers; the oligomerisation domain is the determinant for this process. The autoinhibitory domain contains many basic (positively charged) amino acids and is thought to block the DNA-binding domain, since agents that bind to or alter the charge (phosphorylation) of the inhibitory region activate DNA binding. These agents include synthetic peptides, antibodies, non-specific DNA and protein kinases. Other proteins that regulate p53 function bind to each of these domains (see below). p53 can be phosphorylated (ser/thr) at several sites in both the C- and N-terminal regions. Kinases such as **p**rotein **k**inase **C** (PKC), cycle-dependent kinases and **m**itogen-**a**ctivated **p**rotein (MAP) kinases can catalyse C-terminal phosphorylations, whereas DNA-dependent protein kinase and the ATM kinase coded by the ataxia telangiectasia gene (see Chapter 8) phosphorylate the N-terminal end (see below). Other proteins that regulate p53 function bind to each of the domains (see below).

The three-dimensional structure of the DNA-binding domain indicates a core scaffold region from which three loops extend (Figure 5.12). The first loop, composed of two separate regions of the DNA-binding domain (Figure 5.11), contacts the major groove of the DNA, the second loop contacts the minor groove, and the third loop stabilises the second loop via a zinc atom coordinated to cysteine residues in the loop.

Numerous genes are influenced by p53, mostly but not entirely mediated via the cell's transcription machinery (Figure 5.13). Genes whose transcription is increased by p53 have a response element that specifically binds a p53 tetramer via the tetramer's DNA binding domain. The N-terminal domain recruits additional transcription factors (proteins) required for mRNA synthesis. BAX, p21, **i**nsulin-like **g**rowth **f**actor **b**inding protein **3** (IGFB3), GADD45 and thrombospondin are all increased by this mechanism. Expression of genes such as *Bcl2*, *fos* and *jun* can be inhibited by p53. Such genes do not have a p53 response element, but they do need a transcription factor, the **T**ATA-box **b**inding **p**rotein (TBP) for gene transcription. p53 will bind and inactivate TBP via the C-terminal domain of p53 and thus inhibit transcription from those genes. However, not all inhibitory functions of p53 are mediated by this mechanism. p53 can bind to and influence serine (casein kinase) and tyrosine kinases (*abl* oncogene), calcium-binding proteins (S100b) and excision

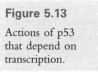

Figure 5.13

Actions of p53 that depend on transcription.

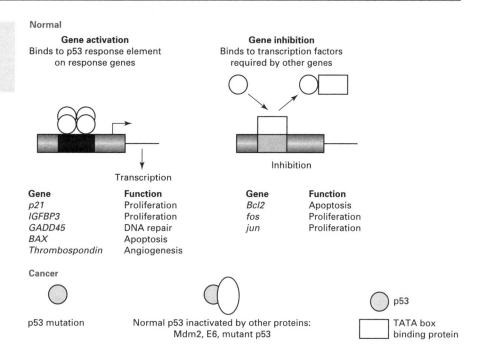

Normal

Gene activation
Binds to p53 response element on response genes

Gene inhibition
Binds to transcription factors required by other genes

Inhibition

Transcription

Gene	Function	Gene	Function
p21	Proliferation	Bcl2	Apoptosis
IGFBP3	Proliferation	fos	Proliferation
GADD45	DNA repair	jun	Proliferation
BAX	Apoptosis		
Thrombospondin	Angiogenesis		

Cancer

p53 mutation

Normal p53 inactivated by other proteins:
Mdm2, E6, mutant p53

p53

TATA box binding protein

repair proteins (XPD, XPB). These non-transcriptional effects could influence functions that are important in carcinogenesis.

Normal cells contain latent p53; the amount and function are influenced by phosphorylation and interaction with other proteins. In such cells, the half-life is low (< 2 min) and the p53 is bound to Mdm2 protein (Figure 5.14). This interaction serves two functions: prevention of transcription activity and acceleration of p53 degradation via ubiquitin-mediated proteolysis. The Mdm2–p53 interaction is regulated by either p53 phosphorylation or sequestration of the Mdm2 protein by the ARF protein. Thus, increasing ARF and using p53 phosphorylation are two independent ways of increasing p53 availability without requiring protein synthesis

Figure 5.14

Regulation of p53 activity.

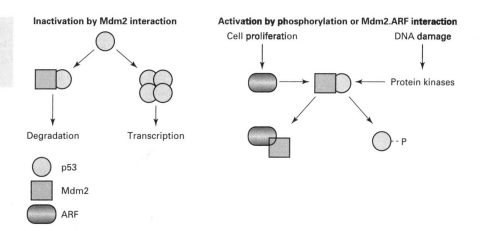

Inactivation by Mdm2 interaction

Degradation

Transcription

Activation by phosphorylation or Mdm2.ARF interaction

Cell proliferation

DNA damage

Protein kinases

- P

p53

Mdm2

ARF

(post-transcriptional regulation). DNA damage activates serine protein kinases, which rapidly phosphorylate p53 and release it from Mdm2, thus increasing cellular levels of functional p53 (up to 100-fold). This feeds through to decreased proliferation and increased apoptosis (see Chapter 9). *In vivo*, mitogen-stimulated proliferation is followed by a smaller wave of apoptosis. Mitogen-induced phosphorylation of Rb results in E2F-activated transcription of the **a**lternate **r**eading **f**rame (*ARF*) gene as well as those that stimulate proliferation (Figure 5.9). The mitogen-activated apoptosis could be a consequence of ARF's releasing p53 from Mdm2.

Four cellular responses are influenced by p53-sensitive genes: cell proliferation, apoptotic death, DNA repair and angiogenesis (Figure 5.13). The important question of how p53 inhibits proliferation without stopping DNA repair in some situations but promotes cell death in others is resolved only partially. One key may be the gene that codes for a **c**ycle-dependent **k**inase **i**nhibitor (CKI), p21, which inactivates the cyclin–cycle-dependent kinase complex essential for DNA synthesis (Figure 9.5); p21 also binds to a protein, **p**roliferating **c**ell **n**uclear **a**ntigen (PCNA), needed for both DNA synthesis and repair. PCNA forms part of the DNA polymerase complex, and PCNA interaction with p21 blocks the synthesis but not repair function of this complex. Hence, p53 might inhibit DNA synthesis while allowing repair to continue. Note that this p21 is different from the similarly named product of the *ras* gene. GADD45 interacts with PCNA, whereas IGFB3 binds and inactivates the growth factors IGF1 and IGF2, and so both of these p53-induced gene products contribute to the inhibition of proliferation.

Apoptosis can be blocked by the products of two other p53-sensitive genes, Bcl2 and BAX (see Chapter 9). Inhibition of Bcl2 and stimulation of BAX expression (Figure 5.13) disrupt this block and apoptosis can proceed.

The *thrombospondin* gene codes for a protein that inhibits angiogenesis and is therefore important in the metastatic process (see Chapter 11).

DNA damage activates p53 function by post-transcriptional and cell-type specific mechanisms. One pathway is by activating protein kinases that phosphorylate p53 (see above and Chapter 7). Binding of short stretches of single-stranded DNA to the autoinhibitory domain is an alternative that relieves the inhibition of the DNA-binding domain and is a possible route whereby damage blocks proliferation and facilitates repair. Whatever the mechanisms, they are very sensitive as they can be triggered by just one double-strand break in the DNA.

The effects of p53 on growth suppression and cell transformation (see Chapter 9) can be divorced because experimental mutants lacking C-terminal sequences are capable of suppressing transformation, whereas growth inhibition requires the presence of both C- and N-terminal regions.

Mutations   These are mostly missense mutations. All the tumour-related mutations are in the DNA-binding domain, albeit dispersed widely between codons 112 and 286 (see Figure 5.11). Importantly, they all disrupt DNA binding, either directly by preventing interaction with DNA bases or indirectly by destabilising the loop structures needed for this interaction (see Figure 5.12). Mutations are sometimes described as *conformational* if they are in the scaffold region or as *contact* if they are present in the loops that directly interact with DNA bases. The most frequent mutation is in codon 248, coding for an arginine that reacts directly with the DNA. This codon is affected not only in somatic cells but also in inherited germline mutations, as in people with Li–Fraumeni syndrome, who get multiple cancers (see Chapter 8). Mutation in the adjacent codon 249, as seen in aflatoxin-induced hepatic tumours, disrupts DNA binding only in an indirect way, indicating how small differences can alter biochemical mechanisms.

The codon and type of p53 mutation vary according to cancer type and even geographical distribution. Mutational hot spots occur at codon 273 in ovarian and pancreatic tumours, but additional hot spots at codons 157, 248 and 249 are seen in lung cancer. Codon 249 mutations are high in liver cancers in China but not in the USA, which correlates with aflatoxin exposure in China but not the USA. Likewise, tobacco carcinogenesis generates different patterns of *p53* mutation in lung and bladder. All these features are discussed further in Chapter 6.

The DNA domain mutations have minimal influence on dimerisation so that mutant and wild-type p53 can heterodimerise but will not bind to the DNA consensus sequence. This is the molecular basis of the dominant-negative effect of a *p53* mutation in only one allele. The autoinhibitory effect of the C-terminal region on the DNA binding domain (see above) can be exploited to reactivate some mutant forms of *p53*. Small peptides corresponding to this domain disrupt the autoinhibitory effect, and in culture they can restore p53-mediated apoptosis to cells containing mutant p53. The concept of reactivating mutant repressors has potential therapeutic benefits.

In normal cells, p53 protein has a very short half-life (minutes) but this can be increased either by mutation or by interaction with other proteins and it thus accumulates within the cell. This feature is exploited clinically to identify cancers with *p53* mutations, but not all mutations are so detected. Wild-type *p53* is destroyed rapidly by Mdm2/ubiquitin-mediated proteolysis, whereas mutant forms are not. Heterodimers of wild-type and mutant *p53*, as occur in Li–Fraumeni cells (see Chapter 8), also have extended half-lives.

Inactivation of normal p53 by protein binding   Adenovirus codes for a protein E1B that binds to the transactivation domain of normal p53 and blocks its transcriptional activity; some human sarcomas have *Mdm2* gene amplifications that have the same end result. The human papilloma virus encodes a protein E6 that binds to the oligomerisation domain and prevents dimerisation, while the HBX protein of hepatitis B virus binds and inactivates p53. Normal *p53* alleles are polymorphic in that the codon for amino acid 72 can code for either a proline or an arginine, depending on which allele is present. This has no obvious effect on any of its normal functions but it does influence the half-life of p53 when complexed with the E6 protein from the HPV virus. The p53arg.E6 complex is degraded faster than the p53prol.E6 oligomer. Women with two copies of the arginine gene have a seven-fold greater risk of developing HPV-associated cervical cancer compared with women homozygous for the proline form. Presumably the increased risk is linked to the faster degradation of p53.

p53 is a nuclear protein in normal and most cancer cells, but in neuroblastomas and some breast cancer cells it is cytoplasmic. Wild-type p53 is present in neuroblastomas, and so presumably something is blocking nuclear retention and thus preventing p53 function.

Oncogenes and tumour suppressors cooperate

Although some oncogenes can generate cancers on their own, the more usual situation is for synergism between cooperating oncogenes. Thus, transgenic mice containing the *neu* oncogene (homologue of the human *erbB2* gene) have a high incidence of breast tumours, whereas either *ras* or *myc* alone is poorly carcinogenic in such mice and a combination of *ras* plus *myc* results in breast tumours in most of the test mice (see Figure 2.4). At a general level, the commonest type of cooperation seen in experimental systems is between an oncogene that will immortalise a cell and an oncogene that changes additional aspects of cell function. Frequently, but not always, this shows up as a complementation between a nuclear and a non-nuclear oncogene (Table 5.6).

Most cooperations between oncogenes have been identified in cell culture as changes in behaviour, such as density regulation and anchorage independence (transformation) (see Chapter 2). They should not be considered in too rigid a manner, although the concept of cooperation has clear relevance to the multiple changes required for human carcinogenesis. Loss of a tumour suppressor gene, as in retinoblastoma, is a frequent event in human cancers, although cooperation between different suppressors or between an oncogene and a tumour suppressor is often observed. The *ras* and *p53* mutations in colorectal cancer are examples of cooperation between different suppressors; *p53* and *Rb* synergisms occur in several cancers. DNA viral carcinogenesis frequently involves production of proteins that inactivate both p53 and Rb. Rb- and p53-mediated functions also intercommunicate in non-viral situations. One such example is phosphorylation of Rb followed by induction of ARF and subsequent activation of p53 (see above). These p53 and Rb examples illustrate the point about not treating the nuclear/non-nuclear cooperation too rigidly as they are both nuclear proteins.

Table 5.6 Cooperation between genes.

Immortalising (nuclear) gene	Transforming (non-nuclear) gene
myc	*ras*
fos	*src*
p53	*erbB2*
Rb	*abl*

Further reading

Brhem, A. and Kouzarides, T. (1999) Retinoblastoma protein meets chromatin. *Trends Biochem Sci* **24**, 142–145.

Chin, L., Pomerantz, J. and DePinho, R.A. (1998) The INK4a/ARF tumour suppressor: one gene–two products–two pathways. *Trends Biochem Sci* **23**, 291–296.

Cooper, G.M. (1995) *Oncogenes*, 2nd edn. Boston, MA: Jones & Bartlett.

Goldman, J.M. and Melo, J.V. (2003) Chronic myeloid leukaemia: advances in biology and new approaches to treatment. *N Engl J Med* **349**, 1451–1464.

Hainaut, P. and Hollstein, M. (2000) p53 and human cancer: the first ten thousand mutations. *Adv Cancer Res* **77**, 81–137.

Hesketh, R. (1997) *The Oncogene and Tumour Suppressor Gene Factsbook*, 2nd edn. San Diego, CA: Academic Press.

Llovet, J.M., Burroughs, A. and Bruix, J. (2003) Hepatocellular cancer. *Lancet* **362**, 1907–1917.

Matheu, A., Pantoja, C., Epeyan, A., *et al.* (2004) Increased gene dosage of Ink-4a/Arf results in cancer resistance and normal ageing. *Genes Dev* **18**, 2736–2746.

Pikarsky, E., Porat, R.M., Stein, I., *et al.* (2004) NF-κB functions as a tumour promoter in inflammation-associated cancer. *Nature* **431**, 461–468.

Savelyeva, L. and Schwab, M. (2001) Amplification of oncogenes and tumour suppressor genes. *Ann NY Acad Sci* **758**, 331–338.

Sherr, C.J. and McCormick, F. (2002) The role of RB and p53 pathways in cancer. *Cancer Cell*, 103–112.

Young, L.S. and Rickson, A.B. (2004) Epstein–Barr virus 40 years on. *Nature Rev Cancer* **4**, 757–768.

6 Chemical and radiation carcinogenesis

KEY POINTS

- Chemicals and radiation can both cause cancers.
- Chemical carcinogens can act by damaging DNA (genotoxic) or by other means (non-genotoxic).
- Genotoxic carcinogens can damage DNA by direct interaction or after metabolic activation.
- Activation commonly requires cytochrome P450-dependent oxygenases.
- A carcinogen is converted to a proximate and then ultimate carcinogen. The ultimate carcinogen forms covalent adducts with purine and pyrimidine bases of DNA.
- Guanine is a frequent target of carcinogenic attack.
- Adduct formation requires electrophilic groups on the carcinogen and nucleophilic centres on DNA.
- Many genotoxic carcinogens that humans may encounter have been identified. They include polycyclic aromatic hydrocarbons, aromatic amines, nitrosamines and alkylating agents.
- Reactive oxygen species, generated naturally or from artificial sources, damage DNA and alter signal transduction.
- Antioxidants such as dietary vitamins can protect against cancer formation.
- Non-genotoxic carcinogens are important for major human cancers. Their mode of action is unclear.
- Laboratory tests that identify putative carcinogens are used widely but are not foolproof.
- Ionising radiation from atomic particles, γ-rays and X-rays generates single- and double-stranded breaks in DNA.
- Several sources of natural and synthetic radiation can cause cancers.
- Ultraviolet light causes skin cancers.
- Partial predictions can be made concerning which agents are involved in human carcinogenesis from the type of DNA damage seen in different cancers. This is called mutational spectrum analysis.

Introduction

A working definition of a carcinogen is 'any agent that can induce cancer'. An enormous range and number of carcinogenic agents have been identified since the original eighteenth-century observation that soot causes scrotal cancer in chimneysweeps. To this list of chemicals has been added atomic radiation, ultraviolet radiation and X-radiation. A feature common to most but not all of these agents is that they damage DNA and generate changes that result in a growth advantage for the affected cell. Agents that damage DNA, either directly or indirectly through metabolic activation, are classified as genotoxic carcinogens; agents that exert their carcinogenic effects in other ways are non-genotoxic carcinogens.

This chapter will deal separately with carcinogenesis mediated by chemicals and by the various forms of radiation. It will then discuss the consequences of changes to DNA structure generated by such agents.

Chemical carcinogenesis

Carcinogenic chemicals range from the simple, such as arsenic and chromium, to the complex, such as aflatoxin from a fungus. As living organisms such as viruses and bacteria are chemical, albeit a complex mixture thereof, they also fall within the definition given at the start of this chapter. Viral carcinogenesis is discussed in Chapter 5. Bacterial involvement is limited to the ancillary role of *Helicobacter pylori* as a co-factor in human gastric cancer. Diet is also a major determinant of human carcinogenesis, which reflects the effects of complex chemical mixtures. The general effects of diet on human cancers are discussed in Chapter 4, but more specific points about antioxidant mechanisms of dietary compounds such as vitamins will be included here.

During the 1930s, identification of carcinogenic chemicals and the chemical features that confer carcinogenicity on a compound were a major emphasis of cancer research and resulted in the identification and elimination from use of many industrial carcinogens. Bladder cancer was common in workers in the dyestuff and rubber industries, the cause being 2-naphthylamine (β-naphthylamine), while lung cancer was linked with the chromium industry. These findings generated a feeling that many human cancers could be eliminated if the causative chemical could be identified. Attention was directed at chemicals in manufactured items such as food, drink, medicines and plastics, and tests were devised to determine the carcinogenic potency of compounds. Such tests became mandatory before a product could be used by humans. This approach ensured that many potentially dangerous products either were not marketed or were withdrawn from use. However, as evidence accumulated about causes of cancer, it became clear that industrial products and food additives accounted for less than 2% of such cancers and that it might not be possible to eliminate cancer by such a route. This 2% value does not include the large number of tobacco-related cancers (lung, bladder, mouth) for which data are available but about which little is done (see Table 4.4).

Although data obtained thus far have had only a minor impact on reducing the major human cancers, chemical carcinogenesis is an important topic because its study has defined pathways by which different classes of chemical can generate inheritable changes in cell function. With this knowledge, it is becoming possible to invert some of the concepts. Instead of defining chemicals that cause DNA base changes, mutations can be identified from which it may be possible to characterise the chemical nature of the causative agents. This approach of mutational spectrum analysis using molecular techniques is being applied to the *p53* suppressor gene and may provide clues as to causative events in major cancers whose aetiology is unclear.

Genotoxic carcinogens

Four major classes of compounds exert their effects by forming covalent adducts with bases of DNA: **p**olycyclic **a**romatic **h**ydrocarbons (PAHs), aromatic amines, nitrosamines and alkylating agents. A feature common to all these compounds is that they have electrophilic (electron-deficient) groups or groups that can be metabolically converted to such. These groups form covalent bonds with nucleophiles (electron–rich groups) such as amino, sulphydryl and hydroxyl groups on other molecules. Nucleophiles are present in proteins, RNA and DNA; although carcinogen interactions with each of these macromolecules have been identified, DNA adducts are the those linked most closely to carcinogenesis.

In non-proliferating cells, the two strands of DNA form a double helix that limits the accessibility of a carcinogen to individual bases. During DNA synthesis, the two strands separate and the DNA becomes especially vulnerable to carcinogenic attack.

Adduct formation distorts the DNA structure, such that DNA replication is disrupted. Normally this can be repaired; if not, then an inappropriate base is introduced into the new strand (a *mutation*). Different carcinogens form different adducts, which in turn generate different mutations. This implies that all mutagens are carcinogens, but this is only approximately true. Some mutagens are so toxic that the cell is killed rather than surviving with a growth advantage over its neighbours (Figure 6.1).

Many genotoxic chemicals must first be activated by the introduction of epoxide or hydroxyl groups catalysed by **cy**tochrome **P**450-dependent enzymes (cyp). The general reaction sequence and terminologies involved are shown in Figure 6.1.

Figure 6.1

Conversion of a carcinogen into a DNA adduct, and the consequences.

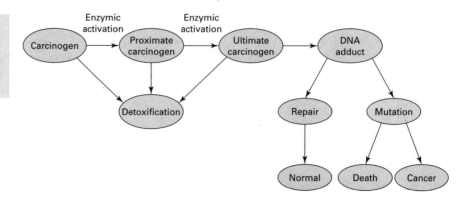

Where activation is required, the administered carcinogen is converted first to a proximate and then to the ultimate carcinogen; the ultimate carcinogen reacts with the DNA.

Environmental carcinogens taken up by the body are excreted eventually, mainly in the urine. As urine is stored in the bladder, any carcinogens present may be in prolonged contact with bladder epithelium, so it is not surprising that bladder cancer commonly results from carcinogen exposure.

Detoxification of carcinogens can also occur by cytochrome P450-dependent hydroxylations as well as by sulphation and glucuronide formation. The genes for some of these enzymes vary from individual to individual and can be detected as restriction length polymorphisms. Some of these polymorphisms indicate altered enzyme activity and could therefore influence carcinogenesis. One such polymorphism in cytochrome P450 2D6 has been implicated in lung carcinogenesis. This hydroxylase was first detected by its ability to metabolise the drug debrisoquine. People with polymorphisms resulting in slower metabolism might not activate carcinogens in tobacco smoke and would thus be less likely to develop lung cancer. Epidemiological evidence supports this concept, but the beneficial polymorphism is rare and so it has little impact in the general population.

Polycyclic aromatic hydrocarbons

Many PAHs have been identified in the environment. This class of compound has been used widely in experimental carcinogenesis models. PAHs were originally characterised as pyrolysis products of oils and biological materials, but they are also generated in tobacco, whisky and grilled meat and by incomplete combustion of fossil fuels such as coal and petrol. These few examples illustrate the potential impact of PAHs on human carcinogenesis.

The fused rings that make up PAHs come in many configurations, but some basic chemical features have been defined that determine whether a compound is carcinogenic. The parent compound is phenanthrene (Figure 6.2), composed of three fused aromatic (benzene) rings. Additional rings and substituents can be added to the inactive phenanthrene structure to convert it into a carcinogen. The minimum requirement for carcinogenicity is (i) three fused aromatic rings in the phenanthrene configuration, (ii) additional fused rings and/or (iii) a methyl group in the bay region.

The additional fused ring is effective only when joined at specific regions of phenanthrene. Thus, the extra ring in benzanthracene (Figure 6.2) yields a very weak or inactive product, whereas dibenzanthracene is a somewhat stronger carcinogen. Addition of two rings in the benzopyrene configuration results in a very potent carcinogen. Addition of one methyl group in the bay region of benzanthracene (12-methylbenzanthracene) generates a moderate carcinogen, while a second methyl group (7,12-**dim**ethyl**b**enz**a**nthracene, DMBA) generates one of the most potent carcinogens known. Much interest centred on the K-region (Figure 6.2) as being important, but this is now known not to be the case, as it can be modified without destroying potency.

There are two naturally occurring derivatives of phenanthrene: the steroid hormones and cholesterol plus its bile acid derivatives. Cholesterol has not been linked with human carcinogenesis, but steroid hormones are involved in the genesis of major cancers such as those of breast, endometrium and prostate. This has led to many

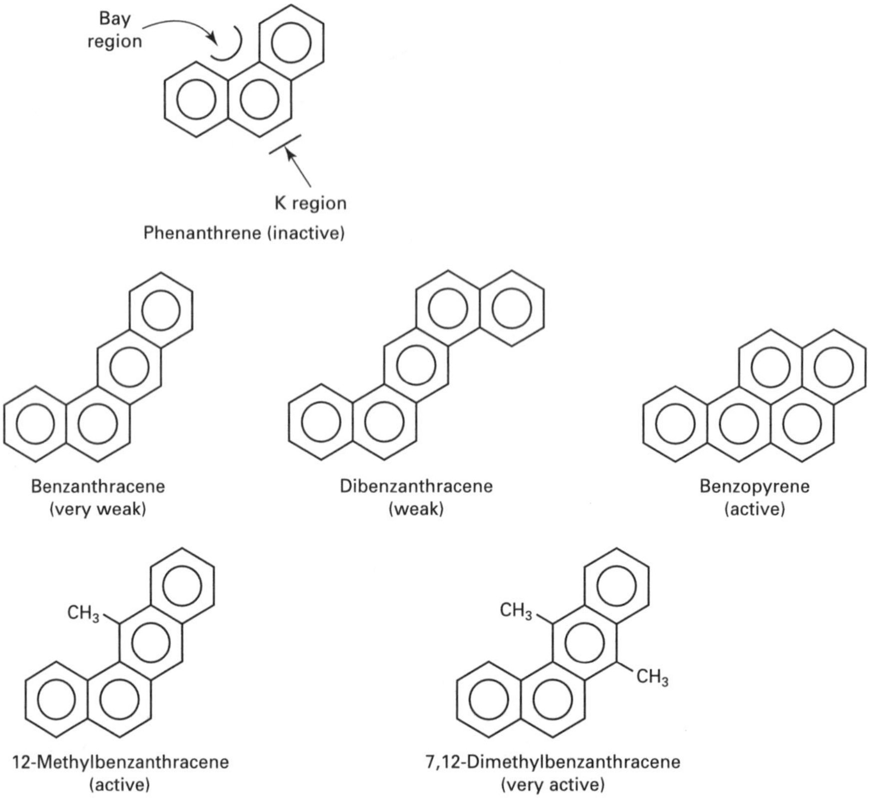

Figure 6.2

Carcinogenic potency of polycyclic aromatic hydrocarbons. Figure 6.3 shows the numbering system.

Bay region

K region
Phenanthrene (inactive)

Benzanthracene
(very weak)

Dibenzanthracene
(weak)

Benzopyrene
(active)

CH_3

12-Methylbenzanthracene
(active)

CH_3

CH_3

7,12-Dimethylbenzanthracene
(very active)

attempts to show analogies between PAHs and steroids, none of which has been productive. In fact, they have very different actions, as steroids are non-genotoxic carcinogens (see below).

PAHs form adducts with purine bases, especially guanine, but only after enzymic activation via proximate and ultimate carcinogens. The example shown in Figure 6.3 is benzopyrene but analogous reactions occur with other PAHs. CYP monooxygenases generate an epoxide that is converted to a diol by an epoxide hydrolase. A second epoxide is then formed, often in the bay region, and this attaches covalently to DNA. This can be to the 2-amino of guanine or the 6-amino of adenine.

Aromatic amines

Aromatic amines, also known as arylamines, were identified as being hazardous through their use in the dyestuff and rubber industries. An example is 2-naphthylamine (Figure 6.4), which has been banned because it caused bladder cancer in the workers who handled it. Another compound, dimethylaminoazobenzene (butter yellow), was so named because it was used to colour margarine in the 1930s. It was withdrawn from use when it was shown to cause liver and bladder cancers in animals.

The carcinogenic action of aromatic amines has been best analysed with 2-**a**cetyl**a**mino**f**luorene (AAF) (Figure 6.5), which causes multiple cancers, such as bladder, liver, ear, intestine, thyroid and breast, in animals. AAF was originally used

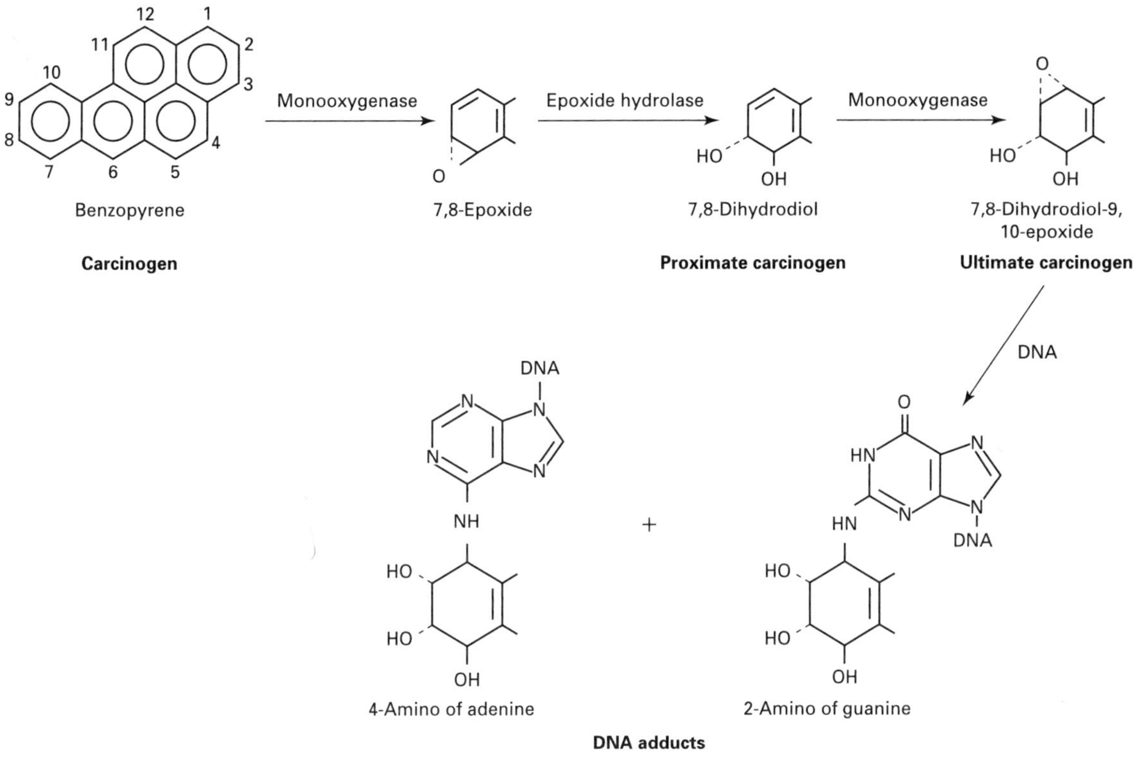

Figure 6.3

Activation of benzopyrene and formation of DNA adducts.

as an insecticide, and related compounds can be detected in cooked meat. This illustrates one of the unresolved problems with carcinogen identification through animal studies and their relevance to humans. Milligram quantities of AAF are needed to generate cancers in rats of body weight about 0.2 kg, whereas one-millionth of that level has been detected in cooked meat to be eaten by much bigger humans (70 kg). Given the differences in both quantities and body volumes through which the carcinogen will be distributed, is it appropriate to say, as some do, that meat-eating may cause cancer (Chapter 2)?

AAF is carcinogenic only after metabolic activation through a CYP-mediated N-hydroxylase and sulphotransferase (Figure 6.5). The first metabolite, N-hydroxy-AAF (proximate carcinogen), will not form DNA adducts, but sulphation or acetylation (not shown) of the N-hydroxyl group generates the ultimate carcinogen that reacts with guanine bases in DNA. There are large variations in the susceptibility of different species to AAF, and this is correlated with the activity of hepatic sulphotransferase and N-hydroxylase in those species. The sulphate and acetyl esters are

Figure 6.4

Carcinogenic aromatic arylamines.

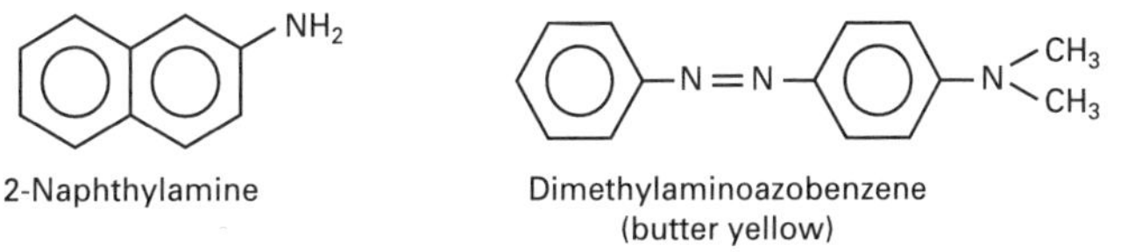

2-Naphthylamine

Dimethylaminoazobenzene (butter yellow)

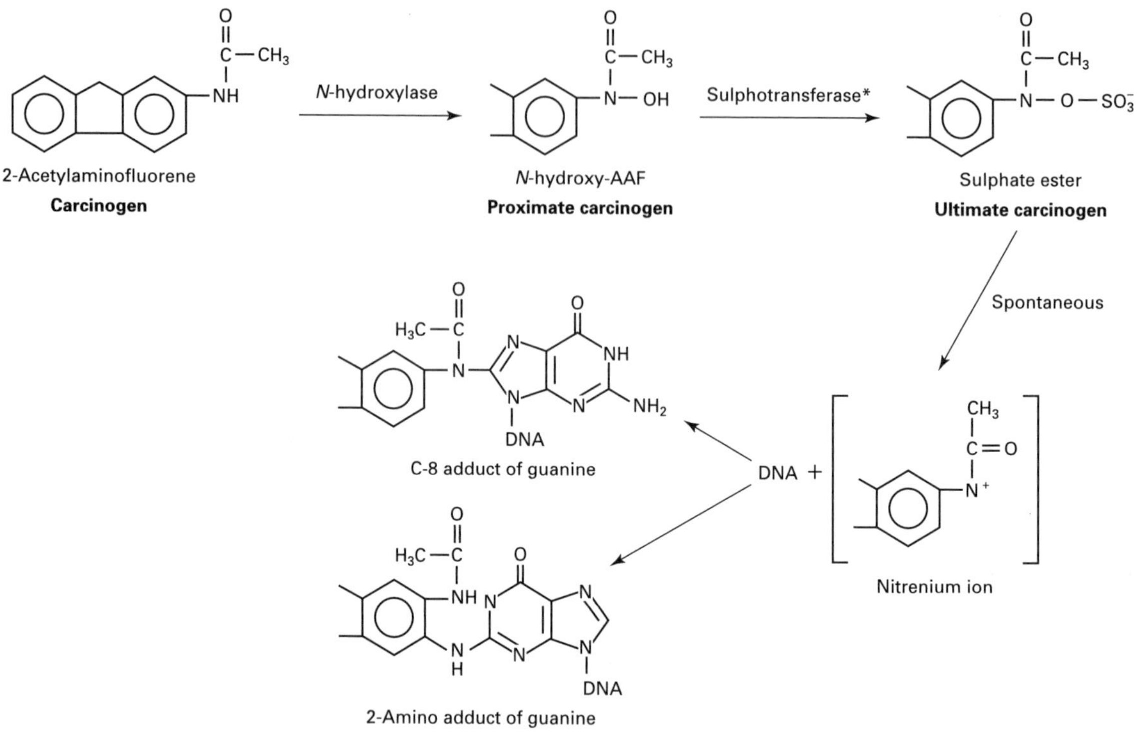

Figure 6.5

2-Acetylaminofluorene (AAF): activation and adducts. *Plus 3′-phosphoadenosine-5′-phosphosulphate.

unstable and undergo a spontaneous reaction to form a nitrenium ion, which generates a qualitatively major adduct via the C-8 and a minor adduct via the 2-amino group of guanine. However, the minor occurrence of the 2-amino adduct is counterbalanced by its longer period of attachment to DNA before being removed. Probably both adducts are important.

Other aromatic amines are activated by analogous mechanisms through hydroxylation and ester formation at their amino group.

Nitrosamines

Humans can be exposed to nitrosamines in a number of ways. Nitrosamines are formed in smoked meats and fish by interaction of natural amines with nitrites added as preservatives, but their most significant presence is in tobacco and its associated products. Nitrosamines in tobacco and its smoke contribute to lung and bladder cancers, while their presence in snuff and chewing-tobacco cause nasal and oral cancers, respectively.

Enzymic activation is required to form ultimate carcinogens that methylate guanines of DNA (Figure 6.6). N^7-methylguanine is the major product but its formation does not correlate with carcinogenicity, whereas the minor O^6-methylated product does. Hence, formation of the latter product reflects the major carcinogenic event. The O-2 of thymine is also a site of adduct formation.

N-methylnitrosourea (Figure 6.6) is a nitrosamine used widely to generate cancers in experimental systems, its advantage being that it spontaneously forms the

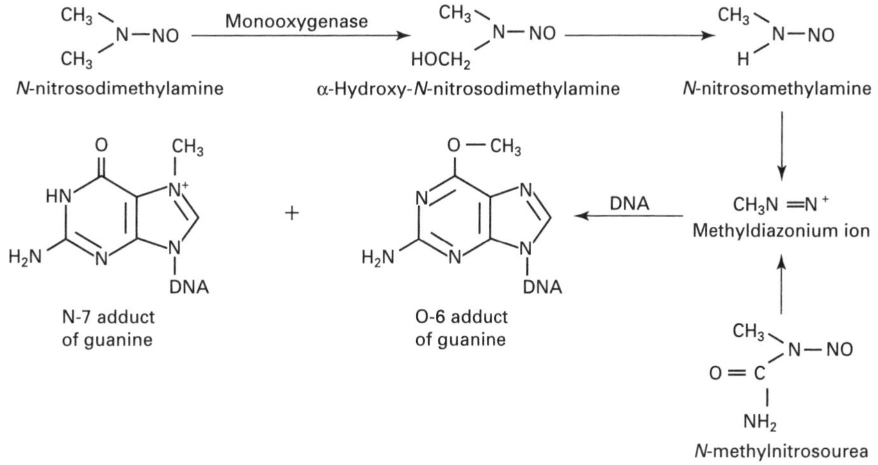

Figure 6.6

N-nitrosodimethyl-amine and *N*-methylnitrosourea: activation and DNA adducts.

methyldiazonium ion without requiring enzymic activation. It is therefore classified as a direct-acting carcinogen, with no metabolic activation being required.

Other alkylating agents

Mustard gas (dichlorodiethylsulphide) (Figure 6.7) was used during the First World War. Affected soldiers subsequently developed a higher than expected incidence of cancers at exposed sites such as nose, bronchus and larynx. Mustard gas is a bifunctional compound, having two chlorine groups capable of reacting directly with nucleophilic amino and hydroxyl groups, as with the nitrosamines. It can therefore form intrachain and interchain cross-links with adjacent bases. It can also form single adducts. Mustard gas is a direct-acting carcinogen as the chlorine groups are sufficiently electrophilic that metabolic activation is not required.

Monofunctional alkylating agents can also be carcinogenic due to adduct formation. An example is vinyl chloride (Figure 6.7), used in the plastics industry as **polyvinyl chloride** (PVC) for products such as food wrappers.

The ability of bifunctional alkylating agents to damage DNA has been turned to beneficial effect in developing drugs for killing cancers. Cyclophosphamide (Figure 6.7), a derivative of dichlorodiethylsulphide in which the S is replaced with N, is used widely for this purpose (see Chapter 12). Cyclophosphamide can, however, cause second cancers (leukaemia, bladder) in a small proportion of patients about 5 years after being treated with the drug (see Appendix A). This side effect is considered minor relative to death from the first cancer.

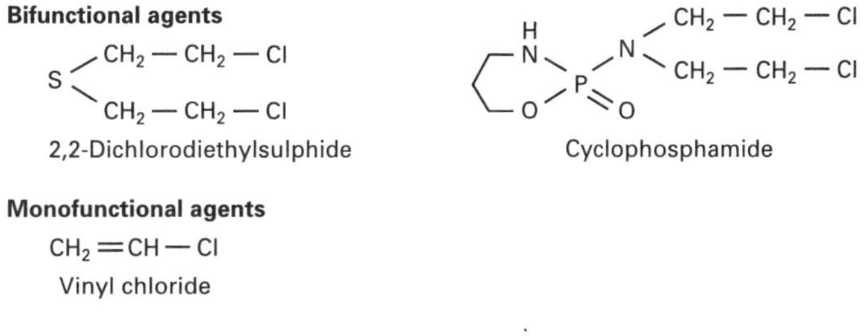

Figure 6.7

Carcinogenic alkylating agents.

Oxidation as a cause of cancer

A considerable number of reactive free radicals or chemicals capable of being converted thereto are generated in cells by normal metabolic pathways. They can oxidise nucleic acids, proteins and lipids, and they have many of the characteristics of carcinogens. They generate structural alterations in DNA, decrease DNA repair by damaging essential proteins and activate signal transduction pathways. It has been suggested that cells are under 'oxidative siege' and it follows that antioxidant mechanisms will correct that siege. The oxidation status of a cell is sometimes known as its redox (**reduction/oxidation**) state. By analysis of urinary metabolites of purine and pyrimidine bases, it has been calculated that, under normal circumstances, DNA in each cell receives 10^4 oxidative hits per day. Most of this substantial number of base changes are repaired, but any that escape the process might alter cell functions and contribute to carcinogenesis. The main source of damaging agents is **r**eactive **o**xygen **s**pecies (ROS), but additional contributions are made by **r**eactive **n**itrogen **s**pecies (RNS).

Reactive oxygen species Several types of ROS exist. They are formed mainly as by-products of mitochondrial electron transport or exposure to ionising radiation, but they can also be produced from other sources such as phagocytic cells and lipid peroxidation. Endogenously produced ROS are important contributors to the natural mutation rate (see Chapter 7). The term 'spontaneous mutation' is often used inappropriately, given that something has to generate the base change.

Oxidative phosphorylation, in which mitochondrial electron transport converts energy into ATP, is the major source of ROS. About 10^{12} oxygen molecules are processed per cell per day, about 1% of which are used incompletely and result in ROS formation. Hence, the 10^{10} potential ROS are more than adequate to explain the 10^4 DNA hits mentioned above. However, superoxide and hydroxyl free radicals travel only short distances ($< 0.1 \ \mu m$) before being destroyed. Given a cell diameter of about 10 μm, it follows that direct interaction of mitochondrial ROS with nuclear DNA is unlikely. Perhaps chain reactions can be initiated by ROS that could transfer effects over longer distances, or ROS may be generated within the nucleus (see DNA damage on p. 98).

The main ROS are superoxide and hydroxyl radicals and hydrogen peroxide produced by electron capture, as shown in Figure 6.8. Hydrogen peroxide, a component of the production pathway, is not a free radical but it is a precursor of such.

Figure 6.8

Production and destruction of reactive oxygen species.

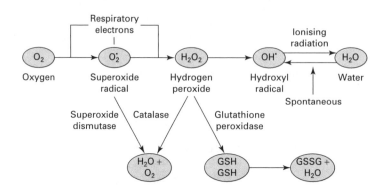

Furthermore, it can have direct oxidative effects of its own on other proteins, such as the transcription factor NFκB. The hydroxyl radical is the most reactive ROS and therefore the most damaging. Given concerns about destruction of the protective ozone layer in the atmosphere and increased risk of skin cancer, it should be noted that ozone (O_3) is converted to oxygen by free radicals. This has the deleterious effect of reducing the amount of atmospheric ozone available to protect the planet from harmful radiation. The protective effect of the ozone is also achieved by a free-radical mechanism. Superoxide dismutase catalyses the conversion of superoxide to hydrogen peroxide; Fe^{2+} and Cu^+ accelerate hydroxyl radical formation from hydrogen peroxide. Hydroxyl radicals can also be produced from water by radiation (see below). ROS are also generated as products of reactions catalysed by cyclooxygenases, lipoxygenases and NADPH oxidase. Oxidising agents in tobacco smoke, such as nitric oxide, could also contribute to carcinogenesis via ROS formation.

The cell contains proteins and other molecules such as glutathione (Figure 6.8) and vitamins A, C and E, all of which are capable of inactivating ROS. Enzymic proteins include catalase and glutathione peroxidase, which convert hydrogen peroxide to water. The other product of catalase is oxygen and, for glutathione peroxidase, oxidised glutathione. Glutathione peroxidase requires selenium, and this might account for selenium's beneficial effects (see Chapter 4). Thioredoxin is a protein with adjacent cysteine residues that can be reversibly oxidised to cystine (Figure 6.9). It can thus act as a sink for ROS, and it is noteworthy that thioredoxin is involved in the NFκB signal-transduction pathway (see below). The protein metallothionine chelates divalent metal ions such as Fe^{2+} and Cu^{2+}, and so it can destroy their role in hydroxyl radical formation.

Reactive nitrogen species These include nitric oxide (NO•), nitrogen peroxide (NOO•) and peroxynitrite (ONOO•) radicals. The nitric oxide radical is not as reactive as the other two. All three can be formed endogenously, but their main interest is as carcinogenic products of the oxides of nitrogen in tobacco smoke.

Antioxidants as protective agents Antioxidants that destroy ROS without damaging cell function are protective. Natural products that fall into this category are ascorbic acid (vitamin C), tocopherol (vitamin E), carotene (a precursor of vitamin A) and glutathione. Each of these compounds will protect animals against the effects of carcinogens. Dietary-supplementation trials with carotene as a means of preventing some cancers in humans are being conducted. Fruit and vegetables are important sources of antioxidant vitamins and polyphenols, which may account for the protective effects of these foods against colorectal and stomach cancer in humans (see Chapters 4 and 13).

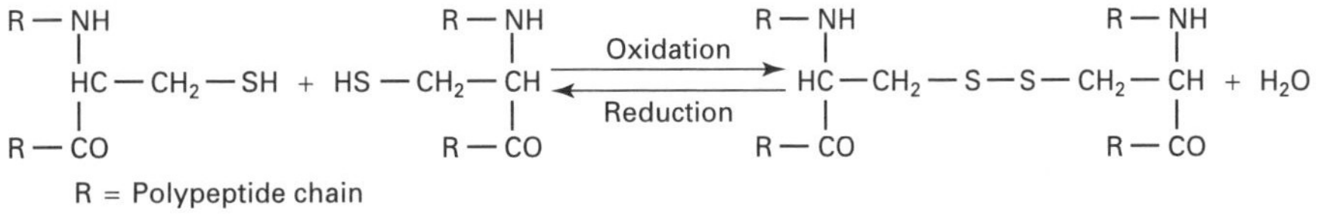

Figure 6.9

Oxidation of cysteine residues in proteins.

Figure 6.10

Types of DNA damage caused by reactive oxygen species.

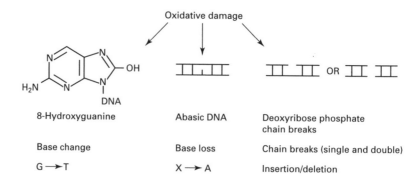

DNA damage Hydroxyl radicals can oxidise guanine to 8-hydroxyguanine and generate abasic sites or strand breaks in DNA (Figure 6.10). 8-Hydroxyguanine is misread as a thymine and therefore paired with an adenine during DNA replication. If the C-1 of deoxyribose is oxidised, then the DNA chain remains intact but the base is lost, with the generation of an abasic site. This is preferentially replaced with an adenine during repair. Oxidation at C-4 of deoxyribose breaks the DNA strand and a single-strand break is formed. Double-strand breaks can also be produced.

Oxidations thus generate various types of change, such as $G \rightarrow T$ point mutations, deletions and insertions; they are described more fully in Chapter 7.

Hydroxyl radicals are so reactive that they do not diffuse far from their site of formation. Their highest concentration is in mitochondria, so the high concentration of 8-hydroxyguanine in mitochondrial DNA is to be expected, but mitochondrial genes code primarily for respiratory-chain proteins in contrast to the much broader spectrum of cell functions coded for by nuclear genes. Although mutations in mitochondrial genes do occur and may increase with increasing age, it is unlikely that they contribute directly to carcinogenesis; inherited defects in mitochondrial DNA exist, but none is linked with an increased risk of cancer. The sources of oxidative mutations in nuclear DNA cannot be identified with certainty, but they undoubtedly exist, since 8-hydroxyguanine is present in nuclear DNA, albeit at much lower levels than in mitochondria. Potential sources of nuclear hydroxyl radicals include precursors formed within the nucleus and extranuclear products like mitochondrial hydrogen peroxide, which, being less reactive, can diffuse within the cell.

Protein oxidations and signal transduction The cysteine–cystine interconversion (see Figure 6.9) was mentioned earlier in relation to thioredoxin function, but other proteins require cysteines for their normal function. Oxidation to cystine alters those functions. When cells are exposed to mitogenic growth factors such as EGF and PDGF, there are two consequences: DNA damage and increased signalling to the nucleus. Several signalling components can be activated (i) at the level of transduction between cell membrane and nucleus via protein phosphorylation/dephosphorylations and (ii) within the nucleus (Table 6.1). Activation of NFκB is indirect in that ROS activate phosphorylation/ubiquitin-dependent proteolysis of the inhibitory factor IκB, which thus releases its cytoplasmic bound NFκB for translocation to the nucleus. ROS can thus act as second messengers in signal-transduction pathways;

Table 6.1 Signal transduction proteins whose activities are altered by ROS.

Protein	Activity	Effect of oxidation
Tyrosine phosphatase	Inhibited	Increased effectiveness of mitogenic tyrosine kinases
Mitogen-activated protein kinase	Activated	Increased effectiveness of extracellular mitogenic signals
Nuclear factor κB	Activated	Increased transcription
AP1 transcription complex for jun/fos sensitive genes	Activated	Ref-1 transcription factor reduces cystines and increases transcription

this effect is achieved at lower concentrations than required to generate mutations in DNA. Another difference between this effect and cysteine oxidation in proteins is that different ROS may be involved; hydrogen peroxide can directly alter the function of proteins such as NFκB but without damaging DNA.

Hypoxia and signal transduction Inadequate oxygen supply (hypoxia) can also influence cell function (see Chapter 11), some features of which are analogous to those just described for ROS. The term 'oxidative stress' is sometimes used to cover both circumstances. The biological consequences of hypoxia are mediated by hypoxia-induced transcription factors (HIFs) and are most relevant during metastasis (induces angiogenesis) and in response to chemotherapy (less effective). These processes are described in Chapters 11 and 12, respectively.

Non-genotoxic carcinogens

The aetiological chemicals of major cancers such as those of breast, prostate and endometrium are hormonal steroids, which do not damage DNA. Hormones are classified as tumour promotors in contrast to initiators, which do react with DNA (see Chapter 2). These hormones are mitogens, increasing cell proliferation by binding to intracellular receptors that are transcription factors. The tumour promotor phorbol ester also binds to its receptor, protein kinase C, thereby activating mitogenic pathways, but the ester is not a naturally occurring agent (see Chapter 10). Proliferation is a risk factor for carcinogenesis; its role in mutation accumulation is discussed in Chapter 2. Another factor linking proliferation with increased cancer risk is that bases in single-stranded DNA are more susceptible to attack by genotoxic carcinogens than when paired with other bases in double-stranded DNA. As regions of single-stranded DNA occur during DNA synthesis, it follows that increased proliferation increases the probability of DNA damage. If that damage is to the DNA repair processes, then an autocatalytic effect would be generated.

Asbestos is a chemically inert silicate that causes a special type of lung cancer, mesothelioma, in exposed workers. How it does this is not clear, but cells can phagocytose the asbestos fibres, which physically damages DNA. Another possibility is that the asbestos may carry bound PAHs. Thus, although asbestos is classified as non-genotoxic because it does not alter DNA bases, that classification may be suspect.

Tests for carcinogens

With so many chemicals having the potential to cause cancer, methods for testing environmental, industrial and nutritional components are important in the drive to reduce human exposure to carcinogens. Tests on humans are ethically inadmissible, so they are carried out on alternative material. These tests fall into three broad categories: tests on animals (tumour induction), tests on cultured cells (DNA damage) and tests on microorganisms (mutability) (Table 6.2). Each type of test has its own advantages and disadvantages, and so reliance should not be placed on data from a single type of test. The overriding principle behind such testing is that it is better to err on the side of caution rather than be wise after the event, even if this means misclassifying some compounds as being carcinogenic when they are not. Government agencies that license compounds for human use establish testing criteria that must be satisfied before a licence is granted. Procedures that test the possibility of tumour induction over the lifetime of experimental animals are considered to be the most reliable.

Animal tests

These tests detect both genotoxic and non-genotoxic agents. The animals used most commonly are rats and mice, for convenience of size, cost and relatively short lifespan. Initially, a maximum tolerated dose is established. Then a range of doses based on the maximum tolerated dose is established and administered to a group of about 50 animals of both sexes. These doses are administered throughout the notional lifespan of the animal (2 years). At the end of the trial, all animals are subjected to post-mortem examination for the presence of tumours and about 40 organs are used in a histopathological investigation for signs of cancer. Any animals dying during the course of the experiment are subjected to the same examinations. Interpretation of results presents problems, because it is difficult to extrapolate data obtained from one species to another, considering the differences in metabolism and longevity (Table 6.3). Such testing is very expensive and takes a long time; therefore, in order to keep up with the flow of chemicals produced by industry, it is useful to have alternative tests that are cheaper and more rapid.

Table 6.2 Methods for testing carcinogenic potential of compounds.

Animals	Tumour appearance
	Abnormal chromosomes in bone marrow
Cell culture	DNA damage
Microorganisms	Reversal of a mutation

Table 6.3 Problems in interpreting animal carcinogenesis tests.

Doses used: very high compared with human exposure

Timescale: short compared with human exposure

Species: relevance of animal studies to humans

Metabolism: activation/deactivation variable in different species

There are several short-form hybrid tests that use animals. One such test uses a range of doses on animals, which are then used to provide samples of bone marrow. These are subjected to cytological examination using criteria such as the presence of micronuclei and chromosome abnormalities. These tests produce results rapidly but are subject to the same criticisms as those based on tumour induction in animals.

Cultured cells

Test compounds are added to the medium of cultured cells, which are monitored for defects of cell function relative to carcinogenesis. Metabolic activation of the test compound may not occur in the culture; therefore, it is standard to add rat-liver microsomes with a supply of NADPH to activate the carcinogens. In practice, it is usual to monitor features indicating DNA damage; these include the appearance of abnormal chromosomes and unscheduled DNA synthesis. The latter involves the incorporation of labelled DNA precursors at inappropriate phases of the cell cycle.

Ability to cause mutations in specific genes is another end point of such tests. A commonly used gene codes for hypoxanthine–guanine phosphoribosyl transferase, mutations in which can be readily detected by altered sensitivity of the cells to anti-proliferative drugs such as 8-azaguanine. This is incorporated into DNA and blocks DNA synthesis. The enzyme is necessary to convert the drug into the nucleoside monophosphate, essential for its incorporation into DNA. If mutant (inactive) enzyme is present, then 8-azaguanine is not incorporated and the cells proliferate, whereas non-mutagenised cells are killed.

The advantage of this type of test is that a result is obtained relatively quickly; the disadvantage is that the test does not detect non-genotoxic carcinogens.

Microorganisms

The most widely employed test is the Ames test, which uses strains of the bacterium *Salmonella typhinurium* that cannot synthesise the amino acid histidine. The bacteria are seeded into histidine-deficient medium together with rat-liver microsomes and a source of NADPH to which the chemical to be tested is added. The test ma-terial is considered carcinogenic if it causes back mutations in the bacteria, enabling it to form colonies in the deficient medium. There are also a number of steps that can be added to the basic procedure in order to increase sensitivity.

The Ames test is straightforward and can produce results rapidly. However, it detects only genotoxic agents. The test also gives rise to a number of false positive and negative results, typically identifying 50–70% of known carcinogens but mis-classifying about a quarter of non-carcinogens. Despite the high error rate and the inability to detect non-genotoxic carcinogens, the Ames test is used widely as a screening test before other forms of assessment.

Radiation carcinogenesis

Several types of radiation can cause cancer in humans. Atomic radiation, such as that produced by radon, a radioactive gas created naturally by the decay of uranium, caused lung cancers in workers mining uranium ore. The dense radiation flux resulting from the atomic bombs dropped on Japan in 1945 and the atmospheric contamination by radionucleides produced by the meltdown of the Chernobyl pile have provided further tragic proof of the carcinogenicity of atomic radiation. Other types of radiation such as X-rays and **u**ltraviolet (UV) light are also carcinogenic (Table 6.4).

Radiation is energy whose power depends on its source and type. There is an overlap of the energy spectra between the different radiation types; the descending order of energy release is as follows: atomic particles > X-rays > UV light > visible light > infrared, microwave and electrical waves. Only the first three of these have been shown to be carcinogenic. Atomic radiation is of several types: α (2 protons + 2 neutrons), β (electrons), neutrons and γ (waveform).

Each of the carcinogenic forms of radiation, except UV light, can generate ions in the media through which they travel and are termed ionising radiation. As ionising and non-ionising radiation cause cancer by different mechanisms, we will consider them separately.

Ionising radiation

The types of cancer generated by such energy sources were described in the previous section; all involve DNA damage. Ionising radiation contain energies much greater than that in chemical bonds, and so chemical bonds can be broken by radiation. Although many molecules are thus affected, water and DNA are the principal compounds involved as far as cancer formation is concerned. The energy released by the radiation as it passes through water produces electrons, which in turn generate reactive radicals in much the same sequence of reactions as those in the mitochondrial electron transport chain (see Figure 6.8). This physical stage of radiation

Table 6.4 Types of radiation that cause cancers in humans.

Agent	Source	Cancer
Ultraviolet light	Sunlight	Skin
X-rays	Medical treatment	Leukaemia, thyroid
Atomic radiation	War	All types
Radon	Mining, geological seepage	Lung

Table 6.5 Biological effects of 1 Gy on cultured cells.

2×10^5 ionisations per cell
100 DNA strand breaks per cell
Start to see chromosome changes
High LET radiation: 1% cells survive
   30 transformations per 1 million cells (0.003%)
Low LET radiation: 90% cells survive
   3 transformations per 1 million cells (0.0003%)

LET, linear energy transfer.

carcinogenesis occurs within a fraction of a second, followed by the chemical stage in which DNA bonds are broken. The consequences of the chemical changes become apparent in the final cell and tissue stage, and this can take years to appear.

Ionising radiations produce single- and double-strand breaks in the DNA, resulting in chromosome damage involving mainly deletions and rearrangements rather than the point mutations generated by chemical carcinogens and UV light. Another difference between the types of carcinogen is that cells are most sensitive to ionising radiations during the G_2/M phases of the cell cycle whereas early S phase is the sensitive period for chemical agents and UV light.

The unit used to define energy release is the **gray** (Gy); 1 Gy is the release of 1 J/kg of tissue. Absorption of energy may be defined in terms of **l**inear **e**nergy **t**ransfer (LET), which is the transfer of energy over the path length of the particle concerned. A given amount of energy released in a short distance does more damage than the same amount over a longer distance. To convert from gray units to low LET values, there is no multiplying factor. But to convert from gray units to high LET values, there is a multiplying factor of up to ten; this is to account for high-LET effects. When a gray unit has been multiplied by this quality factor, the unit becomes a **s**ie**v**ert (Sv). It is usual to refer to high- and low-LET radiation; high-LET radiation is more dangerous than low-LET radiation.

Some approximate indications of the effect of 1 Gy on cultured mammalian cells are given in Table 6.5. The large number of ionisations are more than sufficient to generate the strand breaks observed, which in turn account for the gross chromosome abnormalities that start to appear at this exposure. High-LET radiations, as produced by α particles and neutrons, generate so much DNA damage that the cells die; low-LET radiation (X-rays and γ-rays) is much less cytotoxic. Anchorage-independent growth is a reasonable cell biological marker of carcinogenesis (see Chapter 2); the number of cells acquiring this property (transformants) also increases with LET, although only a small proportion are so affected. To put these values into the context of human exposure, the total lifetime exposure of an average individual is only 0.1 Gy. The majority of cancers in Japanese survivors of the atom bombs occurred in people exposed to more than 1 Gy.

Atomic bombs and nuclear accidents

The most profound proof of the carcinogenic nature of ionising radiation is provided by the survivors of the atomic bombs dropped on Japan in 1945. Survivors

Table 6.6 Predicted carcinogenic effect of the Chernobyl nuclear accident.

Group	Exposure (Gy)	Percentage increase in lifetime cancer risk
Local inhabitants	10^{-1}	2
Europe (except former USSR)	10^{-2}	0.1
USA	10^{-1}	0.0001

who were subjected to high sub-lethal doses of this radiation showed an increase in the incidence of leukaemia. Accidents at nuclear installations are fortunately rare; however, the meltdown of a pile at Chernobyl contaminated very large areas of adjacent territories. The atmospheric plume released from the burning installation contained large quantities of radioactive iodine, and this has caused an increase in the incidence of juvenile thyroid cancer in the Ukraine and adjacent countries (Table 6.6).

Background radiation

Humans are exposed daily to low doses of radiation, both natural and synthetic. The major component of this background radiation is derived from radon seeping from the ground (Table 6.7; see also below). The other major contributor is cosmic radiation reaching the earth from sources in space. The synthetic component is derived from diagnostic and therapeutic X-rays, treatment with radioactive products and residual radiation from the nuclear industries. The natural component of background radiation cannot be regulated, but the synthetic components are regulated by statutory regulation and adherence to recommended dose limits. The lower end of the limit (threshold dose) is almost impossible to define with accuracy. Although there are good

Table 6.7 Human lifetime exposure to ionising radiation.

Source	Percentage of total*
Natural	
Radon gas	55
Cosmic radiation	8
Terrestrial radiation	8
Synthetic	
Medical X-rays	11
Nuclear medicine	4
Consumer products	3
Other	< 1

* Total lifetime exposure = 0.1 Gy.
(Source: Adapted from Table 12.2 in DeVita, V.T., Hellman, S. and Rosenburg, S.A. (eds) (1993) *Cancer: Principles and Practice of Oncology*, Fourth Edition. Philadelphia, PA: Lippincott.)

dose–response curves for high doses of radiation, these cannot be simply extrapolated to zero. Statutory organisations, such as the Radiation Protection Board in the UK, are concerned with determination of annual body burdens of licensed radiation workers in the nuclear industries, medicine, dentistry and the basic sciences.

How much these types of radiation contribute to human cancers is a subject of debate. Individual sources of radiation such as radon and the atomic power industry are considered below; however, part of the debate centres on uncertainty about the biological effects of low levels of radiation. There are good dose–response data for levels greater than 1 Gy to indicate that atomic radiation increases all types of cancer, with leukaemia being the most sensitive. However, these dose–response curves have to be extrapolated back to zero to get the low radiation values encountered in everyday life, and it is not clear what type of extrapolation is valid. Fewer leukaemias seem to occur than predicted from a linear extrapolation, but that may not be true for solid cancers.

Radon

Radon is a radioactive gas produced in very low quantities by the natural decay of elements in the ground. Local atmospheric quantities of radon vary with the nature of the underlying rocks and the built environment. The atmosphere of houses contains more radon than the surrounding open air because houses trap the radon seeping from the ground; people living in these houses then breathe in this radon. As this gas and some of its daughter products are α-emitters (high LET), they are potential radiation hazards. Internal radiation derived in this way has been estimated to cause about 1500 lung cancers per year in the UK and about ten times that number in the USA. Important as these figures are, they should be seen in the context that they represent only a small fraction of the smoking-related cancers.

Nuclear industries

Workers in the nuclear industries might appear to be at risk of an increased background radiation. However, by using personal dosimeters, individual burdens of absorbed radiation are calculated regularly, and thus excessive radiation doses are avoided. Consequently, there is no increase in incidence of cancer in radiation workers, apart from personnel involved in accidents. The finding of a zone of high incidence of childhood leukaemia around the nuclear plant at Sellafield suggested a possible adverse effect of low-grade environmental contamination. However, the geographical distribution of childhood leukaemia tends to occur as local hot spots that move with time; the zone that once occurred around Sellafield has now disappeared.

There remain contentious issues, such as the intentional discharge of low-grade radioactive waste from nuclear plants into adjacent seas acting as an environmental contaminant. Additionally, there is the problem arising from the use of depleted uranium (weakly radioactive) in munitions. Depleted uranium is a very dense metal and can be used in armour-piercing shells. When this metal is subjected to explosive heating, it can form a cloud of metallic oxide, which could be inhaled by combatants and act as a source of internal irradiation. Over the course of time, heavy metals are redistributed in the body and tend to accumulate in bone, and so it follows that depleted uranium incorporated into bone could possibly constitute a carcinogenic hazard.

X-rays

Therapeutic X-ray units deliver high doses of radiation (1–10 Gy) to patients with conditions such as cancer and ankylosing spondylytis. Follow-up data from such therapy indicate a three-fold increase in the incidence of leukaemia and a 30% increased risk of lung and colorectal cancer. Diagnostic X-ray units deliver much lower radiation doses; provided they are not used too frequently, they do not constitute a hazard.

Ultraviolet light

Because of its limited penetration in tissues, the UV component of sunlight affects only skin in exposed regions of the body. The energy spectrum of UV light is divided into three regions according to wavelength: UVA (> 320 nm), UVB (290–320 nm) and UVC (200–290 nm). UVB is the most important fraction for skin carcinogenesis. Most UVB is filtered from sunlight by the atmospheric ozone layer, and so any depletion of the ozone layer is likely to increase the incidence of skin cancer. Pale-skinned people are particularly vulnerable to this type of radiation. Not surprisingly, this group shows a north–south increase in the incidence of malignant melanoma in the northern hemisphere; this gradient is reversed in the southern hemisphere.

Solar damage to the skin is reduced by application of creams containing UV-absorbing organic chemicals such as cinnamates and inorganic pigments containing zinc or titanium oxides. Apart from this, moderate UV exposure induces melanin formation (tanning), which provides protection against further damage by sunlight. Any damage to DNA initiates repair, but this is a delayed response. Intermittent UV exposure is more deleterious than prolonged exposure, as the delayed repair results in the accumulation of DNA damage.

In contrast to its sensitivity to ionising radiation, DNA is most sensitive to UV light during early S phase of the cell cycle, because the pyrimidine bases that are altered by UV are more exposed during this period and therefore subject to attack.

UV radiation has lower energy than ionising radiation and therefore has less potential for breaking chemical bonds. However, it does excite other molecules, making them more reactive. As far as DNA is concerned, this involves the formation of covalent links between adjacent pyrimidines. Thymine–thymine, cytosine–cytosine and cytosine–thymine dimers can be formed. An example of a thymine–thymine dimer is illustrated in Figure 6.11. Cyclobutane dimers are read as thymines, and so mutations result only if cytosine is a component of the dimer. This can result in a C → T transition (Tables 6.8–6.10), sometimes as unique double-tandem mutations. Other photoproducts are formed with only a single bond linking the two

Figure 6.11

UV-induced formation of pyrimidine dimers.

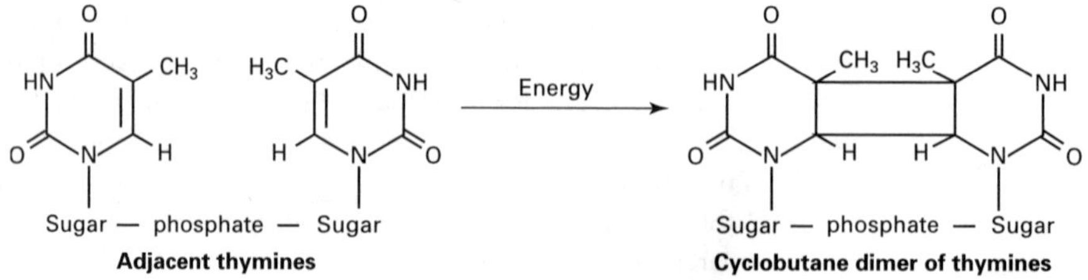

Adjacent thymines   Cyclobutane dimer of thymines

pyrimidines, (6−4) photoproduct and its isomer. All the photoproducts are mutagenic, but the cyclobutane dimer is probably most important in skin carcinogenesis as the other products are repaired more quickly.

Other forms of radiation

It has been suggested that radiation from power lines, transformers and mobile phones might cause cancers. However, there is no clear evidence that this low-energy radiation can do so. Nevertheless, low-energy radiation can influence rates of chemical reactions without breaking covalent bonds, and so adverse effects remain theoretically possible.

Consequences of DNA damage

The three possible consequences of DNA damage are (i) repair and return to normality, (ii) extensive damage leading to cell death and (iii) misreading of modified bases at the next round of DNA synthesis. DNA synthesis generates mutations whose types depend on the nature of the damage (Table 6.8). The commonest result of chemical damage or UV light is a point mutation in which one base is replaced by another. Depending on the base involved and its location within a given region of DNA, such a point mutation can result in no effect (redundant DNA), replacement of one amino acid by another (altered codon), truncated protein (generation of nonsense or stop codon), altered regulation (regulatory sequences) or abnormal-sized protein (altered intron : exon boundaries, chromosome rearrangements). Specific examples of each type of change are given in Chapter 7.

Table 6.8 Mutations caused by DNA-damaging agents.*

Modifying agent	Example	Recognised as	Base pairing	
			Old	New
Small adduct	G → Me.G	A	G : C	A : T
Large adduct	G → G.BP	T	G : C	T : A
Ultraviolet light	Cytosine dimers	T	G : C	A : T
Oxidation	G → 8-OH.G	T	G : C	T : A
Oxidation	Strand breaks		Deletions	
Ionising radiation	Strand breaks		Deletions	
Spontaneous	C/MeC deamination	T	G : C	A : T

* These are the major mutations; others occur with each agent.
A, G, C, T, DNA bases; BP, benzopyrene; Me, methyl.
(Source: From Table 1 in Greenblatt, M.S., *et al.* (1994) Mutations in the p53 tumor suppressor gene: clues to cancer etiology and molecular pathogenesis. *Cancer Research*, **54**, 4855–78. Copyright © 1994 Reproduced with permission from the American Association for Cancer Research.)

Ionising radiations generate a wider spectrum of alterations, with deletions being frequent and point mutations being less common.

Base transitions and transversions

Small adducts, such as the O-methylguanine generated by N-methylnitrosourea, are treated as an adenine and become paired with a thymine rather than the normal cytosine at the next round of DNA synthesis. Subsequent divisions generate A : T pairs instead of the original G : C pairs. This G → A mutation is referred to as a 'transition', a term used when a purine is substituted by a different purine or a pyrimidine with a pyrimidine. Oxidative damage commonly produces a G → T mutation, as does the presence of a bulky adduct such as benzopyrene or aflatoxin on guanine. This change from purine to pyrimidine is called a 'transversion'. The changes listed in Table 6.8 are those associated most frequently, but not exclusively, with the carcinogens mentioned.

Relevance of model changes to real genes

Given that only a small fraction of the bases in DNA have a coding or regulatory role, it follows that the majority of mutations are silent and have no functional effect. Therefore, it is important to show that the adducts and base changes determined by experimental interaction of carcinogens with DNA have relevance to functional DNA in whole cells. To do this, cultured human cells have been exposed to different carcinogens and a housekeeping gene, adenosyl phosphoribosyl transferase, has been sequenced to see what mutations have occurred. The results (see Table 6.9) fit the predictions from model experiments with non-specific DNA (see Table 6.8), but in the gene analysis there were 30−40% of mutations besides those that had been predicted. Thus, the G → T transversion predicted for benzopyrene accounts for 62%

Table 6.9 Mutations in adenosyl phosphoribosyl transferase gene generated in cultured cells.

Agent	Most frequent change	Percentage of all mutations
Spontaneous	G → A	71
Benzopyrene diol epoxide (large adduct)	G → T	62
Nitrosamines	G → A	63
Ultraviolet light	C → T	61
Ionising radiation	Deletions	31
	G → A	19
	A → C	19

(Source: Reproduced from Table 2 in Greenblatt, M.S., *et al.* (1994) Mutations in the p53 tumor suppressor gene: clues to cancer etiology and molecular pathogenesis. *Cancer Research*, 54, 4855–78. Reproduced with permission from the American Association for Cancer Research.)

of mutations, with G → C transversions accounting for another 14%. More information is required in order to identify the molecular basis of those other mutations.

Deletions predominate with ionising radiations, but some point mutations are also observed. Agreement also occurs if an oncogene rather than a housekeeping gene is analysed. In rat *N*-methylnitrosourea-induced bladder cancers, *H-ras* is activated by a G → A transition, as predicted for the formation of a small alkyl guanine (see Table 6.8). A carcinogen such as 3-methylcholanthrene forms a bulky adduct with the consequential G → T transversion at codon 12 of *H-ras*. Mutations in the tumour suppressor gene *p53* are discussed in the next section.

Predicting the type of carcinogen by mutational spectrum analysis

As types of mutation can be predicted by knowing the carcinogen, the logic should be reversible, i.e. the type of carcinogen can be identified from mutations detected in cancers. This approach is being used with some success, even though certain problems have still to be resolved. Epidemiological methods have been the main approach in identifying carcinogenic risks in humans, and so 'molecular epidemiology' is the name given to molecular methods such as gene sequencing that are used for epidemiological purposes (see Chapter 4).

The approach is to select a gene known to be involved in many cancers and then to analyse the types of mutation (mutation spectrum) in those cancers. The gene coding for the suppressor protein p53 has generated most information because the majority of human cancers contain aberrant p53 and several thousand mutations have been identified. These can be looked at in a general way by determining the proportion of transversions and transitions in different cancers, and in a more specific way through the actual bases involved.

Transversions and transitions in p53

The pattern of change is different in each of colon, lung, breast and liver cancers (Figure 6.12), suggesting that different carcinogenic events are involved in each case. Transversions predominate in lung cancers and their number increases with

Figure 6.12

p53 in human cancers: transitions and transversions. (Source: Adapted from Figure 4 in Levine, A.J., *et al.* (1994) *British Journal of Cancer*, 69, 409–16. Copyright © 1994. Reprinted with permission of Macmillan Publishers Ltd.)

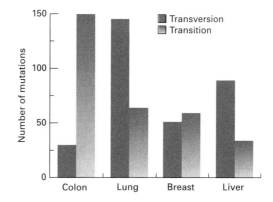

number of cigarettes smoked. Liver cancer follows a similar pattern to lung cancer, but transitions are the dominant feature in colorectal cancer. The mixed pattern seen in breast cancers suggests a complex aetiology. Non-genotoxic female sex steroids are the major known factor for breast carcinogenesis. It is not clear why these steroids are carcinogenic, but increased proliferation and generation of genetic instability is a possibility (see above). Such general mechanisms might be expected to generate diverse mutational changes.

Specific base changes in p53

The data just described indicate that different pathways of carcinogenesis are operative in the relevant cancers. Identifying the specific base changes involved can provide clues as to what might be causing those changes in the *p53* gene (see Table 6.10). Lung cancers caused by smoking have a high transversion of $G \rightarrow T$, compatible with both bulky adduct formation and oxidations. Potential adducts such as benzopyrene and oxidants such as nitric oxide have been identified in tobacco smoke. Smoking also increases bladder cancer, and $G \rightarrow T$ transversions of the lung type are present, but there is also a high frequency of $G \rightarrow C$ mutations. This suggests that other carcinogens are carried by body fluids to the bladder. The high $G \rightarrow T$ transversion rate in liver cancers (see Table 6.10) is compatible with bulky adduct formation such as from aflatoxin in foodstuffs (see Figure 4.7). The high $G \rightarrow A$ transition pattern in colorectal cancer might indicate involvement of carcinogens generating a small DNA adduct. Skin cancers exhibit the anticipated $C \rightarrow T$ transition expected from pyrimidine dimer formation, and there are some double transitions in adjacent cytosines. Such double mutations have been observed only in cancers induced by UV light.

Not only do certain types of base change occur in different cancers but also the affected codon within the *p53* gene can vary (see Table 6.10). This could be due to differential access of carcinogens to specific bases in various cancers. With the *ras* oncogene, another situation arises in that the same codon (codon 12) is affected in lung and bladder cancer but different bases within that codon are altered. In bladder cancers, $G \rightarrow T$ transversions predominate, whereas $G \rightarrow A$ transitions are more

Table 6.10 *p53* mutations in human cancers.

Cancer	Most frequent		
	Mutation	**Codon**	**Predicted agent**
Lung	$G \rightarrow T$	273	Benzopyrene, oxidations
Colon	$G \rightarrow A$	175, others	Small adduct
Liver	$G \rightarrow T$	249	Aflatoxin
Skin	$C \rightarrow T$	–	Ultraviolet light
	(plus tandem double mutations)		

common in lung cancers, again pointing to different tobacco-related carcinogens being involved at the two sites. Interestingly, not all the *p53* mutation hot spots identified in model systems *in vitro* coincide with those reported for human tumours *in vivo*. This may be due to faster repair *in vivo* at some sites than at others, masking some of the hot spots detected *in vitro*.

Conclusions

These examples of mutational spectrum analysis indicate the potential of the approach, but refinements are required in order to make the predictions more accurate for identifying human carcinogens. Both large adducts and oxidative damage generate $G \rightarrow T$ transversions and so at present it would not be possible to distinguish between these two sources of mutation. However, they can be distinguished from small adducts. A $G \rightarrow A$ transition characteristic of this type of carcinogen also occurs with UV light (secondary to the causative $C \rightarrow T$ mutation), but this is characterised by dual tandem mutations because of its cross-linking effect.

Further reading

Blancher, C. and Harris, A.L. (1998) The molecular basis of the hypoxia response pathway: tumour hypoxia as a therapy target. *Cancer Metastasis Rev* **17**, 187–194.

Darby, S., Whitley, E., Silcocks, P., *et al.* (1998) Risk of lung cancer associated with residential radon exposure in south-west England: a case control study. *Br J Cancer* **78**, 394–408.

Dogliotti, E., Hainaut, P., Hernandez, T., D'Errico, M. and DeMarini, D.M. (1998) Mutation spectra resulting from carcinogen exposure: from model systems to cancer-related genes. *Recent Results Cancer Res* **154**, 97–124.

McGregor, D.B., Rice, J.M. and Venitt, S. (1999) *The Use of Short- and Medium-Term Tests for Carcinogens and Data on Genetic Effects in Carcinogenic Hazard Evaluation.* Lyons: IARC Press.

Noshchenko, A.G., *et al.* (2001) Patterns of acute leukaemia occurrence among children in the Chernobyl region. *Int J Epidemiol* **30**, 125–29.

Rouse, J. and Jackson, S.P. (2002) Interfaces between the detection, signalling and repair of DNA damage. *Science* **297**, 547–551.

Ryan, K.M., Phillips, A.C. and Vousden, K.H. (2001) Regulation and function of the p53 tumour suppressor protein. *Curr Opin Cell Biol* **13**, 332–337.

7 Mutations, DNA repair and genetic instability

KEY POINTS

- DNA is continually exposed to endogenous and exogenous damaging agents. It is repaired efficiently in normal cells so that errors (mutations) are not inherited by daughter cells.
- Cancer cells acquire defects in the repair process that accelerate the mutation rate.
- Genetic instability is a consequence of defective repair.
- The damaged region of DNA is detected and excised, together with adjacent nucleotides; then the correct nucleotides are inserted. Several mechanisms exist to do this, each having different abilities to handle specific types of damage.
- Repair processes can be strand-specific or strand-independent.
- Strand-specific mechanisms can repair errors caused by the introduction of bases into the newly synthesised strand that do not pair with bases on the template strand. This is termed mismatch repair.
- Instability of microsatellite DNA is a common feature of cancers. It is an index of genetic instability due to inefficient mismatch repair.
- Strand-independent mechanisms such as nucleotide excision repair, which are less specific about the type of damage, can cope with damage caused by carcinogens, ionising radiations and UV light.
- Strand-independent mechanisms exist to remove oxidised or methylated guanines. This is called base excision repair.
- DNA damage activates p53, which then inhibits proliferation and promotes DNA repair and apoptosis.
- Several clinical conditions are due to an inherited defect in DNA repair. People with these conditions have an increased risk of developing specific types of cancer.
- Lynch's syndrome is due to an inherited defect in one allele of genes required for mismatch repair. Cancer results from loss of the second allele.
- People with Li–Fraumeni syndrome develop cancers at several sites caused by an inherited mutation in the *p53* gene.
- People with xeroderma pigmentosum have an inherited defect in nucleotide excision repair that results in an increased risk of skin cancer.

Introduction

Cancer results from changes in DNA sequence called mutations. The mutations are reflected in proteins, which have an altered amino acid sequence. These altered proteins ultimately change the cell function. DNA changes are generated by normal intracellular metabolic events and by external factors such as diet, lifestyle and solar radiation. It is therefore important to identify the mechanisms whereby cells minimise adverse effects of mutations. The preceding chapters have discussed the various agents capable of causing and propagating mutations; this chapter will deal with mechanisms used to repair altered DNA sequences. Repair of damaged DNA is an important defence mechanism that prevents most people developing cancers. The original clues came from bacteria in which repair defects increased the appearance of mutations. This link between repair and mutations also became evident from observations that people with rare inherited diseases such as Bloom's syndrome, ataxia telangiectasia and xeroderma pigmentosum, which have the common feature of deficient DNA repair, have an increased risk of developing certain cancers (see Chapter 8). The importance of DNA repair defects has now widened to include cancers such as those of colon and breast.

Decreased efficiency of repair is now viewed as being an important event in the succession of changes required for cancer formation, because such defects accelerate the rate of genetic change. This opinion developed from several data sets. Spontaneous mutation rates were too small to explain the speed with which multiple changes occurred that resulted in a cancer. The concept of a 'mutator phenotype' arose, in which cells with a faster mutation rate gained a survival advantage over their neighbours. Defective DNA repair could be the molecular engine for such a process because the inability to normalise damaged DNA would accelerate the accumulation of errors in DNA bases (mutations). If the defect was in the repair process itself, then an autocatalytic process would be generated. Such defects have been identified in a subtype of inherited colorectal cancer, hereditary non-polyposis coli cancer (HNPCC; see Chapter 2), and shown to be present in a number of spontaneous cancers. However, there is debate as to whether the accelerated accumulation of mutations is solely a characteristic of cancer cells. Mutation rates also increase with age in normal cells, and it may be a normal phenomenon, with carcinogenesis being a normal consequence of the ageing human lifecycle. Regardless of whether the mutator phenotype reflects normal or abnormal events, there must be causative agents. There has been an emphasis on external agents as the most important, but these may be supplemented by spontaneous events generated through normal cell metabolism. The human data are supplemented by animal information such as the observation that mice develop cancers much more readily, have a higher spontaneous mutation rate and have a less active DNA repair system than humans.

The elucidation of DNA repair mechanisms is a good illustration of the multidisciplinary contributions to cancer biology. Many of the molecular characteristics of the repair processes were first elucidated in microorganisms and subsequently shown to have relevance to human cells. Characterisation of the cellular defects in people with xeroderma pigmentosum required the expertise of clinicians, geneticists and molecular biologists, as did investigations on the people with HNPCC.

Cell biologists contributed by isolating cultured cells possessing the molecular characteristics of the parent tissues, thereby facilitating analysis of the cellular defects.

Although a decreased ability to repair DNA is an important factor in carcinogenesis, many cancers have defects not in the repair processes themselves but in ancillary pathways concerned with regulation of repair and/or the transfer and accumulations of DNA defects to daughter cells. Cell proliferation is the prime determinant of the accumulation; over time, the number of mutations accumulated per cell is proliferation-dependent. For this reason, proliferation has been defined as a risk factor for cancer. For similar reasons, cell death is also part of the equation that determines whether sufficient mutations accumulate to generate a cancer.

Cells have several repair pathways capable of dealing with various types of abnormal base sequence which are described below. Additionally, a special type of DNA repair is used to correct changes to telomeric ends of chromosomes (see Chapter 9).

Mutations

Changes in DNA base sequence advertise themselves in several ways: single or multiple bases can be changed, deleted or inserted. Sophisticated molecular techniques may be required to detect such changes, but the changes can sometimes appear as gross changes in DNA content per nucleus (ploidy), as chromosome rearrangements or as gene amplifications. Data are sparse on mutation rates in normal human cells, but three factors are clearly important in determining that rate: age, cell type and DNA characteristics (Table 7.1). The higher frequency in kidney epithelium relative to that in blood lymphocytes is important because it might account for the high frequency of cancers in epithelial cells. Little is known about why some somatic

Table 7.1 Mutation frequencies in normal human cells.

	Mutations per 1 million cells*	
Cell type and age of individual		
Kidney epithelium	40 (young)	250 (old)
Lymphocytes	3 (young)	8 (old)
DNA type		
Microsatellite	10 000	
Hypoxanthine phosphoribosyl transferase gene	10	
Other factors		
Potent carcinogen	100-fold increase	
Theoretical value to account for age–incidence data	1000-fold increase	

* Approximations from a wide range of values.
(Source: Based on data from Simpson A.J.G. (1997) *Advances in Cancer Research*, 71, 209–40. Copyright © 1997. Reproduced with permission of Elsevier.)

cells have higher mutation rates than others, but rates are probably set during embryonic development. Efficiency of DNA repair is one factor that influences mutation rates, but additional components related to a cell's redox state may also be involved. A cell with a high incidence of free-radical production may be more vulnerable than a cell with minimal production of these DNA-damaging agents. Answers to these points might solve the question of why cancers are more common at some sites than at others. The increase in mutation rate with age is analogous to the age-dependent incidence of common cancers (see Chapter 2); this comparison between mutation rate and cancer incidence has another similarity, in that both increase in an exponential manner rather than a linear manner.

Mutations are more likely to occur in stretches of DNA containing repeat sequences because of misalignment of multiple repeats on the template and daughter strands than in a gene with few such repeats. This accounts for the higher number of mutations in microsatellite DNA, which consists of these sequences, than in the hypoxanthine phosphoribosyl transferase gene.

From the data for normal epithelial cells given in Table 7.1, it is possible to calculate theoretical mutation rates for a suppressor the size of the crucial colorectal cancer gene, *APC* (see Chapter 2). The spontaneous mutation frequency for one allele would be one per thousand cells per generation; for both alleles, the figure would be one per million cells. This is not a large number of cells, being the equivalent of a sphere about 1 millimetre in diameter. A similar number emerges from a different data set – normal urinary excretion of metabolites of purine and pyrimidine bases – suggesting that about 10 000 bases are destroyed per cell per day. If DNA repair of this damage is 99% efficient, then 100 mutations per cell per day would result. Such calculations are subject to major errors and should not be overinterpreted, but they do indicate that spontaneous mutations could generate initial carcinogenic changes in normal cells.

Genetic instability

In cell culture, potent carcinogens such as *N*-methylnitrosourea increase mutation rates between 10-fold and 100-fold (see Table 7.1), but sufficient concentrations of such potent compounds are unlikely to be encountered *in vivo* in human tissues. It has been calculated that if DNA repair is working properly, then the spontaneous mutation rate would have to be increased more than 1000-fold in order to account for the relatively short time necessary to generate the seven rate-limiting mutations necessary for colorectal carcinogenesis (see Chapter 2). However, if DNA repair is defective, and if an ancillary process such as proliferation increased or if cell death decreased, then mutations that conferred selective advantages on the cells would accumulate at an accelerated rate.

A different form of instability becomes evident at later stages of carcinogenesis, especially during progression to more aggressive cancers. This involves gross increases in DNA content per nucleus (ploidy changes) or multiple amplifications of specific regions of certain chromosomes. Thus, the chromosome region containing the dihydrofolate reductase gene can be amplified more than 1000-fold in advanced cancers, so it becomes visible as a homogeneous staining region in chromosome preparations (see Chapter 12).

Types of DNA damage

Figure 7.1 illustrates the main types of damage suffered by DNA, which, if not corrected, could result in the substitution of abnormal bases. Damaging agents can be categorised according to whether they are of endogenous (intracellular) or environmental origin. Chapter 6 details the mechanisms whereby oxidation, ionising radiation, UV light and chemical carcinogens modify DNA structure; the mutational consequences are listed in Table 6.8. They will only be summarised here, but the additional processes identified in Figure 7.1 will be discussed.

Oxidation of guanine by reactive oxygen free radicals generated by ionising radiation or cell metabolism produces 8-hydroxyguanine (8-oxoguanine); DNA polymerase reads this as a thymine at the next round of synthesis (see Figure 6.10). Ionising radiation also induces single- and double-strand breaks, which create deletions and gross chromosome abnormalities. UV light cross-links adjacent pyrimidines (cytosines or thymines; see Figure 6.11), which are read as thymines. The effect of adducts consequent to carcinogen exposure is determined by the carcinogen involved. Small

Figure 7.1

Types of base change induced by different agents.

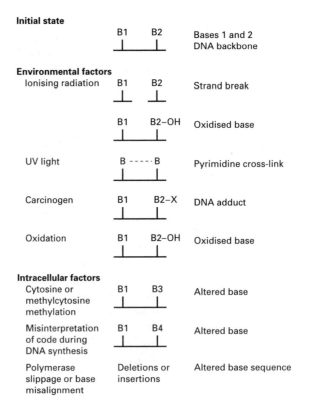

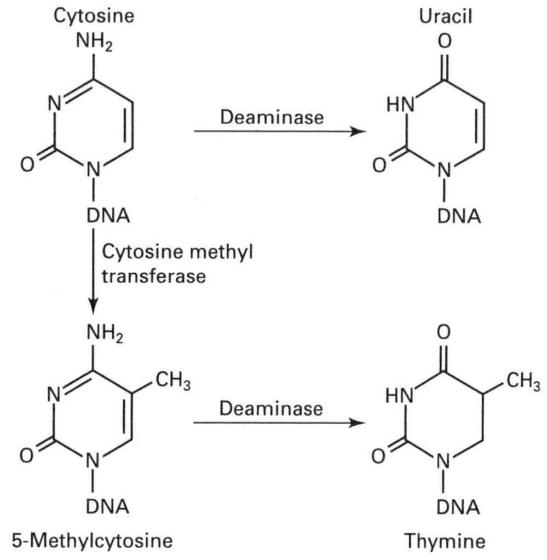

Figure 7.2

Deamination of cytosine and 5-methylcytosine as mutational events.

adducts such as those formed between guanine and dimethylnitrosamine (see Figure 6.6) are read as adenines, whereas bulky guanine adducts such as those formed with benzopyrene (see Figure 6.3) either can be treated as thymines or can distort the DNA structure so much that strand breaks occur. Several intracellular metabolic events generate mutations. Free radicals were mentioned above, but a common change is the deamination of cytosine to form uracil or 5-methylcytosine to form thymine (Figure 7.2); both are interpreted as thymines. DNA synthesis is an efficient process, with the base sequence of the template strand being converted with high fidelity (one error per 10^{10} nucleotides) into a complementary sequence on the daughter strand. This is due largely to the $3'-5'$ exonuclease (phosphodiesterase) activity of some of the DNA polymerases involved (see Box 5.1 for explanation of DNA terminology).

The commonest error of this type is a G pairing with a T instead of the normal G : C pattern. This is aptly called the proof-reading function of DNA polymerase. At least four DNA polymerases are involved in DNA synthesis (see Box 8.1), two of which (α and β) have no attendant nuclease activity and therefore no proof-reading ability. Polymerases α and β can generate more than 100 errors for every 1 million nucleotides incorporated. Fortunately, polymerases δ and ϵ have efficient exonuclease activities with good proof-reading functions, and the result is fewer than 20 errors per 1 million nucleotides. Even if the overall fidelity of base incorporation were 99.99%, then for a human genome of 10^9 base pairs there would be 10^5 misincorporated bases per cell at each round of DNA synthesis in the absence of additional repair processes. Given the other sources of damaged DNA, the experimental figure seems reasonable – 10^4 bases per cell being repaired.

Replication of repeated base sequences presents special problems for the machinery responsible for their synthesis. The DNA polymerase can 'slip' on runs of similar base sequences and either incorporate additional bases into the daughter strand or leave out bases from the template strand. In each case, the outcome is misaligned single-strand loops of unpaired bases. If the loop is on the template strand, then the daughter strand will contain a deletion; if the loop is on the daughter strand, then the daughter strand will contain an insertion.

Gene amplifications

In advanced cancers, large regions of DNA can be replicated several thousand-fold. Thus, the dihydrofolate reductase gene (see Chapter 12) can be amplified together with large adjacent stretches of DNA. This complex process involves formation of multiple abnormal replication forks during DNA synthesis.

Clinical evidence that links DNA repair and carcinogenesis

Several inherited conditions exist that link DNA repair defects to a high risk of cancer. They are listed in Table 8.3 and described in Chapter 8. People with these inherited diseases often present with an ill-assorted collection of symptoms; these diseases were originally called syndromes to hide our ignorance about their causes. Bloom's syndrome, ataxia telangiectasia and Franconi's syndrome have each been linked with increased risk of leukaemia and lymphoma. Xeroderma pigmentosa is associated with a 2000-fold increased risk of skin cancer. These conditions all result in chromosome fragility, and the molecular basis of the symptoms has been identified as inherited defects in genes coding for proteins that regulate DNA repair. Three other inherited conditions associated with DNA repair are linked with a different pattern of cancers, albeit at specific sites. People with Li–Fraumeni syndrome are at increased risk of bone cancers (sarcomas), breast cancers and brain cancers, whereas people who have HNPCC (Lynch's syndrome) exhibit a different pattern of cancers – colorectal, endometrial (uterus), ovary and stomach. Inheritance of mutations in the breast cancer genes *BRCA1* or *BRCA2* confers yet another pattern of increased breast, prostate, ovary or colorectal cancers (see Chapter 8). Compared with the general population, cancers appear at an earlier age in people with such defects. This fits with faster accumulation of errors because, having inherited the first mutation in a gene linked to DNA repair, other mutations will arise more rapidly. The defects are transferred to offspring through the germ cells (eggs or sperm), so all cells in the body carry the error; it is not clear, therefore, why cancer does not occur everywhere but occurs only at a limited number of specific sites, which can vary with the defect. The repair processes involved are common to all cells, which emphasises our ignorance about why the cell selectivity for cancer risk occurs. It might reflect repair efficiency or the number and type of damaging events to which the cell is subjected.

People with HNPCC have defective mismatch repair (see below), whereas people with Li–Fraumeni syndrome carry inactivating mutations in the *p53* gene. This gene is not an immediate component of DNA repair, but the p53 protein indirectly facilitates it. In normal cells, genotoxic damage such as ionising radiation increases the p53 content; this blocks proliferation and allows DNA repair to proceed. p53 also activates apoptosis, a suicide method of eliminating defective DNA (see Chapter 9). Defective p53 does not block proliferation and apoptosis, and so damage accumulates in daughter cells. The functions of the *BRCA* genes are not understood fully, but defective cells are sensitive to ionising radiation and genotoxic carcinogens; repair of strand breaks may be one of the normal actions of proteins from the *BRCA* genes (see Chapter 8).

Mutations in the retinoblastoma (*Rb*) tumour suppressor gene can also contribute to error accumulation. When one *Rb* allele has mutated, the chance of the second allele becoming defective is increased (see Chapter 8); when that occurs, the G_1 block to the cell cycle is relieved, thereby decreasing the time available for repair (see Chapter 9).

Repair mechanisms

With one exception (alkyl transferase), repair mechanisms use the principle of detection and excision of the damage followed by refilling the gaps. The main types of damage rectified by each of the following mechanisms are listed in Table 7.2.

Base excision repair

Basic excision repair is the primary way of removing nucleotides damaged by intra-cellular processes such as free-radical oxidations and deamination of cytosine and 5-methylcytosine. Base excision repair will also handle bases alkylated by exogenous agents such as nitrosamines. A family of *N*-glycosidases can hydrolyse the glycoside link between the N-9 of the purine base and deoxyribose, thereby releasing the damaged base and leaving an abasic site (**ap**urinic/**ap**yrimidinic, AP site) in the DNA chain (Figure 7.3). The deoxyribosephosphate chain is cleaved 5′ to the damaged base by an AP endonuclease and on the other side by exonuclease activity of DNA polymerase β. If an oxidised base is to be removed, then a four-nucleotide section is excised. The glycosidase responsible for excising 8-OH guanines is often deleted

Table 7.2 Repair mechanism and damage type.

Mechanism	Type of damage
Base excision repair	Abasic sites
	Free radical oxidations
	Deamination of cytosine/methylcytosine
	Alkylations
Base mismatch repair	Small adducts
	Free radical oxidations
	Insertions/deletions
Nucleotide excision repair	Large adducts
	UV cross-links
Exonuclease component of DNA polymerase	Code misinterpretation (proof-reading function)
Alkyl transferase	Small alkyl adducts
Homologous recombination	Strand breaks
DNA end-joining	Strand breaks

Figure 7.3

Base excision repair: general situation. In the specific case of removing an 8–OH guanine, this is accompanied by removal of three additional nucleotides 3′ to the damaged site.

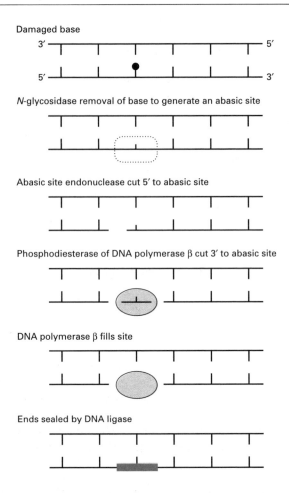

Damaged base

N-glycosidase removal of base to generate an abasic site

Abasic site endonuclease cut 5′ to abasic site

Phosphodiesterase of DNA polymerase β cut 3′ to abasic site

DNA polymerase β fills site

Ends sealed by DNA ligase

in lung cancers. DNA polymerase β fills the single-nucleotide gap with a nucleotide determined by the sequence of the other strand; DNA ligase seals the nucleotide into the DNA strand.

The *N*-glycosidases repair uracil substitutions better than they repair thymines, which means that methylated cytosines are potentially more mutagenic than the parent cytosine. The relevance of this to DNA methylation, differentiation and carcinogenesis is discussed in Chapter 9.

Alkyl transferase (ATase)

A second type of base repair removes bases with small adducts such as O^6-methylguanine produced by alkylating mutagens such as *N*-methylnitrosourea (see Figure 6.7). Although known as an enzymic mechanism, this is incorrect, since the methyl group transferred to a cysteine on the protein renders the protein inactive (Figure 7.4).

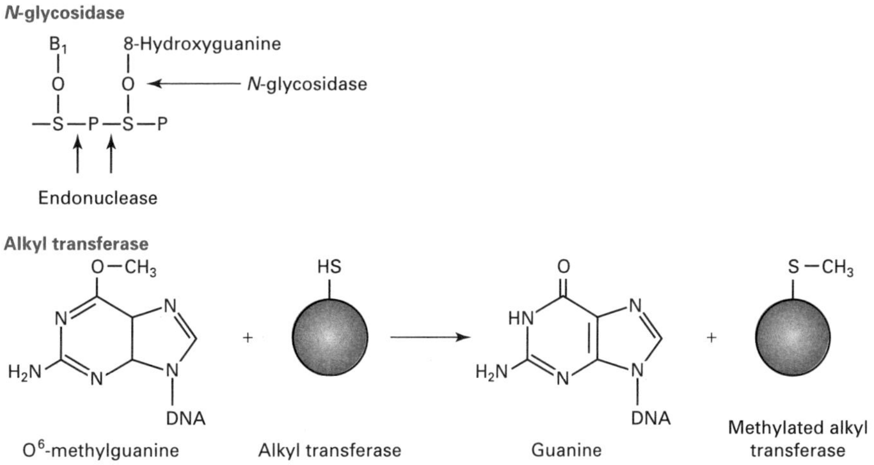
N-glycosidase
B1
8-Hydroxyguanine
O
O
N-glycosidase
—S—P—S—P
Endonuclease
Alkyl transferase
O−CH3
HS
O
S−CH3
N
N
H2N
N
N
DNA
HN
+
+
O6-methylguanine
Alkyl transferase
Guanine
Methylated alkyl transferase

Figure 7.4
Base excision repair.

Nucleotide excision repair

Compared with base excision, nucleotide excision has a different specificity: it can remove mismatches as well as UV-induced pyrimidine dimers (see Figure 6.11) and bulky adducts such as polycyclic aromatic hydrocarbons (see Figure 6.4) and aflatoxin. In fact, it is the only method of removing bulky DNA adducts (see Table 7.2).

The process is complex, involving proteins capable of recognising damaged regions and removing the defective segment. The remaining single-stranded unaffected section is then used as a template to fill in the gap (Figure 7.5). All of this takes time, and so proliferation is stopped by p53-mediated processes to allow repair to occur (see below). Interestingly, the repair mechanism uses the protein TFII, more usually associated with mRNA synthesis; thus, the damaged cell can divert other functions to achieve repair.

The processes involved have largely been identified with cells obtained from people with xeroderma pigmentosum or related disorders such as Cockayne's syndrome (Figure 7.5). The presenting symptoms are due to hypersensitivity of skin to light, but affected individuals also have a high probability of developing leukaemias and lymphomas. Xeroderma pigmentosum is a family of disorders in which one or more of the 20–30 proteins needed for nucleotide excision repair are defective. About 80% of people with xeroderma pigmentosum have defects in at least one of seven proteins, labelled XPA to XPG, needed in the early stages of repair. Recognition and melting of the double-stranded damaged region is initiated by the DNA-binding proteins XPA and XPC.

XPA is a DNA-binding protein that reacts with a second protein RPA (**r**eplication **p**rotein **A**); RPA interacts with single-stranded DNA. XPC is then recruited to the damaged site. The small region of single-stranded DNA is then enlarged by the **t**ranscription **f**actor **IIH** (TF-IIH) complex of six to nine proteins that includes XPB and XPD. The latter proteins unwind the DNA helix (helicase activity) to

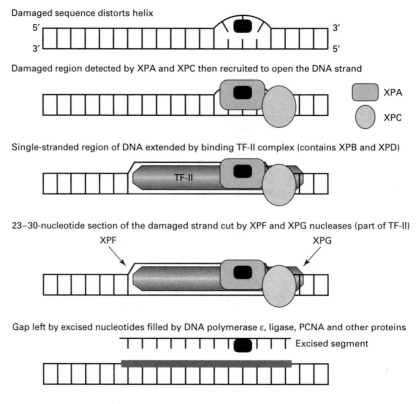

Figure 7.5

Nucleotide–excision repair.

generate the open region spanning 23–30 nucleotides. As the name implies, TF-IIH is also needed for gene transcription. This interrelationship between two important cell functions – repair and gene transcription – has beneficial functional relevance in that genes being transcribed at the time of damage are more likely to have rapid adverse effects on cell function. It is therefore helpful that actively transcribed genes are repaired rapidly, because the damage blocks RNA polymerase function and repair is facilitated by having TF-IIH already present at the site of damage. The single strand of damaged DNA is then excised by the endonuclease activities of XPF and XPG. Full nuclease activity of XPF requires the **e**xcision **r**epair **c**ontrol **c**omponent (ERCC1) protein. XPE participates with TF-IIH in repairing UV damage. The gap left by the excised nucleotides is then filled by a combination of DNA polymerase δ and/or ε, DNA ligase, **p**roliferation **c**ontrol **n**uclear **a**ntigen (PCNA) and other proteins.

The remaining 20% of people with xeroderma pigmentosum have normal XPA–XPG proteins but have variants (XPV) defective in later stages, possibly due to an abnormal DNA polymerase subunit.

Mismatch repair

The repair processes described thus far are capable of repairing either DNA strand. If a mismatched base is incorporated into a newly synthesised daughter strand, it

Figure 7.6

Mismatch repair. Symbols with graduated tints indicate proteins altered in cancers.

Mismatched bases recognised by MSH6 (or MSH3). MSH2 heterodimer PMS1 and MLH1 then bind

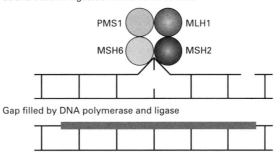

Strand cut and digested with an exonuclease

Gap filled by DNA polymerase and ligase

can be repaired by mismatch repair (Figure 7.6). This is called post-replication repair. It can cope with a broad spectrum of small damage types. Misincorporated bases, alkyl adducts, small insertions or deletions, and oxidations can be repaired, but bulky adducts and UV cross-linked pyrimidines (Table 7.2) cannot. The mismatched bases are recognised by a multiprotein complex, short regions of DNA sequence digested from the newly synthesised strand, and the gap filled by DNA polymerase δ and ligase. Recognition of the incorrect base(s) requires four proteins, two of which (MSH2, MLH1) cause HNPCC (see Chapter 8) and are also altered in some sporadic cancers; PMS1 may even be a third. It is not known how strand specificity is achieved, but initial recognition of the damage is by binding of an MSH2.MSH6 (or MSH3) protein heterodimer. MSH6 was called GT-binding protein because it has selectivity for guanine : thymine mismatches. MSH6 is preferentially recruited to single-base errors and MSH3 to those involving two to four bases, but there is overlap of activities. PMS1 and MLH1 bind to the MSH2.MSH6 dimer, and repair is effected by exonuclease cleavage and digestion of a limited number of nucleotides followed by gap-filling with DNA polymerase and ligase. PCNA, which plays a coordinating role in DNA synthesis (see Box 9.1), interacts with MLH1.PMS1 heterodimers, thus providing a link with the machinery needed to fill the excised gap.

HNPCC is an autosomal recessive condition in which both alleles of the affected gene must be inactivated. Normal cells from a person with HNPCC have a mismatch repair function 100 times better than cancer cells from the same person. A single normal allele in an affected individual can result in effective mismatch repair; but when that normal allele is lost by somatic mutation, the repair mechanism is lost. This example of the two-hit model of carcinogenesis also provides evidence of a causal association between defective DNA repair and increased cancer risk. Over

40 different mutations have been identified in *MLH1* and *MSH2*; only a single family has been identified with a *PMS1* defect; and no *MSH6* or *MSH3* mutations have been detected. In most cases, the mutations result in truncated proteins or inactivating amino acid substitutions.

Microsatellite instability

The multiple two- to four-base-pair repeats in microsatellites are subject to mis-alignment during replication (see above). In normal cells, they are repaired by mismatch repair. Thus, defective mismatch repair increases the length of microsatellite sequences (microsatellite instability), which can be detected by gel electrophoresis. Microsatellite instability is a surrogate marker for defective mismatch repair; it is sometimes known as the **r**eplication **e**rror **r**epair (RER) phenotype.

DNA strand breaks

Both single- and double-strand breaks occur as a consequence of ionising radiation and bulky adduct distortions of the DNA helix. If not repaired, the open-ended broken strands form promiscuous liaisons with inappropriate strands, which leads to chromosome abnormalities. Double-stranded breaks are particularly difficult for the cell to handle, but they can be repaired either by homologous recombination with the undamaged second chromosome (see Box 8.1) or by DNA end-joining of the broken strands.

Homologous recombination

Diploid cells contain two double helices of DNA (sister chromatids). A double-strand break occurs in only one helix, leaving the sister helix intact. Homologous recombination requires extensive regions of base homology on the undamaged helix to provide a template for repair (Figure 7.7). 5′-3′ exonucleases digest damaged strands to expose single-stranded regions either side of the break. A complex series of proteins (RAD proteins) promote the sensing of homologies between single-stranded damaged DNA and homologous bases in the same region of the undamaged helix; resynthesis of the excised sequences is then determined by the base sequence of the undamaged strand of the sister helix. The functions of the RAD proteins are unclear, but RAD51 polymerises on to the single-stranded DNA and searches for the homologous sequence on the undamaged helix. The other RAD proteins plus the single-stranded DNA-binding protein RPA facilitate cross-over between the strands (strand exchange). DNA polymerase, ligases and accessory proteins synthesise and ligate the four strands to reform two helices. RAD51 will also interact with p53, BRCA1 and BRCA2 proteins, providing a mechanistic link with proteins known to be involved in DNA repair. Cells deficient in any of these proteins are sensitive to agents such as ionising radiation that generate double-strand breaks and chromosome abnormalities (see Chapter 8). There may be a role for the enzyme **p**oly(**A**DP-**r**ibose) **p**olymerase (PARP) in repair of strand breaks. PARP is recruited to the breaks and undergoes an autocatalytic modification by synthesis of poly(ADP-ribose). This plays an undefined indirect role in repair.

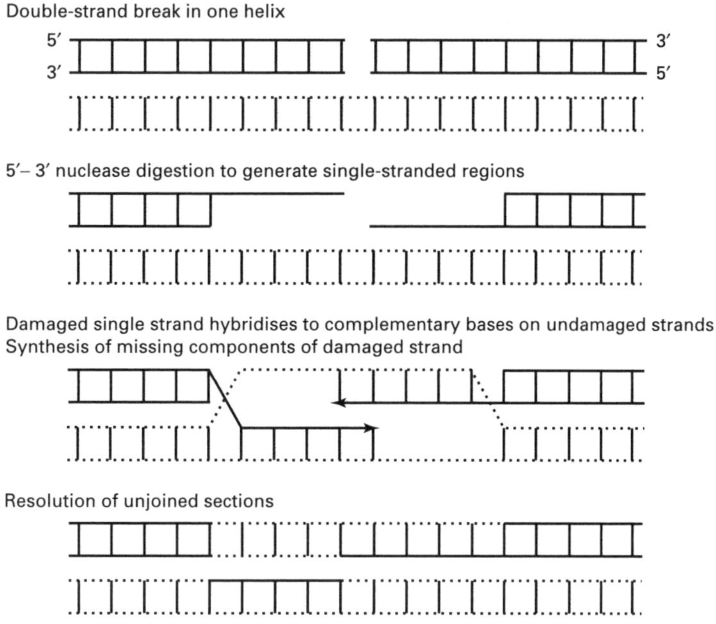

Figure 7.7

Repair of DNA double-strand breaks by homologous recombination.

Double-strand break in one helix

5′–3′ nuclease digestion to generate single-stranded regions

Damaged single strand hybridises to complementary bases on undamaged strands
Synthesis of missing components of damaged strand

Resolution of unjoined sections

DNA end-joining

This needs only limited homologies to rejoin juxtaposed ends of broken strands; only the damaged helix is involved (Figure 7.8). Damaged strand ends are detected by protein heterodimers (KU70 plus XRCC5), which then recruit a **DNA**-dependent serine **p**rotein **k**inase (DNAPK). Additional proteins are incorporated into the complex, phosphorylated by DNAPK and rejoin the broken strands. The *ATM* gene, defective in ataxia telangiectasia, also influences strand repair and other types of repair, although the mechanism is unclear. The ATM protein is a protein kinase that is vaguely said to regulate a signalling cascade responsive to DNA damage. It is activated by certain types of damage and is involved in p53 activation (see below).

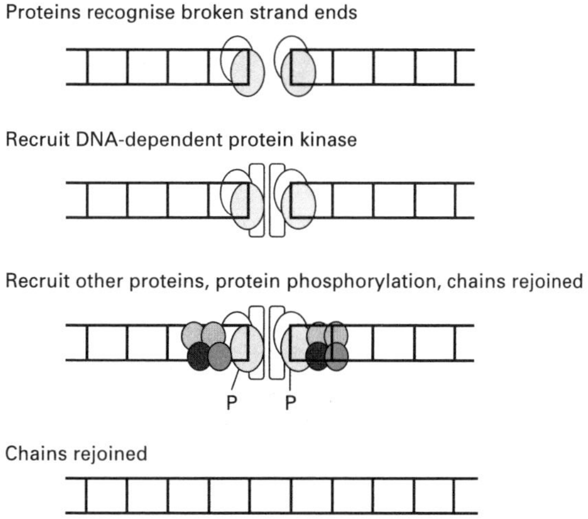

Figure 7.8

Repair of DNA double-strand break by DNA end-joining.

Proteins recognise broken strand ends

Recruit DNA-dependent protein kinase

Recruit other proteins, protein phosphorylation, chains rejoined

Chains rejoined

Coordination of DNA repair, proliferation and apoptosis

DNA repair, proliferation and apoptosis work in a coordinated fashion to ensure that damaged DNA does not adversely affect cell function. Damage inhibits proliferation; if the damage is too great to be repaired, then the cell 'commits suicide' by apoptosis. DNA damage activates the p53 suppressor protein that plays a major role in coordinating these functions; it warrants the title of 'guardian of the genome'. Different types of damage activate p53 by different pathways (Figure 7.9), although post-transcriptional methods are used in each situation; protein synthesis is not required. Mechanistic details are sparse. Ionising radiation activates both DNAPK and ATM kinases, and ATM-deficient cells exhibit only a slow response to such radiation. The N-terminal phosphorylation sites of p53 are involved, but it is not clear whether there are direct or indirect interactions between the components shown in Figure 7.9. UV light-induced damage affects both N- and C-terminal domains of p53, although current details are confusing. The N-terminal phosphorylations generated by UV light are independent of ATM kinase, although the C-terminal changes require this enzyme. However, some of the C-terminal changes activated by UV light may eventually be mediated by a protein phosphatase that removes an inhibitory serine phosphate besides activating phosphorylations at other sites. Chapters 5 and 9 describe events downstream of p53 activation.

In normal cells, transient expression of p53 enables it to fulfil multiple functions primarily, but not exclusively, through its role as a transcription factor. It increases transcription from genes involved in the inhibition of DNA replication (*p21*, *Gadd45*) but has opposing effects on *BAX* and *Bcl2*, the two genes that regulate apoptosis. There is increased expression of the pro-apoptotic *BAX* and inhibition of

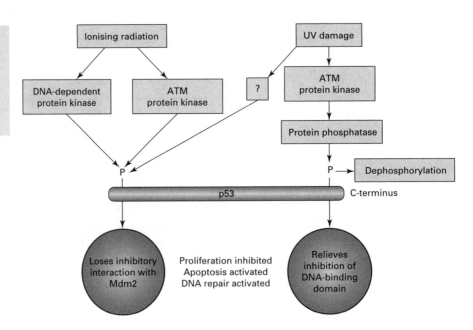

Figure 7.9

Activation of p53 by DNA damage. UV damage also results in C-terminal phosphorylation (not shown).

the anti-apoptotic *Bcl2*. This alteration in *BAX* : *Bcl2* ratio relieves a block in the apoptosis pathway. The net result is blocked proliferation, which enables repair to proceed, and increased apoptosis, which eliminates cells with damaged DNA.

The p21 protein is an inhibitor of the cyclin-dependent kinases that are essential for progression through the cell cycle (see Chapter 9). It also binds to PCNA, part of the active DNA polymerase complex required for both synthesis and repair. The p21–PCNA interaction inhibits DNA synthesis but not repair functions; this achieves coordinate inhibition of synthesis while allowing repair to proceed. p53 also facilitates repair by binding to two of the XP proteins (D and B).

Bcl2 inhibits apoptosis, whereas BAX stimulates it, so in normal cells a p53-mediated block of *Bcl2* and stimulation of *BAX* gene transcription synergistically promotes apoptosis. Mutated *p53* has none of these functions, and so proliferation continues in the absence of apoptosis and mutations are passed on to daughter cells.

Inactivation of *p53* in cancer cells can be achieved by mutation of the gene or by interaction with other proteins (see Chapter 5). The overall effect of such inactivation is loss of growth control and decreased repair of DNA damage. The biological effectiveness of this process is illustrated by the fact that cultured cells from people with Li–Fraumeni syndrome are genetically unstable and are more sensitive to DNA-damaging agents than their normal counterparts. It is not known how p53 senses the damage, but p53 inactivation favours genetic instability. There may be an autocatalytic loop operative such that codons in the *p53* gene that are important for normal function of the protein are repaired only slowly. Therefore, mutations in these codons are more likely to escape repair and decrease the efficiency of subsequent repair processes.

Further reading

Benhamou, S., and Sarasin, A. (2000) Variability in nucleotide excision repair and cancer risk: a review. *Mutat Res* **462**, 149–158.

De Boer, J., and Hoeijmakers, J.H. (2000) Nucleotide excision repair and human syndromes. *Carcinogenesis* **21**, 453–460.

Evan, G.I. and Vousden, K.H. (2001) Proliferation, cell cycle and apoptosis in cancer. *Nature* **411**, 342–348.

Hoeijmakers, J.H. (2001) Genome maintenance mechanisms for preventing cancer. *Nature* **411**, 342–348.

Pedroni, M., Sala, E., Scarselli, A., *et al.* (2001) Microsatelite instability and mismatch-repair expression in hereditary and sporadic colorectal carcinogenesis. *Cancer Res* **61**, 896–899.

Pierce, A.J., Stark, J.M., Araujo, F.D., *et al.* (2001) Double-strand breaks and tumourigenesis. *Trends Cell Biol* **11**, S52–S59.

Poirier, M.C. (2004) Chemical-induced DNA damage and human cancer risk. *Nat Rev Cancer* **4**, 630–637.

Simpson, A.J.G. (1997) The natural somatic mutation frequency and human carcinogenesis. *Adv Cancer Res* **71**, 209–240.

Venkitaraman, A.R. (2002) Cancer susceptibility and the functions of BRCA1 and BRCA2. *Cell* **108**, 171–182.

8 Familial cancers

KEY POINTS

- Mutations inherited through germ cells contribute to a minority of cancers.
- At least two rate-limiting changes (hits) are required for tumour development. If the first hit is inherited through a germ cell, then the cancer occurs earlier than if generated in a somatic cell.
- Germline mutations occur in suppressor genes that can act in a recessive or dominant-negative way.
- Sporadic cancers often acquire mutations in the same genes as inherited cancers. In such situations, data from familial cancers have relevance to sporadic cancers. This is not universally true.
- Dissimilar germline mutations in one cell type can have a common end result: a cancer.
- Within one gene, germline mutations occur at different loci in different families.
- Germline mutations generate cancers only in selected cell types and in a limited number of cells of a common type.
- Defective DNA repair results in increased cancer risk.

Introduction

Three categories of cancer can be defined according to the degree to which inherited features are involved (Table 8.1). The great majority of cancers are of the sporadic type with no evidence of inherited links in cancer incidence within members of a family. These arise by mutations in somatic cells. However, a small percentage of the common cancers arise because of inherited defects, and a high proportion of rare cancers can result from inherited mutations. The inherited defects are passed from parents to offspring via the egg or sperm. These germline mutations are confined to tumour suppressor genes. The probability of inheriting the same rare defect from both parents is very low, and so the offspring from one affected parent are heterozygous, carrying one defective allele and one normal allele. The germline mutations are in genes coding for suppressor proteins, and so usually both alleles must

Table 8.1 Categories of cancer.

Familial involvement	Percentage of all cancers	Examples
None (sporadic)	> 90	All types of cancer
Involved	5–10	Colorectal, breast
Well-defined	0.1	Retinoblastoma, Wilms' (kidney)

be inactivated before an effect is seen (see Chapter 5). Hence, the one normal allele inherited from the unaffected parent must also be inactivated by a somatic cell mutation. The somatic cell mutation is usually different from the type present in the germ cells, although the gene and end effect are common.

Despite the rarity of familial cancers, genetic information obtained from their study is relevant to sporadic cancers. Thus, the *Rb* tumour suppressor gene was first identified by its absence in familial retinoblastoma and is now known to be a negative regulator of proliferation in many cell types (see Chapter 9) and *Rb* mutations occur in several sporadic cancers. Likewise, the inherited mutation in the **a**denomatous **p**olyposis **c**oli (*APC*) gene is involved in both familial and sporadic forms of colorectal cancer (see Chapter 2), but such generalisations cannot be taken too far. The germline mutation in genes linked to familial **br**east **c**ancer (*BRCA1* and *BRCA2*) genes is unaffected in sporadic cases. Before examining these points, consider some of the terms used to describe chromosome details (Box 8.1).

Box 8.1	**Chromosome nomenclature and structure**

The normal diploid human genome is composed of two copies of each of 22 *autosomal* chromosomes plus two sex chromosomes, X and Y (male) or X and X (female). Chromosomes are numbered in descending order of size. Each chromosome has a short arm (p) and a long arm (q) either side of the *centromere*, which is the point of attachment of mitotic spindles (Figure 8.1). These tubulin-containing spindles retract the chromosomes into daughter cells

Figure 8.1

Chromosome structure.

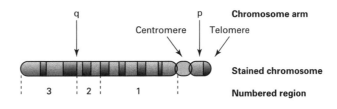

129

at mitosis. Each chromosome has a characteristic staining pattern that is used to divide a chromosome arm into numbered regions; for example, the *Rb* gene on the long arm of chromosome 13 at position 14 is defined as having location 13q14. There is one copy (allele) of each gene per chromosome. Diploid cells have two alleles of each gene and are termed *homozygous*. When one allele is lost and the other is unaffected, the cell is *heterozygous* for that allele. If the second normal allele is lost, there is *loss of heterozygosity* (LOH). This is illustrated in Table 8.2. At the end of each chromosome is a *telomere* made up of a large number of *tandem* (head-to-tail) TTAGGG repeats. These tandem repeats play an important role in determining the lifespan of cells (see Chapter 9). The number, size and shape of a cell's chromosome complement define its *karyotype*.

One DNA double helix extends the length of the chromosome and is condensed into coils and supercoils; the lowest common denominator is the *nucleosome*, in which 200 **b**ase **p**airs (bp) of DNA are wound around a histone protein core. The internucleosome bridges of DNA are sites of DNAase digestion during apoptosis (see Chapter 9). Other proteins and RNAs are wrapped around the nucleosomes to form *chromatin*, sometimes called *interphase chromatin* in non-mitotic cells. At mitosis, the chromatin rearranges into chromosomes. Interphase chromatin is attached to a cytoskeleton, the *nuclear matrix*. About 3% of human DNA base sequences code for proteins; the other 97% have complex regulatory and other poorly defined roles. One type of

Table 8.2 Retinoblastoma characteristics.

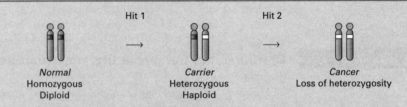

Two forms: one (unilateral) or both (bilateral) eyes affected
Unilateral cancer: acquired both hits; sporadic form
Bilateral cancer: inherited first hit (germline); acquired second hit (somatic cell)

Familial form: up to ten cancers per eye, each with a different mutation; clonal origin

Low probability of first hit, high probability of second hit; first hit generates genetic instability

Chromosome 13q14, *Rb* tumour suppressor gene 30 kb, coding region 3 kb
Deletions common, mutations less frequent
Mutations of the second allele can be of a different type from mutations of the first allele
Rb gene produces a 110 kDa serine/threonine phosphoprotein that inhibits the cell cycle

non-coding sequence, *microsatellite DNA*, consists of tandem 2–4 bp repeats, and their length can increase if DNA mismatch repair is defective (see Chapter 7); this is called *microsatellite instability*.

The sequence of bases in DNA can be altered in several ways, collectively known as *mutations*. Not all mutations have functional significance for the cell. Non-significant mutations are called *silent mutations* or *neutral mutations*. Chromosome *translocations* occur commonly in cancers, especially leukaemias. *Heterologous* or *non-homologous recombination* involves exchanging segments of one chromosome with segments from a different chromosome. *Homologous recombination* between similar regions of two identical chromosomes is used to repair DNA strand breaks. Chronic myeloid leukaemia is characterised by a reciprocal translocation between chromosomes 22 and 9 (see Chapter 2) and is defined as having a t(9;22)(q34,q11) karyotype; the first set of parentheses contains the chromosome numbers and the second set contains the breakpoints. The **t** indicates a translocation; **del** indicates a deletion and **inv** an inversion. Sometimes, DNA deletions and inversions are large enough to be detected by *cytogenetic* methods (chromosome staining). *Nonsense* and *frame-shift mutations* involve base changes that alter the coding sequence to a non-coding sequence and prematurely terminate transcription; *truncated proteins* are then produced. This can occur with *Rb* in retinoblastoma. Single *base substitutions* can result in the gene coding for a different amino acid (point mutations); this new amino acid may then alter the function of the overall protein. In colorectal cancer, a guanine-to-adenine mutation in the *ras* oncogene leads to replacement of the normal glycine by aspartate and permanent activation of the ras protein (see Figure 5.6). Not all base changes have adverse effects. *Polymorphisms* are neutral variations in base sequences between individuals and have little effect on function. At a cleavage site for a restriction enzyme, polymorphisms alter the digestion pattern; this forms the basis of *restriction fragment length polymorphism* (RFLP) analysis for detecting mutations. RFLP changes also can be generated by any of the mutation types just described. Other relevant definitions are given in Box 9.1.

Strong familial link

Rare cancers that occur in childhood with high frequency in affected families are due to the inactivation of both alleles of key tumour suppressor genes. In Chapter 2, the tendency for common cancers to occur in older people was explained as being due to the time taken to accumulate the several genetic changes required for cancer formation. It follows that a cancer occurring in children indicates fewer changes. This is true for retinoblastoma (eye), the incidence of which can be explained by a two-hit model in which each allele is inactivated independently. Another, less well characterised, more complex familial example is Wilms' tumour (kidney).

Retinoblastoma

Retinoblastoma occurs in unilateral and bilateral forms, with the bilateral form appearing in younger children. Over 90% of bilateral cases are diagnosed before the age of 2 years, whereas the same point is reached by age 4 years with unilateral cancers. Children with bilateral cancers have a familial connection with retinoblastoma, whereas the unilateral cases do not. These differences are explained by the number of mutations (hits) required to generate a cancer. Two hits are needed for both types of retinoblastoma, but the first one is inherited in bilateral cases and acquired in unilateral cases (Table 8.2). The familial form is also characterised by having up to ten individual cancers in each eye, each with a different type of second *Rb* mutation. This indicates that each cancer arose independently and provides evidence of the clonal origins of these cancers. With germline mutations, all cells in the body contain the first hit, which raises questions as to why many more cancers do not appear in such individuals given that *Rb* is so important in regulating proliferation of all cells (see Chapter 9). The retina contains about 10^8 retinoblasts, but even a severely affected child has fewer than ten tumours; therefore, some unknown inhibitory influences must be operative. The same applies to other cell types. People with familial retinoblastoma are at increased risk of developing bone cancers but not other types of cancer. On the other hand, once the first *Rb* allele has been inactivated, there is a high probability of the second deletion occurring in the other copy. With 10^8 target cells, each with 10^9 nucleotide bases, random hits at a specific locus are extremely improbable. The first hit must generate genetic instability so as to increase the probability of generating the second event. This has been described as the creation of a mutator phenotype. How this is achieved is unclear, but disruption of the balance between DNA synthesis, repair and cell death may be involved (see Chapter 9).

A normal individual has cells with two *Rb* alleles (homozygous), whereas a carrier has only one copy (heterozygous) (see Table 8.2). Loss of the remaining allele returns the cell to a homozygous state, albeit a different state than for a normal individual. If retinoblastoma cells are compared with normal cells from a carrier of the germline mutation, then the retinoblastoma cells have no copies of the *Rb* gene whereas the normal cells have one copy each. This provides convincing evidence that the cancer is due to loss of the second allele.

Rb was localised to chromosome 13q14 by means of karyotypic markers. Familial retinoblastoma cells were compared with normal cells from the same individual and were found to have lost a number of markers from region 13q14 including the *esterase D* gene. Three separate retinoblastoma families were identified, each with a different chromosome 13q14 deletion. Two of the families had additionally lost the esterase gene whereas the third had not, thereby allowing precise localisation of *Rb*.

In normal cells, *Rb* codes for a phosphoprotein that inhibits proliferation at the G_1/S boundary of the cell cycle by binding to the transcription factor E2F (see Chapter 9).

Rb alterations have been detected in other, non-familial cancers such as those of bone, breast, lung and bladder. Thus, identification of the *Rb* tumour suppressor gene through a rare familial cancer has provided important clues about other cancers.

Wilms' tumour

This kidney tumour is the commonest abdominal tumour in children and exhibits some genetic similarities with retinoblastoma. It occurs in familial and sporadic forms, it is inherited as an autosomal trait, and two hits are required for tumour formation. Furthermore, the sporadic form affects only one kidney, whereas the inherited defect has bilateral effects. However, several forms of inherited defect have been identified, with most information being available about the **W**ilms' **t**umour (*WT1*) gene on chromosome 11p13. This gene codes for a 49 kDa DNA-binding transcription factor that is expressed only in cells of the kidney and possibly the gonads, which contrasts with the widespread distribution of *Rb*. Another difference from retinoblastoma is that the *WT1* gene can act in a dominant-negative way similar to that observed with *p53* (see Chapter 5), so that both alleles need not be deleted. Genes influenced by WT1 include those for cytokines such as **i**nsulin-like **g**rowth **f**actor **II** (*IGF-II*), **e**pidermal **g**rowth **f**actor (*EGF*) and **p**latelet-**d**erived **g**rowth **f**actor (*PDGF*); cytokine receptors for IGF-I and transforming growth factor β; and other functions such as apoptosis (*Bcl2*). WT1 inhibits expression of both IGF-II and the IGF-I receptor through which that cytokine works (see Chapter 10), which is one route through which WT1 could suppress growth.

Weaker familial link

Most cancers in this category involve genes that are implicated directly in the carcinogenic process, although some function indirectly through processes such as immune response and metabolic defects.

There are families whose members have an elevated risk of developing one of several different types of tumour. In one example, a mother who eventually died of liver cancer had 12 children, nine of whom developed cancers or preneoplastic lesions of the breast (six cases), cervix (two cases) and bladder (one case). Although increased risk may relate predominantly to one cell type, other cell types can be affected. This is not surprising if the gene in question regulates a pathway common to many cell types, such as cell proliferation or transduction of signal from outside the cell to the nucleus, but it is important not to take too simplistic a view of a complex phenomenon. Thus, p53 is a regulator of cell proliferation, but knocking out both alleles in all cells of a mouse generates abnormalities in only a limited range of cell types, and a similar cell-specific phenomenon is associated with Rb loss in humans (see above).

Conversely, it is clear that different genes contribute to formation of the same cancer (Table 8.3), implying that disruption of alternative pathways can generate the same apparent end result. The word 'apparent' is used because it has long been a view in clinical circles that a specific cancer, e.g. breast cancer, is really a collection of diseases with some common features.

Several familial conditions are known that carry an increased risk of getting specific multiple cancers. Many such cancers have the same morphological classification as sporadic cases, although their natural histories may be different. Thus, familial forms

Table 8.3 Inherited cancer syndromes caused by a single genetic defect.

Condition	Gene	Chromosome	Cancer*	Function
Retinoblastoma	*Rb*	13q	Eye	Proliferation control
Wilms' tumour	*WT1*	11p	Kidney	Transcription
Familial adenomatous polyposis coli	*APC*	5q	Colon	Cell recognition
Hereditary non-polyposis colon cancer	*MSH2*	2p ⎫	Colon	DNA mismatch repair
	MLH1	3p ⎭		
Familial breast cancer	*BRCA1*	17q	Breast ⎫	DNA repair
	BRCA2	13q	Breast (male and female) ⎭	Transcription?
Li–Fraumeni syndrome	*p53*	17p	Breast	Transcription
Neurofibromatosis 1	*NF1*	17q	Neurosarcoma	Signal transduction
Multiple endocrine neoplasia type 1	*MEN1*	11q	Parathyroid, pancreas, anterior pituitary	?
Familial melanoma	*INK4A*	9p	Skin	Proliferation control
Xeroderma pigmentosum	*XP(A–D)*	Several	Skin	DNA excision repair
Ataxia telangiectasia	*AT*	11q	Leukaemia, lymphoma	DNA repair
Bloom's syndrome	*BLM*	15q	Leukaemia, lymphoma	DNA repair
Drug metabolism	*CYP2D6*		Lung	Drug metabolism

* Not all listed here; see Table 8.5.

of breast cancer and colorectal cancer occur at earlier ages than their sporadic counterparts as anticipated from the acquisition of one of the required mutations through the germ cells.

The multiple endocrine neoplasias and neurofibromatosis are poorly understood but others listed in Table 8.3 are informative.

Colorectal cancer

This is a good example of the multiple routes to cancer formation because more than three inherited defects have been identified in different families in addition to the sporadic cases. Their natural history is detailed in Chapter 2, but some of the points relevant to this chapter will be repeated here.

People with **f**amilial **a**denomatous **p**olyposis **c**oli (FAP) inherit a defective *APC* tumour suppressor gene that results in multiple benign polyps within which cancers develop. The *APC* gene codes for a protein that mediates intracellular signalling pathways from contacts with other cells (see Chapter 10). A second familial type of colon cancer is **h**ereditary **n**on-**p**olyposis **c**olon **c**ancer (HNPCC, Lynch's syndrome), in which polyp formation is not observed. Three subgroups of HNPCC have been identified depending on whether they have germline mutations in the *MSH2* gene, the *MLH1* gene or neither. The majority of people with HNPCC have inherited mutations in the *MSH2* gene, with smaller numbers in the *MLH1* and other genes. The genes involved code for nuclear proteins directly required to repair mismatched bases in the DNA double helix (see Chapter 7). Different genetic disorders such as

Gardner's syndrome, Peutz–Jeghers syndrome and flat-cell adenoma syndromes of unknown cause also increase the risk of developing colorectal cancer.

Breast cancer

Two main variants and several minor variants have been shown to increase risk. The important ones, familial breast cancer and Li–Fraumeni syndrome, make up less than 5% of all breast cancers.

Familial breast cancer

Familial breast cancer is characterised by early age of onset and greater than 80% probability of developing breast cancer. This compares with the 10% lifetime risk of developing sporadic breast cancer. Two genes, **br**east **ca**ncer **1** and **2** (*BRCA1* and *BRCA2*) are the inherited culprits. Inheritance of either gene also confers an increased risk of developing cancer at other sites, which differ according to the gene concerned (see Table 8.5 below). The function of both alleles is lost in cancers, indicating that *BRCA1* and *BRCA2* are tumour suppressor genes.

Whereas the *APC* gene advertises its presence by the many polyps and associated symptoms, the familial breast cancer genes generate no such phenotypic traits. *BRCA1* was identified by detailed screening of DNA samples from different breast-cancer families to identify the region common to each family. Figure 8.2 shows the pedigree of one such family, in which both daughters and four of five granddaughters developed breast cancer. Epidemiological evidence has shown a two- to three-fold increased risk of developing breast cancer if a mother or a sister has the disease; this can increase to ten-fold if several of the first-degree relatives are affected. *BRCA1* is autosomal and can therefore be inherited from either mother or father; note that one male descendant in the above example developed breast cancer.

The proteins encoded by *BRCA1* and *BRCA2* are involved in DNA repair. The BRCA1 protein binds preferentially to branched DNA and may function in homologous recombination by colocalisation with other DNA repair factors at sites of double-strand breaks through direct interaction with RAD50. Many different mutations have been found in families carrying *BRCA1* mutations, the majority being deletions, insertions, nonsense mutations and splice variations, which result in a

Figure 8.2

Inheritance of the *BRCA1* gene in one family. Solid symbols indicate people with breast cancer.

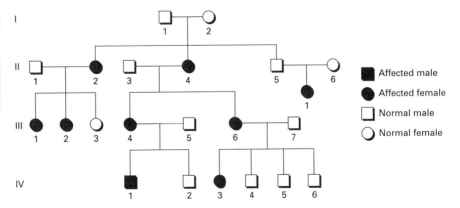

truncated protein being synthesised. In experimental systems, complete deletion of the *BRCA1* gene is lethal, whereas incomplete loss resulting in the production of a protein truncated at the C-terminal end is not. The truncated protein can support some development, albeit of an abnormal type. This suggests that different regions of the protein serve different functions. Ashkenazi Jewish families have a high incidence of specific point mutations in *BRCA1* and *BRCA2*. The close associations within this community have ensured that the initial mutation has remained common within the population.

The BRCA2 protein binds to single-stranded DNA and stimulates a RAD51-mediated reaction (see Chapter 7).

BRCA1 is expressed in many normal cells such as testis, breast and ovary, and in cell culture the expression is increased in the G_1 phase of the cell cycle by proliferative stimuli such as growth factors and the female hormone oestradiol. This is important given the stimulatory role of oestradiol in the genesis of breast cancer (see Chapter 4), but the hormonal effect is indirect because the *BRCA1* gene does not have a response element for the oestradiol receptor. Furthermore, *BRCA1* expression can be elevated by mitogens in oestradiol-insensitive cells. It is not clear why increased expression of the BRCA1 suppressor protein results in increased rather than decreased proliferation. One explanation for this anomaly is that BRCA1 is not part of the DNA synthesis/mitosis pathway but regulates other processes, such as DNA repair, associated with faithful replication of the DNA. Increased BRCA1 expression in normal cells would facilitate repair, whereas loss would enhance damage accumulation. The decreased BRCA1 expression accompanying the transition from *in situ* to invasive breast carcinoma would fit with this hypothesis, as would the observation that *BRCA2* mutations disrupt DNA repair but do not affect cell proliferation or apoptosis.

BRCA2 has been identified on a different chromosome to that of *BRCA1*. Loss of *BRCA2* confers a modest increase in the risk of ovarian cancer plus an increased risk of breast cancer in men and women.

Li–Fraumeni syndrome

This disorder is due to germline mutations in the *p53* gene, resulting in breast cancers and sarcomas but not other cancer types. The functions of p53 are described fully in Chapters 5 and 9, but its universal involvement in normal pathways of proliferation and death raises the question of why its loss results in so few cancers. We do not know the answer to this question; nor do we understand why an inherited *Rb* mutation results quickly in eye cancers whereas *p53* mutations take much longer to develop. Familial eye cancers arise within 2 years of birth whereas Li–Fraumeni breast cancers take at least 20 years to appear.

The pattern of *p53* mutations in Li–Fraumeni cells is different from the pattern seen in somatic cells (see Figure 4.6).

DNA repair defects

DNA is subject to daily insults that require efficient repair mechanisms for their correction. Damaging agents include cosmic radiation, free radicals, UV light and a variety of chemicals (see Chapter 6). There are familial conditions in which repair is defective and which are linked to increased cancer risk (see Table 8.3). The HNPCC condition (see above) is in this category. Xeroderma pigmentosum is a complex condition caused by loss of a DNA-binding protein that identifies damaged regions of DNA before excision repair (see Chapter 7). Affected people have a 1000-fold greater risk of getting skin cancer when young, due to increased sensitivity to sunlight. Individuals with Bloom's syndrome and ataxia telangiectasia also have defective repair mechanisms, Bloom's patients because of DNA ligase deficiency and ataxia patients because of defective damage surveillance. The ataxia gene codes for a protein kinase involved in DNA repair (see Chapter 7). The net result of these mutations is increased genomic instability and elevated error accumulation. Leukaemias and lymphomas arise most commonly in such people, but skin cancer can also be a problem in individuals exposed to sunlight.

Gene–environment interaction

People with deficiency in the P450 enzymes CYPD26 and CYP2A6, which are involved in the metabolism of nicotine, smoke fewer cigarettes and can give up smoking more easily than people with the normal version of these enzymes. It follows that polymorphism of these genes might affect the behaviour of individuals relative to smoking and, thus, with cancer.

Connection with sporadic cancers

Mutations in the *Rb* gene are responsible for both familial and sporadic forms of retinoblastoma. The same is true for *APC* in colorectal cancer, but for other examples the picture is more complex (Table 8.4). The inherited HNPCC defects are found only in some sporadic colorectal cancers, whereas mutations in the *BRCA* genes are not seen in sporadic cancers. These examples reinforce the point about the existence of multiple ways to generate one type of cancer. However, absence of mutations does not mean that the gene plays no role in sporadic carcinogenesis;

Table 8.4 Inherited defects that also occur in sporadic cancers at the same site.

Familial cancer	Gene	Altered in sporadic cancers
Retina	*Rb*	Yes
Colon	*APC*	Yes
	HNPCC	13% of cases
Breast	*BRCA1, BRCA2*	No
Melanoma	*INK4*	Yes

Table 8.5 Gene mutations identified in specific familial cancers that are changed in sporadic cancers at other sites.

Gene	Familial cancer*	Sporadic cancer
Rb	**Eye**, osteosarcoma	Many
APC	**Colon**, brain, thyroid	?
MSH2, MLH1	**Colon**, endometrium	Some
BRCA1	**Breast**, ovary, colon	None
BRCA2	**Breast (both sexes)**, prostate, ovary	None
INK4A	**Melanoma**	Many
p53	**Breast**, sarcoma	Most

* The major cancer associated with each defect is shown in bold type.

BRCA1 expression does decline in some cases (see above), and so gene regulation rather than structure may be influential.

A different but related question is whether the genes identified from familial studies are relevant to sporadic cancers at sites other than the familial ones. In many cases the answer is yes, but there are exceptions (Table 8.5).

Further reading

Bartsch, H., Nair, U., Risch, A., *et al.* (2000) Genetic polymorphism of CYP gene, alone or in combination, as a risk modifier of tobacco-related cancers. *Cancer Epidemiol Biomarkers Prev* **9**, 3–28.

Bishop, D.T. (2005) Inherited susceptibility to cancer. In *Introduction to the Cellular and Molecular Biology of Cancer*, ed. M. Knowles and P. Selby. Oxford: Oxford University Press.

DiCiommo, D., Gallie, B.L. and Bremner, R. (2000) Retinoblastoma: the disease, gene and protein provide critical leads to understanding cancer. *Semin Cancer Biol* **10**, 255–269.

Fearnhead, N.S., Britton, M.P. and Bodmer, W.F. (2001) The ABC of APC. *Hum Mol Genet* **10**, 721–723.

Ponder, B.A.J. (2001) Cancer genetics. *Nature* **411**, 336–341.

Scharnhorst, V., van der Eb, A.J. and Jochemsen, A.G. (2001) WT1 proteins: functions in growth and differentiation. *Gene* **273**, 141–161.

Tutt, A. and Ashworth, A. (2002) The relationship between the roles of *BRCA* genes in DNA repair and cancer predisposition. *Trends Mol Med* **8**, 571–576.

9 Growth: a balance of cell proliferation, death and differentiation

- Growth can be altered by changing proliferation, apoptosis or differentiation.
- Different cancers use different options to achieve uncontrolled growth.
- Proliferation is regulated at several checkpoints in the cell cycle.
- The G_1 checkpoint is the focus of negative and positive extracellular signals.
- In normal cells, hypophosphorylated Rb blocks transit through the checkpoint. This inhibition is relieved by cyclin-dependent serine/threonine protein kinases (CDKs).
- CDKs are subject to stimulatory (cyclin) and inhibitory (CKI) controls mediated by protein–protein complexes. Protein phosphorylations modulate these interactions.
- The cell cycle is regulated at different stages by altered activities of specific CDKs, CKIs and cyclins.
- Alterations in cyclins and CKIs have been detected in cancers.
- There are two types of cell death: apoptosis (programmed cell death) requires RNA and protein synthesis, but necrosis does not.
- Apoptosis is activated by DNA damage, withdrawal of growth-stimulatory cytokines or addition of death-promoting cytokines.
- Diverse apoptotic signals converge to alter mitochondrial function. Pro-apoptotic (BAX, Bad) and anti-apoptotic (Bcl2) proteins regulate the release of mitochondrial cytochrome C.
- Apoptosis can be regulated by altering the relative proportions of pro-apoptotic and anti-apoptotic proteins.
- Cytochrome C activates proteases of the caspase family.
- Proliferation and apoptosis are integrated by mechanisms involving p53 and Rb.
- Leukaemias result from blocked differentiation.
- Methylation of cytosine bases in regulatory regions of DNA contributes to differentiation.

Introduction

Growth is a general term indicating alteration in size of a cell mass and is the end product of several interrelated influences, such as proliferation, differentiation, cell death, cell contacts and blood supply. This chapter will deal with three of those influences: proliferation, death and differentiation. If the time taken for cultured cells to double their number is compared with the time required for a tumour to double its volume in a patient, then there is a discrepancy: cultures double in days whereas months or years are required in patients (Table 9.1). Regulatory processes are present in solid cell masses but are absent in dispersed cells in culture. Cell culture conditions have been designed to maximise proliferation and minimise negative influences such as cell death. In patients, changes in cell number represent a balance between proliferation and death, so alteration of either parameter can influence the size of a cellular mass. Additionally, if cells differentiate, their proliferation potential decreases, and so differentiation has a negative influence on growth kinetics. Thus, in a normal tissue, cell number remains constant because of a balance between proliferation, death and differentiation (Figure 9.1). In abnormal situations, increased cell number can result either from blocked death and/or differentiation or from increased proliferation with no change in the other two properties. Each of these routes is involved in carcinogenesis.

Cancer cells are often said to proliferate faster than their normal counterparts, but this is far from true. Proliferation rates of well-differentiated tumours are not dissimilar to those seen in progenitor normal cells. What is different is the lack of stop signals in the cancer that maintain normal tissue stasis. As tumour cells progress from differentiated to dedifferentiated, the situation changes and proliferation rates increase. This is seen in the much shorter doubling times of metastases compared with those of primary tumours (Table 9.1).

Two types of cell death exist: necrotic and apoptotic. Necrotic cell death is passive whereas apoptotic cell death requires macromolecular synthesis. A third mechanism, whereby cancer cells are lost from a tumour mass, is migration of live cells into blood and lymphatic vessels during metastasis.

Table 9.1 Doubling times of human tumour cells.

Cell type	Tumours	Doubling times (days)	
		In patient★	**Cell lines**
Colon	Primary	700	3
	Metastasis	100	
Breast	Primary	200	3
	Metastasis	20	
Lymphoma		5	1

★ Numbers given are averages that cover a wide range of values.

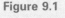

Figure 9.1

Growth can be regulated by altering proliferation, death or differentiation.

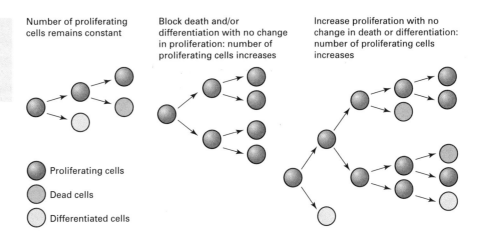

Number of proliferating cells remains constant

Block death and/or differentiation with no change in proliferation: number of proliferating cells increases

Increase proliferation with no change in death or differentiation: number of proliferating cells increases

Proliferating cells

Dead cells

Differentiated cells

As cells multiply, they accumulate errors in their DNA, resulting in senescence after about 40 doublings. If this was the only factor involved, then all cells would eventually die. However, in some cases, cell division is asymmetrical in that one daughter cell proceeds along the development and senescence pathway while the other retains the potential of unlimited proliferation and is called a stem cell. Thus, in the small intestine, epithelial stem cells are located in the base of the crypts; the number of proliferating cells decreases as they differentiate and move towards the mouth of the crypt. The molecular mechanisms behind this asymmetric division are unknown.

This chapter will consider each of the processes mentioned above on the assumption that a single cell type is involved and that factors such as the **extra**cellular **m**atrix (ECM) do not contribute to regulation. Although this is incorrect, it is a necessary simplification. The influence of cell–cell and cell–ECM interactions on growth are dealt with in Chapters 10 and 11. Most of the biological and molecular features of growth control in mammalian cells have been elucidated with experimental systems involving cell culture and animal models. These data have been very informative, but sometimes caution is required when the data are applied to cancers in patients. Cultured cell lines proliferate much faster than cancers in people (Table 9.1) – tumours doubling in size once per year may have additional mechanisms to those detected in cells doubling once per day.

Normal proliferation and its regulation

The cell cycle

For a cell to divide, the DNA must be replicated and distributed equally to the daughter cells. These processes of DNA synthesis and mitosis are separated by gaps, during which RNA and protein are made and the cell reorganises itself for the next round of division. This series of events is called the cell cycle; the first letters of

Figure 9.2

The cell cycle and its regulation. In rapidly dividing cells, the various phases have the following durations: M, 1 h; G_1, 8–30 h; S, 8 h; G_2, 3 h. The whole cycle lasts 20–50 h.

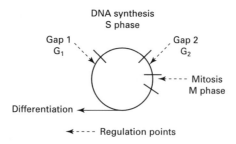

each of these events are used for its description (Figure 9.2). The first gap (G_1) is sometimes divided to include a G_0 phase in order to distinguish quiescent cells from those preparing to enter the next phase of the cycle. Differentiation takes cells out of cycle and can be represented as an exit from G_1. Normal cells have a diploid DNA content; as DNA content doubles during the next phase of the cycle, exit beyond G_1 generates non-diploid cells. For example, exit in the second gap (G_2) between DNA synthesis and mitosis produces tetraploid cells. During the complex series of events leading to cancer formation, chromosomal (DNA) changes occur that generate DNA contents per cell that are simple multiples of those in diploid cells. Such cells are said to be polyploid. Frequently, the altered DNA content is not a simple multiple and the cells are said to be aneuploid. Although doubling the amount of DNA is the major biochemical feature of normal cell proliferation, the other components that contribute to the mass of a single cell must also be coordinately replicated so that the two daughter cells are viable.

Careful regulation is needed for the complex series of events by which cells amplify their synthetic machinery (G_1) in preparation for the synthesis of DNA and other macromolecules (S) and then reorganise their interphase chromatin into chromosomes (G_2) before mitosis (M). Three main checkpoints have been identified in G_1, G_2 and M that must be traversed in order for accurate cell reproduction to occur. For simplicity, these will be dealt with as though they were single entities, which is not the true situation. Thus, within the G_1 checkpoint, different controls exist for commitment to DNA synthesis and transition of the G_1/S boundary.

G_1 transition requires a critical level of regulatory macromolecules, some of which relieve the inhibitory effect of the Rb suppressor protein. Growth stimuli such as hormones, growth factors and cell contacts act via this checkpoint. These stimuli increase the probability that cells cross this barrier, and as such the event is said to be stochastic. The G_1 checkpoint or regulation point ensures two functions: adequate machinery for future events and accurate transmission of genetic information. Adequate machinery involves relief of Rb inhibition by sequential and synchronised changes in gene activity, resulting in protein synthesis. Phosphorylation of serine and threonine hydroxyl groups by protein kinases is a key feature of these regulatory events. Fidelity of genetic information transfer is maintained by three mechanisms for detecting and eliminating damaged DNA. Cells have a delay process mediated by the p53 suppressor protein, which is activated when DNA damage is detected. On the other hand, cells with irreparable DNA are killed. In fact, p53 and Rb act in concert to ensure transition through this stage of the cycle.

The G_2 checkpoint ensures the elimination of damaged cells that may have escaped G_1 control or that have not duplicated their DNA accurately. The spindle assembly checkpoint in the M phase monitors accurate chromosome alignment and retraction into the two daughter cells.

Each stage of the cell cycle will be described separately.

G_1: the first gap phase

G_1 is the most variable of the cycle phases, its length being the major determinant of cycle time. It is also the period in which future commitment to division, differentiation or death is made and is the focal point for important regulatory signals. It follows that if these signals are altered, then the cell cycle is affected. Many changes in gene products have been identified in G_1 and it is convenient to classify these changes into early and late events. Late events include enzymes such as the DNA polymerases and those needed for nucleotide synthesis, e.g. dihydrofolate reductase, and whose levels increase at the G_1/S boundary. The stimuli for these changes come from earlier events, and typically there is a time interval of several hours between addition of a proliferation signal like serum to cultured cells and the onset of DNA synthesis. This delay reflects the time required for both signal transduction from the cell membrane to nucleus and the altered gene activity that results. Transcriptional changes in early genes such as *c-fos* can be detected within minutes of adding serum, indicating that the signalling pathway from membrane to nucleus is fast and the overall lag in DNA synthesis is due to other events. Other examples of early gene activation common to most cell types include the oncogenes *c-myc* and *c-jun*, which code for transcription factors that amplify regulatory signals (see Chapter 10). Jun is a component of several signalling pathways, including the ras pathway (see Figure 10.11), whereas the transcription factor formed by heterodimerisation of myc and max directly activates genes required for DNA synthesis (ornithine decarboxylase, carbamyl phosphate synthetase) or cyclin-dependent kinase activation (Cdc25, a tyrosine phosphatase). Additional cell-specific oncogene products such as c-myb in haemopoietic cells can also be detected at this time. It should be noted that regulation is not confined to the transcriptional level, since the half-life of c-fos mRNA can be extended and the activity of its protein product modulated by phosphorylation (see below).

Primary regulation of the G_1 checkpoint involves three protein families: (i) cyclins, (ii) **c**yclin-**d**ependent serine/threonine protein **k**inases (CDKs) and (iii) **c**yclin-dependent **k**inase **i**nhibitors (CKIs) (Figure 9.3). Their molecular features are detailed later, as they are also important at the G_2 and M checkpoints. The kinases alter the biological functions of regulatory proteins; thus, phosphorylation is one general way of regulating function, the other being the presence of activating (cyclin) and inhibitory (CKI) proteins that enable fine-tuning of this checkpoint. In fact, CKIs have all the properties of suppressors.

One key substrate of the kinase is the protein product of the retinoblastoma gene *Rb*. This protein blocks cell proliferation at the G_1 checkpoint; this suppression is released by protein phosphorylation and regained by dephosphorylation via protein phosphatases. The phosphorylation/dephosphorylation cycle therefore provides a rapidly reversible switch mechanism for altering proliferation rates (see later).

The second element of G_1 regulation involves DNA repair. DNA damaged by UV light or X-irradiation (see Chapter 7) is detected by a mechanism involving the

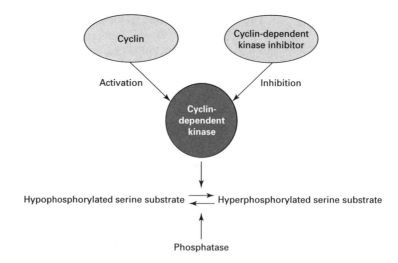

Figure 9.3

Cyclin–dependent protein kinase system.

suppressor protein p53, which blocks cycle progression until repair is completed. In normal cells, p53 levels are low, but its transcription is increased by DNA damage.

DNA synthesis and telomere length

DNA synthesis

Double-stranded DNA has a polarity; one strand is oriented in a 5′ to 3′ direction and the other strand in a 3′ to 5′ orientation. (Box 5.1 gives details of DNA structure and base pairings to form the genetic code.) DNA replication requires opening and unwinding of the helix to generate single-stranded regions of DNA (Figure 9.4). DNA polymerases join the deoxyribonucleotides to form the new chains; the base sequence of the chains is determined by the base sequence of the *parent* strand, also called the *template*, *coding* or *non-transcribed* strand. DNA polymerases add nucleotides to hydroxyl groups only at 3′ ends, which is fine for the new *daughter* (*primer*) strand, being lengthened in a 5′ to 3′ direction; this is called the *leading* strand. The other daughter strand, the *lagging* strand, has the wrong orientation to be made in a 5′ to 3′ direction; it is synthesised as discontinuous small (30–50 nucleotide) 5′ to 3′ segments called *Okazaki fragments*. The Okazaki fragments are then joined by ligases.

The protein complex involved in this series of events is the *replisome* situated at the *growing fork* of the DNA. The replisome contains enzymes and structural components. The enzymes include helicases that generate single-stranded DNA regions, DNA polymerases that synthesise the daughter strands, DNA ligases that join the Okazaki fragments into a continuous strand, and topoisomerases that release conformational constraints generated during passage

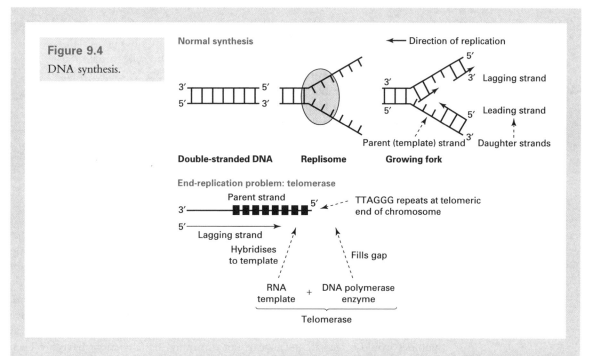

Figure 9.4
DNA synthesis.

of DNA strands through the replisome. At least five DNA polymerases (α, β, γ, δ, ε) are used in different circumstances (see Chapter 5), but the δ and ε enzymes are involved primarily in chain elongation during DNA synthesis. DNA polymerases δ and ε possess 3′ to 5′ exonuclease activities that remove incorrect misaligned bases in order to minimise errors (mutations) of base insertion during synthesis; this is called the *proof-reading* function.

The structural components provide a scaffold to which other regulatory proteins can attach; one of these proteins is **p**roliferating **c**ell **n**uclear **a**ntigen (PCNA). As its name implies, it is detected only in the nucleus of proliferating cells. One of its scaffolding functions is to hold together replicated double-stranded DNA; as the protein is ring-shaped, the DNA passes through the central hole. PCNA has additional functions mediated through its binding of regulatory proteins such as p21 (a cyclin–dependent protein kinase inhibitor), GADD45 (regulation of proliferation), MSH2 and MLH1 (DNA excision repair), several cyclin/cyclin–dependent protein kinase complexes (cell-cycle control) and DNA polymerases (DNA synthesis). The involvement of PCNA with these proteins makes it a key player not only in DNA synthesis but also in cell-cycle control and DNA repair. It is unclear how these processes are coordinated by PCNA.

Telomeres and the end-replication problem

DNA polymerase initiates synthesis by hybridisiation of its RNA with the 3′ regions of the parent strand. This creates a problem at the final 3′ end of the lagging strand: when the RNA is released, a single-stranded stretch of parent strand nucleotides remains at the *telomeric* end of the chromosome (see Box 7.1). It is known as the end-replication problem. Embryonic cells contain the enzyme *telomerase*, consisting of an RNA template and a DNA polymerase; telomerase completes the 3′ chain elongation so the length of the telomere remains constant (see Figure 9.4). If telomerase is inactivated, as in normal adult cells, then the single-stranded region is removed at each round of DNA synthesis and the telomere shortens; the consequences include chromosome instability, senescence and death.

S: the DNA synthesis phase

DNA synthesis is controlled largely at the level of its initiation and the build-up of enzymes, regulatory proteins and nucleotide triphosphates at the G_1/S boundary provides that control. During S, when the DNA strands are separated, bases are exposed and therefore are sensitive to external agents such as drugs and mutagens, and so it is understandable that synthesis should be completed as fast as possible once it has started. Given the fundamental importance of DNA replication, defects in synthesis would be lethal, and so it is not surprising that alterations have not been detected that lead to cancers. On the other hand, many cancer treatments are directed at disrupting DNA synthesis (see Chapter 12). A related process, DNA repair, occurs in S and plays an important role in preventing the more widespread generation of cancers (see Chapter 7).

G_2: the second gap phase

Several reorganisational and synthetic events occur in G_2. The double complement of DNA and chromatin proteins formed during S condense and are packaged into sister chromatids. DNA synthesis also leads to unwanted intertwining of chromosomes, which must be untangled by topoisomerases. Mitosis can be blocked by unreplicated DNA or by damaged DNA that has escaped repair, and so these defects must also be rectified; p53 is involved in monitoring this checkpoint. All of these processes are monitored at the G_2 checkpoint, probably in different ways, but the cyclin/CDK/CKI system is required.

M: mitosis

Sister chromatids must be aligned correctly so that they are retracted to opposite poles of the dividing cell; this is monitored at the spindle assembly checkpoint. Limited data indicate that regulation is achieved at the point of attachment of microtubules to the centromere. This occurs through a chromosome structure known as a kinetochore, which attaches to the microtubules. If any centromeres are not attached to microtubules, then mitosis is delayed. Additional regulation occurs if inappropriate tension or abnormal dynamics of the microtubule are detected. Once again, CDKs are required for these events. If any of these events go wrong such that cells traverse S but not M, increases in ploidy occur.

The cyclin-dependent kinase system

ATP-dependent phosphorylation of serine/threonine residues in proteins such as Rb alter the function of the protein. Changes in activity of protein kinases can therefore regulate the cell cycle. The kinases involved in this control are called cyclin-dependent kinases because they are activated by cyclins. Another family of regulatory proteins, the cycle-dependent kinase inhibitors (CKIs), have the opposite effect. Interactions between these three classes of protein regulate the checkpoints of the cell cycle.

Each of the three components of the kinase system represents a family of molecules, the members of which are activated at different periods of the cell cycle (Figure 9.5). Cyclins E, A and B are highest in late G_1, G_2 and M, respectively, and their presence contributes to checkpoint regulation during those periods. Cyclin D, on the other hand, rises early in G_1 and remains constant thereafter. Cyclins are increased through the transcriptional machinery and destroyed by ubiquitin-mediated proteolysis. CDKs are inactive on their own because their catalytic site, where ATP and substrate bind, is blocked by the C-terminal tail of the CDK; cyclin binding relieves that block. Phosphorylation of CDKs also has an important but poorly understood role in that a threonine phosphorylation activates enzyme activity and tyrosine phosphorylation inhibits enzyme activity. Each cyclin binds preferentially to specific CDKs, as illustrated in Figure 9.5. The presence or absence of specific cyclins and CDKs at different periods of the cell cycle determines which kinase is active during any one period.

An important protein substrate for CDKs is Rb, which, in its hypophosphorylated state, binds to and inactivates the E2F transcription factor. Phosphorylation releases E2F, which is thus available to increase transcription from genes such as DNA polymerase α, and thymidine kinase (Figure 9.6; see also Figure 5.9). Rb phosphorylation also releases blocks on the synthesis of other RNA species required to increase the mass of a cell (see Figure 5.10).

CDKs are activated by mitogenic growth factors such as PDGF (see Chapter 10), which rapidly (5 min) activates the oncogene *fos*. The fos nucleoprotein associates with jun protein to form a complex. Both the fos and the jun proteins form dimers,

Figure 9.5

Changes in cycle-dependent kinases during the cell cycle. (Source: Adapted from Figure 1 in Peters G. (1994) *Nature*, 371, 204–5. Copyright © 1977. Reprinted by permission of Macmillan Publishers Ltd.)

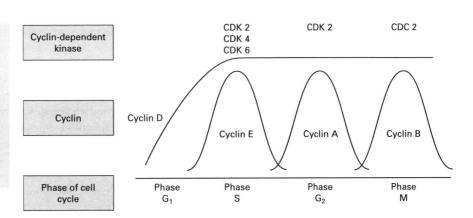

Figure 9.6

Inhibition of cell cycle by p53 and Rb. Each of the 'boxed' proteins can be altered in cancers.

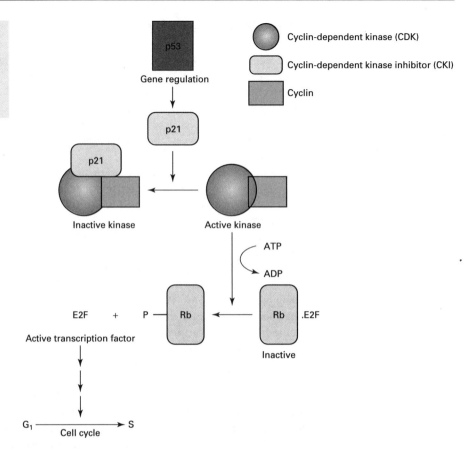

both heterodimers and homodimers. It is probably the combination of Fos with Jun that determines the transcriptional specificity of the complex. The complex binds to regulatory DNA sequences known as AP1 sites. Activation of genes containing an AP1 site results in increased cyclin and CDK function (Figure 9.7).

Inhibitory signals involve the CKI family of proteins, with different signals using different methods to increase CKI activity. There are two main families of CKIs, both of which block the kinases involved in the G_1 checkpoint. The INK4 (**in**hibitor of cyclin-dependent **k**inase **4**) family proteins (p15, p16, p18, p19) bind specifically to CDK4 and CDK6, thus preventing attachment of the cyclin. The other family of proteins (p21, p27, p57) have a wider specificity and bind to the cyclin–CDK complex rather than the CDK alone. Expression of the various CKIs is cell-type-specific. Thus, strong expression of p21 occurs in colon and prostate epithelium, whereas p57 predominates in kidney and skeletal muscle. Figure 9.6 shows an important example of how a CKI functions when binding to a cyclin–CKD complex. The p53 protein blocks proliferation by switching on the synthesis of a 21 kDa CKI (p21, *not* the same as the ras p21 product). This binds and inactivates the cyclin D–CDK4 complex that phosphorylates Rb.

The Rb protein is the product of the retinoblastoma gene, which is mutated in the condition of the same name (see Chapter 8). In spite of the name, this protein

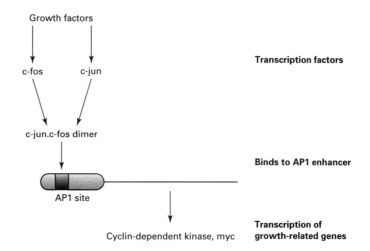

Figure 9.7

Growth factor stimulation of growth-related genes.

occurs in all cells and plays a key role in the regulation of the G_1 checkpoint. Thus, p53 activation results in hypophosphorylation of Rb, which binds and inactivates the E2F transcription factor; growth stimulatory genes are switched off (see Chapter 5). Rb phosphorylation/dephosphorylation provides the chemical basis of the G_1 checkpoint. Phosphorylation is activated by growth factors (see above). An example of the INK family of CKIs is provided by p16, which interacts specifically with CDK4 and CDK6, thus preventing the CDK6 from interacting with cyclins. p16 is involved in a novel mechanism, whereby the INK4 gene can code for two completely different proteins, $p16^{INK4}$ and $p19^{ARF}$ (Figure 9.8). The *INK4* gene can be transcribed into mRNA at two different start sites; the larger transcript codes for a 19 kDa protein and the smaller transcript codes for a 16 kDa product. Some of the DNA base sequences coding for p19 are also used for p16, but because the

Figure 9.8

$INK4^{ARF}$: one gene, two products that inhibit different functions.

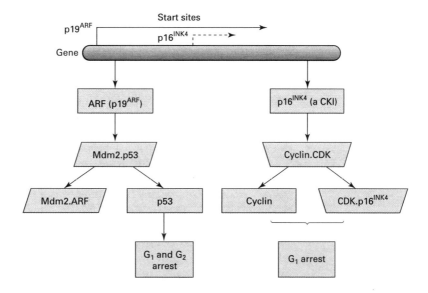

sequences have separate start sites the bases are read in different reading frames (see Box 5.1) and the two products do not have the same amino-acid sequence. This creates terminology problems. The proteins are named according to their size but sometimes are categorised further with superscripts. p16^{INK4} indicates that p16 is a product of the *INK4* gene, whereas p19^{ARF} indicates that p19 is produced from an alternate reading frame (ARF) within the *INK4* gene. The situation is confused further in that p19 is the size of the rodent product whereas in the human it is smaller (p14). The term ARF will be used here for both p14 and p19. Important features of the *INK4* gene structure are that the two mRNAs are regulated independently and the protein products have different functions. p16 is a CKI that blocks Rb phosphorylation, whereas ARF has a different function. It binds Mdm2, thereby releasing p53 bound to Mdm2; p53 is activated by this process (see Figure 5.14). One gene transcript can thus generate products that enhance Rb inhibitory effects and augment p53 responses.

This is reminiscent of some of the carcinogenic DNA viruses that code for proteins influencing both pathways. Any agent that alters both Rb and p53 responses will have major effects, and so it is noteworthy that deletions in the *INK4* gene have been detected in many cancers (see below). Further molecular details of Rb and p53 interactions are given in Figures 5.9 and 5.13, respectively.

Part of the growth inhibitory effect of the cytokine TGF-β (see Chapter 10) may be mediated by stimulation of a member of the INK family of CKIs. Also, cell–cell contacts (contact inhibition; see Chapter 2) inhibit proliferation by a CKI-mediated process, whereas differentiated cells with limited proliferative potential often have high levels of the p27 CKI.

Cancer cells

Proliferation of cancer cells

Cancer cells are characterised by their unregulated proliferation; this means they have a lower requirement for growth factors and they do not respond to negative environmental stimuli such as contact with other cells. These changes, detailed in Chapter 10, feed into the system mainly via the G_1 checkpoint, and many of the mechanistic variations used by different cancers occur in those pathways. Figure 9.9 shows examples of changes in CDK/cyclin/CKI/Rb that have been detected in human cancers and that illustrate the general point that different cancers use alternative pathways to achieve a similar end result, in this case increased Rb phosphorylation. Mechanistic details of these events are given in Figures 9.6 and 9.8. Cyclin and CKI changes are common, whereas activating mutations in CDKs are rare (melanoma, sarcomas, gliomas). The *CDK4* mutation in some melanomas destroys its p16^{INK4} CKI-binding property. The *cyclin D* gene is rearranged in human parathyroid adenomas and amplified and overexpressed in a proportion of breast and oesophageal cell tumours, thereby providing a method of upregulating proliferation. Inactivating changes in the p16^{INK4} CKI are common, particularly in pancreatic cancers and gliomas.

Figure 9.9

Changes of levels of cyclin, CDK and CKI in cancers.

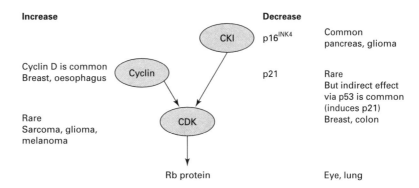

They are mainly deletions and mutations. Such changes could diminish inhibitory signals.

Alterations in *cyclin* and *CKI* genes are important for the genesis of certain cancers but the two genes most frequently altered in cancers are *p53* and *Rb*, especially *p53*. Functional inactivation of the *p53* and *Rb* genes can be achieved by mutation or deletion of the gene itself, or by binding of the normal product to other proteins. At a simplistic level, changes in *p53* are more dangerous because alteration of only one allele will result in derepression due to the dominant-negative effect of heterodimerisation (Chapter 5).

Several features of the cell cycle, especially during the S and M phases, are exploited in the treatment of cancers (Chapter 12).

Senescence, cell mortality and telomerase

A major distinction between cancer cells and normal cells is that, before senescence, cancer cells undergo more cycles of proliferation than normal cells (see Figure 2.7). Cancer cells are said to be immortal, although this is not strictly true as they do die eventually. This prolonged life provides more time in which to accumulate genetic errors, with their attendant effects on cell function. Normal cells must therefore have a mechanism for limiting the life of a cell lineage that is lost in cancers. A major component of this process is the enzyme telomerase that fills the single-stranded gaps at the 3′ ends of newly synthesised lagging strands of DNA (see Figure 9.4 and Box 9.1). In germ cells, foetal somatic cells and adult stem cells, enzyme activity is high, with no problem in completing the full resynthesis of DNA. In adult somatic cells, telomerase declines (Figure 9.10) with the consequence that telomere length shortens progressively at each round of DNA synthesis. This results in chromosome instability, which, at a telomere length of about 4 kb, disrupts cell function sufficiently to cause senescence.

In this state, the cells are alive but arrested in the G_1 phase of the cell cycle. There is not an absolute block to their transition into S phase (see Figure 2.7) until the further telomere shortening results in apoptotic cell death. The term 'crisis' is sometimes used to define this stage; it originated when cultured cell lines (prolonged

151

Figure 9.10

Telomere length and cell function in culture.

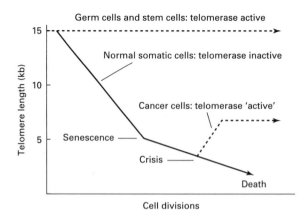

lifespan) were being produced from primary cultures (limited lifespan). The primary cultures eventually stopped proliferating (senescence), but foci (clones) of cells would spontaneously be reactivated and could be recultured as cell lines. These cell lines were said to have passed through 'crisis' and been immortalised. We now know that successful transition of the crisis period is associated with reactivation of telomerase. The link between this enzyme and chromosome instability is exemplified by the fact that primary cell cultures often become polyploid.

In cancer cells, telomerase is frequently reactivated by unknown mechanisms, although not to the levels seen in germ cells. This extends their lifespan by preventing further loss of telomeric repeats but does not lengthen those repeats to the original levels. Hence, a degree of chromosome instability remains. It is unclear as to what stage of carcinogenesis is linked to elevated telomerase. It is high in malignant colon but undetectable in polyps and adenomas at that site. On the other hand, about half of gastric adenomas and pre-invasive prostate cancers are telomerase-positive compared with all their invasive counterparts. The enzyme is also elevated in pre-invasive lung and neck cancers. If a telomerase-positive cell is hybridised with a normal cell that is telomerase-negative, then the hybrid has a normal phenotype; normal cells have a mechanism for inhibiting telomerase. That mechanism remains obscure, although inactivation of a suppressor process is involved. Important regulatory processes are usually controlled by multiple pathways, and so it is not surprising that telomerase-independent mechanisms exist for maintaining telomere length. The exact nature of those mechanisms and their importance are still unknown.

It is not clear why single-stranded 3′ ends of DNA should result in chromosome instability, although there is a causal link between the two processes. The link is vaguely described as being due to 'sticky ends' causing abnormal separation of DNA strands or chromosomes. The term 'sticky' refers to the single strand being able to hybridise inappropriately with single strands on other chromosomes. Cytogenetic abnormalities frequently accompany senescence and crisis. Senescence is associated with polyploidy, whereas chromosome aberrations and aneuploidy characterise the crisis period.

The biochemical consequences of these major chromosomal changes are defined poorly. Senescent cells are arrested in the late G_1 stage of the cycle but there is no clear picture for the cause of that arrest. Growth factors (serum) can still elevate transcription of some growth-related genes such as *myc* and *jun*, but not *fos*, in senescent cells. Receptors for growth cytokines such as epidermal growth factor and platelet-derived growth factor are normal, but signal transduction therefrom may be impaired. Cyclin–CDK complexes actually accumulate at senescence but downstream phosphorylations do not occur.

In cultured cells, senescence (the stable growth arrest resulting from telomere attrition) can be provoked by various stresses, including the enforced expression of cancer-promoting genes. This oncogene-induced senescence is linked to several known cancer pathways (ARF-p53 and p16^{INK14a}-RB pathway). It was thought initially that cell senescence could be an artefact caused by unusual culture conditions. However, it has now been shown that this occurs *in vivo* and should be considered as real. Naevi (skin moles, the benign precursors of melanomas) have clear expression of senescence markers and do not proliferate. However, in melanoma cells, senescence does not occur and proliferation is accelerated. In mouse models of prostate cancer, inactivation of *p53* does not produce a cancer phenotype, and inactivation of the tumour suppressor gene *Pten* triggers a non-lethal invasion only after a long latency (*PTEN* is thought to regulate *p53* stability and *p53* to enhance *PTEN* transcription). However, inactivation of both *Pten* and *Trp53* results in rapid invasion and death.

Ploidy changes and gene amplification

Advanced cancers often have an increased DNA content per nucleus. Unbalanced DNA synthesis and incorrect separation of chromosomes to daughter cells during mitosis are two contributing factors, but amplification of specific DNA segments also occurs. The net result is a DNA content per cell that is not a simple multiple of two (diploid) or four (tetraploid). This is known as an aneuploid DNA content. Aneuploid tumours kill their host faster than do diploid tumours, and amplification of growth factor receptors like those for epidermal growth factor (see Chapter 10) and amplification of the multidrug-resistance gene (see Chapter 12) have been recorded in many tumours. These DNA changes occur because of errors in mitosis or because of unscheduled DNA synthesis.

Cell death

Cell death is a normal process that serves two functions: tissue remodelling and removal of damaged cells that might otherwise harm the rest of the body. DNA is constantly being damaged (see Chapter 6), and although efficient repair mechanisms exist, they are not wholly effective. To prevent unwanted consequences, cells have a method of detecting such defects and committing suicide. In embryogenesis, extensive remodelling occurs in which some cells are removed and others expanded. Removal is achieved by cell death and the process continues into adult life. In skin, the basal keratinocyte stem cells proliferate; as they move towards the surface, proliferation

Table 9.2 Features of apoptotic and necrotic cell death.

	Apoptosis	**Necrosis**
Causes	Programmed tissue remodelling, cell turnover, DNA damage, withdrawal of growth signals	Hypoxia, nutrient shortage, changes in pH and temperature
Morphology		
Affected cells	Single	Groups
Cell volume	Decreased	Increased
Chromatin	Dense	Fragmented
Lysosomes	Intact	Abnormal
Mitochondria	'Normal'	Abnormal
Inflammatory response	No	Yes
Cell fate	Apoptotic bodies	Lysis
Molecular changes		
Gene activity	Required	Not required
DNA cleavage	Specific	Random
Intracellular Ca^{2+}	Increased	No change
Ion pumps	Retained	Lost

stops, differentiation (keratin production) occurs and the cells die, leaving the keratin. Integration of proliferation and death is essential for normal homeostasis and the processes are linked tightly such that death occurs even in rapidly proliferating cells. Conversely, regressing tumours contain mitotic cells. It follows that if the equilibrium between proliferation and death is altered, then abnormal growth occurs. In carcinogenesis, unregulated proliferation or decreased cell death will generate a tumour. The objective of cancer treatments, whether chemical or physical, is to achieve the converse.

There are two types of cell death, apoptosis and necrosis, with different morphological and molecular features (Table 9.2).

Apoptosis

Also called programmed cell death or cell suicide, apoptosis requires mRNA and protein synthesis. Apoptosis is a normal process involved in any situation requiring tissue remodelling. An extreme example is embryogenesis, but adult tissues undergo the same process. Growth stimuli tend to be of variable strength, which leads to periods of low and high exposure. The consequences of this variability are best illustrated with cultured cells (Figure 9.11) in which addition of a growth factor stimulates proliferation. If that was all that happened, then stimulus withdrawal would result in a cell-number plateau, but actually the cell number falls; cell death by apoptosis is increased. An analogous phenomenon occurs *in vivo*, in that waves of proliferation are always followed by a pulse of apoptosis. Thus, cells must have the ability

Figure 9.11

Effect of growth factor on cell number.

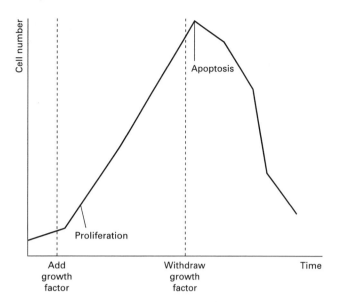

to coordinate proliferation and apoptosis in response to external stimuli. This occurs in both normal cells and cancer cells, but in many cancers the gene changes lead to decreased apoptotic death, which contributes to an increase in cell numbers. In tumours, apoptosis is still a major determinant of size, with individual cells being eliminated in about 3 hours; in regressing tumours, volume can decrease by about one-quarter in 1 day. However, apoptosis is not confined to regressing tumours and it is a balance between proliferation and death that determines whether a cancer gets bigger or smaller. Apoptosis is also important in determining response to treatments like chemotherapy and radiation (see Chapter 12).

Cellular features of apoptosis

The main cellular features of apoptosis are listed in Table 9.2. Under the microscope, the most striking features are the pattern of chromatin condensation and the appearance of membrane-bound apoptotic vesicles representing cell remnants that are removed by phagocytosis. A major biochemical feature of apoptosis is the sequential activation of the caspases (see below), a family of proteases whose substrates include large protein precursors of enzymes capable of destroying DNA (endonucleases); lamin and actin (proteases); and proteins involved in DNA repair, RNA splicing, signal transduction and transcription factors. Endonuclease digestion at internucleosome bridges generates a ladder of DNA fragments that are multiples of 200 bp units characteristic of a nucleosome (Figure 9.12). The nucleases involved are sensitive to Ca^{2+} ions; an increase in Ca^{2+} is another characteristic of apoptosis.

The Ca^{2+} released from mitochondria may be a consequence of their altered permeability (see below). Lamin, a component of the nuclear matrix, provides a structural framework for chromatin, so its loss leads to chromatin condensation. Cytoplasmic collapse and decreased cell volume result from loss of cytoskeletal elements such as actin-containing microfilaments. The membrane-bound apoptotic

Figure 9.12

Pathways promoting apoptosis.

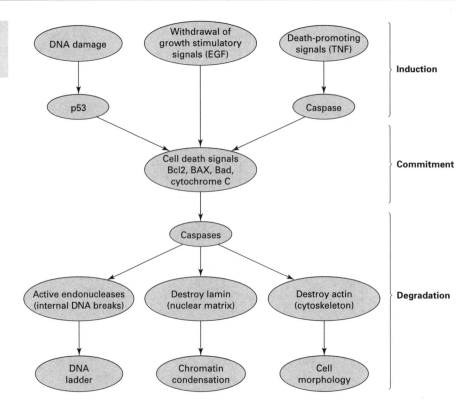

vesicles are unusual in that phosphatidylserine, normally occluded within the vesicles, becomes exposed on the surface, which marks them for elimination by phagocytosis.

A wide range of external events activate apoptosis, such as withdrawal of growth cytokines (TGF-α, IGF, PDGF), addition of apoptotic cytokines (TNF), ionising radiation (via free radicals), genotoxic chemicals (via DNA damage) and drugs used for chemotherapy (disruption of various cell functions).

Untransformed cells in culture require a substrate on which to grow (monolayer culture) plus growth factors. Anchorage is commonly prevented by putting cells into suspension culture (see Chapter 2); they stop in G_1 and eventually undergo apoptosis. This may reflect the conflicting signals received by the cell. The positive signals from the serum conflict with the negative signals due to lack of substratum. In solid tumours, confusion can arise because unregulated proliferation is in conflict with a lack of synchrony between the multiple signalling pathways involved.

Apoptosis can be divided into three phases (Figure 9.12). The induction phase is initiated by diverse pathways described elsewhere – radiation and genotoxic agents (see Chapter 6), cytokines and anchorage independence (see Chapter 10), chemotherapy (see Chapter 12) – although the pathways are outlined below (see Figure 9.16). These pathways converge to a common series of molecular events required for cell death signals to be translated into morphological changes. After induction, the cells enter a commitment phase, with no obvious morphological features, in which they are committed to apoptosis but from which they can be rescued.

Figure 9.13

Caspase activation.

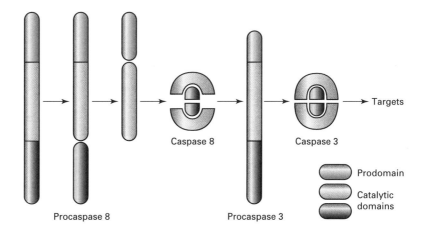

They then pass into the irreversible degradation and execution phase with the morphological changes described in Table 9.2.

A process as important as apoptosis has to be carefully regulated and integrated with other cell functions. How this is achieved requires an understanding of the molecular events involved, primarily related to two categories of protein: caspases, with proteolytic functions, and regulatory proteins of the Bcl2, BAX and Bad families capable of dimerising with themselves and with each other.

Molecular features

All the essential signals for apoptosis arise outside the nucleus, although the culminating event is nuclear destruction. The induction phase ends with the activation of a family of proteases called caspases, so called because they all need a **c**ysteine at their catalytic site and their substrates are cleaved at **asp**artate residues (Figure 9.13). These caspases alter mitochondrial function to release cytochrome C into the cytoplasm, where it activates additional caspases and initiates the final degradation phase.

Caspases   These proteases are synthesised as large inactive precursors (procaspases) from which the active enzyme is released by cleavage at aspartate residues. This means that the activating proteases are themselves caspases, so a cascade of proteolytic events occurs with the sequential appearance of different caspase activities. An example is given in Figure 9.13. Two successive autocatalytic cleavages release the prodomain polypeptide plus two proteins that aggregate to form the active caspase 8. This catalyses a similar set of events on procaspase 3, which can either alter mitochondrial function (Figure 9.14) or activate other caspases. The mitochondrial changes (see below) release cytochrome C that activates procaspase 9 by binding to **ap**optosis-**a**ctivating **f**actor (Apaf). This complex of procaspase 9, Apaf and cytochrome C is called an apoptosome. Caspase 9 activates downstream caspases responsible for the degradation phase; caspase 1 digests actin, caspase 6 digests nuclear lamin, and caspase 3 cleaves and activates a protein, which then activates DNAase.

Mitochondrial events: Bcl2, BAX and cytochrome C   These proteins form the core of the commitment phase of apoptosis. The mitochondrial membranes enclose

Figure 9.14

Commitment to apoptosis.

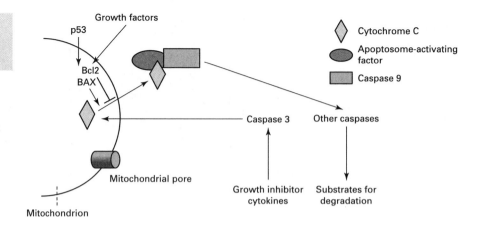

proteins that either activate apoptosis (pro-apoptotic proteins, BAX) or inhibit apoptosis (anti-apoptotic proteins, Bcl2). These proteins are important, along with cytochrome C and the formation of mitochondrial pores, but certain aspects are unclear. The increased mitochondrial permeability is associated with cytochrome C release into the cytoplasm, but it is poorly understood how upstream signals generate that release. Cytokines such as TNF signal via caspase 3, but it is not clear how caspase 3 releases cytochrome C. Likewise, p53 and growth factor withdrawal alter the balance of Bcl2 and BAX, such that BAX stimulates cytochrome C release, but details of this link are unknown. Similarly, we do not understand the inhibitory effect of Bcl2 on cytochrome C release (see Figure 9.14). Bcl2 was first identified in a **B-c**ell **l**ymphoma as a chromosome translocation that moved the *Bcl2* gene from chromosome 18 to 14 (t14;18), adjacent to a strong immunoglobulin promotor, analogous to events in Burkitt's lymphoma with *c-myc* (see Figure 5.5). The *Bcl2* gene codes for a 26 kDa protein found mainly in the outer mitochondrial membrane, although the protein is coded by a nuclear rather than a mitochondrial gene. Bcl2 can also be detected in nuclear-envelope membranes and endoplasmic reticulum. Constitutive overexpression of Bcl2 blocks apoptosis and thus protects cells against ionising radiations, UV light, viral infection and chemotherapeutic agents. A consequence of this effect is that cancers with elevated Bcl2 are resistant to drugs used for treating cancers (see Chapter 12). Skin melanocytes, whose function is to make melanin as a protection against UV damage, express high levels of Bcl2 protein, and so they are resistant to the killing effect of the UV light. Mice in which both alleles have been destroyed would be expected to die *in utero* because of excess apoptosis. Somewhat surprisingly, this does not happen, but they do die within a few weeks of birth, with extensive destruction of lymphoid cells and kidney disease.

Like so many growth regulators, Bcl2 is just one member of a family that includes proteins that either block or induce apoptosis. Members of the anti-apoptosis group include Bcl2 and Bcl_x, and BAX, Bad, Bak and Bik form the pro-apoptosis members. Whether apoptosis is induced or blocked depends on the ratios among family members and reflects the dimerisation state of those members (Figure 9.15).

Figure 9.15

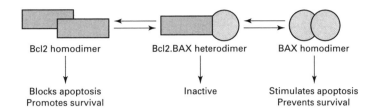

Bcl2 homodimer   Bcl2.BAX heterodimer   BAX homodimer

Blocks apoptosis
Promotes survival   Inactive   Stimulates apoptosis
Prevents survival

Response is determined by the dimerisation state of Bcl2 and BAX. Relative concentrations of Bcl2 and BAX determine the dimerisation state. The pro-apoptotic protein Bad (not shown) influences this equilibrium by forming heterodimers with Bcl2.

Homodimers of Bcl2 block apoptosis, whereas BAX homodimers elicit the opposite effect; Bcl2.BAX heterodimers are inactive. The relative proportions of the two proteins in the cell determine the nature of the response; high Bcl2 blocks apoptosis and favours cell survival, whereas high BAX levels have the opposite effect.

Pro-apoptotic Bad forms heterodimers with anti-apoptotic Bcl2, decreasing the concentration of active Bcl2 (see below). This stimulates apoptosis by altering the equilibrium in favour of BAX dimers. This has important consequences for the regulation of apoptosis, because alterations in relative levels of the two proteins can determine whether apoptosis occurs. It is known that apoptosis is activated more easily in some cells than in others. Thus, cortical lymphocytes are very sensitive to apoptotic signals, whereas medullary lymphocytes are not. The different sensitivities could be explained by a chemostat mechanism in which different cell types have different settings at which apoptosis is switched on or off. The relative levels of Bcl2 and BAX could provide the molecular basis for such a chemostat.

p53 activates transcription from the *BAX* gene and inhibits transcription from the *Bcl2* gene (Figure 9.16; see also Figure 5.13). The net result is that the equilibrium alters in favour of the pro-apoptotic BAX complex. Cell death triggered by withdrawal of growth stimulatory factors is mediated by a third member of the family, Bad (Figure 9.16). In proliferating cells, phosphorylated (serine) Bad is bound to a cytoplasmic protein, enigmatically named 14-3-3, which removes Bad from the apoptosis picture. Growth-promoting factors indirectly promote Bad phosphorylation via a pathway involving phosphoinositols and protein kinase B (Akt; see Figure 10.14). Growth factor withdrawal results in Bad dephosphorylation, dissociation from 14-3-3, heterodimerisation with Bcl2 and blockade of Bcl2's inhibitory effect on cell death. The end result of growth factor removal is Bcl2 inactivation and apoptosis. Growth factor addition reverses these changes and cell survival is enhanced.

Necrosis

Necrosis is commonly seen in the central regions of solid tumours. This is caused by an impoverished nutrient supply resulting from poor vascular supply. This inadequacy leads to disruption of energy-dependent membrane-mediated ion channels, an increase in cell volume, loss of membrane integrity and release of lysosomal enzymes such as proteases and nucleases. Cell lysis is also accompanied by the inflammatory response associated with the cell damage (see Table 9.2).

A link between blood supply to solid tumours and their growth is also seen in the early stages of their development (see Chapter 2) and during metastasis (see Chapter 11).

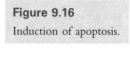

Figure 9.16

Induction of apoptosis.

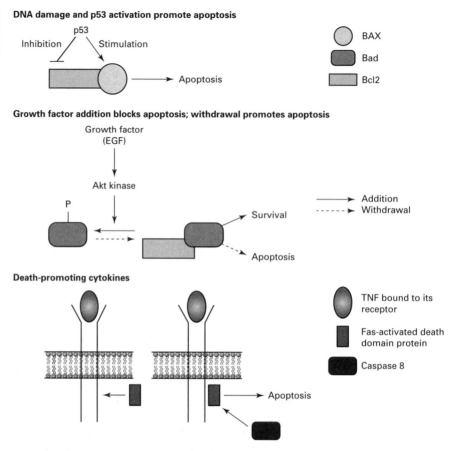

Apoptosis and cancer

Apoptosis is important at several stages of carcinogenesis, some of which have been described already. Transgenic mice that overexpress Bcl2 develop normally but exhibit hyperproliferation of haemopoietic cells and eventually succumb to lymphomas due to the absence of apoptosis. This example of malfunctioning apoptosis in the early stages of carcinogenesis is complemented by the p53 data indicating that genetic defects predispose towards high cancer risk (see Chapter 8). Loss of the p53 brake on the cell cycle to allow apoptotic removal of abnormal cells results in cancer.

Apoptotic defects are also influential in established cancer. In both solid (e.g. prostate) and disseminated (e.g. leukaemia) tumours, Bcl2 overexpression indicates a poor prognosis, presumably because of proliferation in the absence of death. It is also involved in treatment responses. An approximate but far from universal observation is that tumours with high Bcl2 expression are resistant to chemotherapy (see Chapter 12). An ironic example of generalities about cancer being wrong is that the original cancer in which Bcl2 overexpression was detected (follicular B-cell lymphoma) is in fact chemosensitive!

Integration of proliferation, apoptosis and DNA repair

In normal adult tissues, proliferation, apoptosis and DNA repair are in equilibrium and maintain a steady-state level of healthy cells. However, the DNA in these tissues is constantly being damaged (see Chapter 6). The damaged DNA can be repaired or, if damage is extensive, cells enter the apoptotic death pathway (Figure 9.17). For repair to occur, proliferation is stopped to ensure that the damage is not transmitted to daughter cells. If repair is successful, then additional cells are not required, whereas cell death warrants further proliferation to maintain a steady-state mass of cells. Molecular mechanisms exist to ensure that the equilibrium is not altered. If the number of cells in a mass is increased by altering control of proliferation, of death or both, then hyperplasias or benign lumps, but not a malignant cancer capable of invasion and metastasis, will result (see Chapter 3).

For carcinogenesis to proceed, the link between DNA repair and blocked proliferation must be broken so that errors in the DNA base sequence are passed on to daughter cells. If such an error blocks DNA repair, increases proliferation or inhibits apoptosis, then further errors will be propagated. An autocatalytic loop will have been created, which could be the engine (see Chapter 5) that generates the additional changes associated with the malignant phenotype. Different cancers use different options to achieve error propagation, and frequently one cancer will acquire changes in each of the three properties at different stages of carcinogenesis. Thus, the primary driving force for retinoblastoma formation is increased proliferation (see Figure 5.9 and Chapter 8); in hereditary non-polyposis colon cancer it is defective repair (see Chapter 7); and one form of B-cell lymphoma results from decreased apoptosis (see above). In sporadic colorectal cancer, altered proliferation, DNA repair and apoptosis are acquired sequentially (see Chapter 2).

The p53 suppressor protein is a key factor in integrating responses to DNA damage in terms of either stopping the cell cycle and initiating DNA repair or inducing apoptosis (Figure 9.18). It follows that the control of p53 is of great importance in the regulation of these pathways. The type and magnitude of the p53 response to genotoxic insult depends on many factors, which can be divided broadly into general regulators and apoptosis-specific regulators. The general regulators such as

Figure 9.17

The link between DNA damage, repair, proliferation and apoptosis.

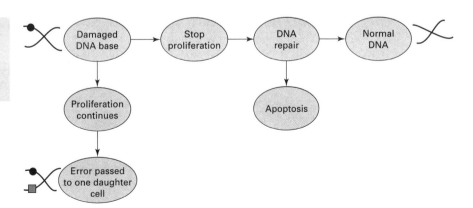

Figure 9.18

Coordination of DNA synthesis, repair and apoptosis.

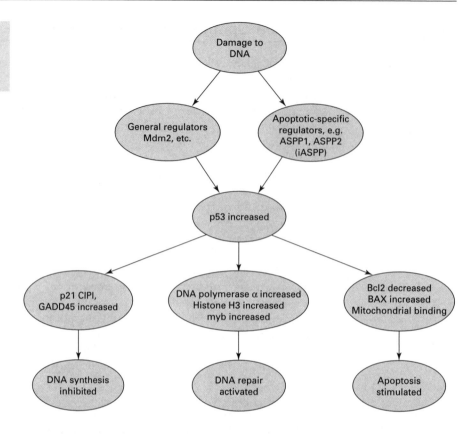

Mdm2, MdmX and E2F are concerned with cell-cycle arrest and the initiation of DNA repair, while the apoptotic-specific regulators control the ability of p53 to initiate apoptosis. The best examples of the latter group are the **a**poptosis-**s**timulating **p**roteins of **p**53 (ASPP); ASPP1 and ASPP2 increase apoptosis. Cotransfection of ASPP1 and ASPP2 increases the transactivation of pro-apoptotic *p53* genes such as *Bax* but has no effect on other *p53* target genes such as *Mdm2* and *cyclin G*. A third member of the ASPP family, iASPP, acts as an inhibitor of ASPP1 and ASPP2 and is therefore a regulator of this pathway. Normal p53, acting as a transcription factor for several genes, inhibits proliferation by inducing p21, a cyclin-dependent kinase inhibitor; this stimulates DNA repair by increasing DNA polymerase, histone H3 and myb and promotes apoptosis by the pathway already mentioned. Provided that these three pathways are intact, DNA damage elicits the coordinated changes just described, allowing the formation of normal daughter cells at mitosis. Defective p53 disrupts all three downstream pathways; its deleterious effects are enhanced by the fact that it is a dominant-negative gene, so only one allele needs to be damaged in order to generate a functional effect (see Chapter 5).

Alterations to the DNA repair pathways can explain the carcinogenicity of genotoxic agents such as tobacco smoke and ionising radiation, but more problematic are non-genotoxic agents such as the sex hormones associated with increased risk of common cancers such as breast and prostate. Oestrogens (breast) and androgens (prostate) are potent mitogens (see Chapter 11) and may disrupt the repair/proliferation/death equilibrium by this route. But proliferation alone will not generate malignant cells; additional changes are required. It is significant that inheritance of the *BRCA* genes greatly increases the risk of developing breast cancer as compared with the normal population, and these genes may be involved in DNA repair (see Chapter 5). The additional changes needed for the formation of sporadic breast cancers are of unknown origin.

These views on how disruption of these pathways contributes to carcinogenesis are backed by a solid body of experimental evidence, but they do not rule out the involvement of other processes. Several experiments involving genetic alterations in key genes in the above pathways indicate that we do not have all the answers. If defective p53 is so carcinogenic for all cells, then why is it that patients with inherited p53 defects in all their cells (Li–Fraumeni syndrome) get cancers in only a few cell types such as breast and fibroblasts (sarcomas)?

The same question arises from studies on p53 null ($p53^{-/-}$) knock-out mice. As anticipated, such mice are prone to tumour formation, but certain types predominate, lymphomas in one strain and sarcomas in another. Additional unknown controls clearly exist to prevent cancers appearing everywhere. Another anomaly has been identified in Rb-regulated pathways. This protein exerts its antiproliferative effects by inhibiting the E2F transcription factor (see Chapter 5), and so genetic elimination of E2F expression would be expected to result in hypoproliferation and malfunctions of embryogenesis. In fact, embryogenesis is completed and some cell types are actually hyperplastic. Once again, answers that are too simplistic usually prove to be wrong when generalised to cancers.

Differentiation

The inverse relationship between differentiation and proliferation is valid if we compare the two features at the beginning and end of a developmental sequence, although they can occur simultaneously at intermediate stages. Thus, in the haemopoietic system, the pluripotent stem cell commits itself to certain cell lineages at an early stage but those cells must be amplified (Figure 9.19). A similar process occurs in solid tissues such as mammary gland, which during pregnancy undergoes differentiation in readiness for milk production and proliferation to generate the requisite number of specialist cells. As illustrated below with leukaemias, this temporary synergy of increased proliferation plus differentiation can be achieved by the production of growth factors. Cells at one stage of differentiation are sensitive to one growth factor, while cells at another stage are stimulated by a different growth factor. These comments are relevant to the early stages of carcinogenesis whereas in later stages, where established tumours progress to dedifferentiated or anaplastic states, there exists the simpler relationship of faster growth and poorer differentiation.

Older models of carcinogenesis referred to reverse differentiation, but this is inappropriate because differentiation is an irreversible process. The dedifferentiation seen in many tumours reflects loss of functions by mechanisms different from those involved in their acquisition.

Figure 9.19

Cytokines and myeloid cell differentiation. Changed differentiation status is represented by altered tinting of the cell symbols.

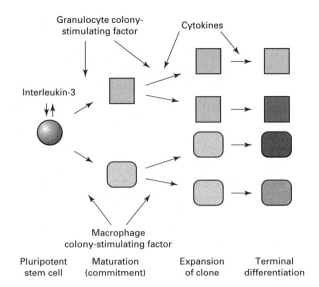

Leukaemias result from blocked differentiation (see below) and the same may be partially true for some of the solid tumours. Thus, a full-term pregnancy in young women (< 30 years) protects against later development of breast cancer, which is compatible with differentiation (pregnancy) hindering carcinogenesis. Cows, despite having a large number of potential target cells, do not get breast cancer because of continuous maintenance of the udder in a differentiated milk-producing state. Another notable example of the inverse link between carcinogenesis and differentiation comes from the loss of tumour properties when a cancer cell is hybridised with a normal cell. The differentiation properties of the normal cell are retained by the hybrid until, with chromosome loss, return of tumorigenicity is accompanied by loss of differentiation (see Figure 2.6).

Leukaemia as a model for blocked differentiation

The several forms of leukaemia can be explained in developmental terms as manifestations of blocked maturation at various stages of differentiation. Each step in the normal differentiation represents a balance between self-renewal and maturation. Leukaemias result from increased self-renewal at the expense of maturation. In normal haemopoiesis, a family of glycoprotein growth factors has been identified that integrate the proliferation and differentiation signals (Figure 9.19). These growth factors are collectively known as cytokines, individual members having names that describe their functions, e.g. **c**olony-**s**timulating **f**actors (CSFs) and interleukins. These proteins alter cell kinetics by reacting with specific cell-membrane receptors. In the case of myeloid cell differentiation, the pluripotent stem cell proliferates under the autocrine influence of **i**nterleukin **3** (IL-3), also known as multi-CSF because of its broad cell specificity. More specific CSFs are switched on that initiate both differentiation and proliferation: granulocyte CSF promotes granulocyte development whereas macrophage CSF induces a macrophage lineage. The crucial events in the genesis of leukaemia occur at this maturation stage; the exact point at which the abnormality occurs determines the resultant type of leukaemia (see Figure A.5).

Autocrine production of cytokines is an important feature of self-renewal, but it does not entirely explain carcinogenesis. For unknown reasons, chromosome translocations are a common cause of leukaemias, although none of the translocations involves cytokine genes, and overexpression of cytokines generates hyperplasias not cancers. Cytokines act via cell-surface receptors (see Chapter 10), at least one of which, c-fms, the proto-oncogene receptor for macrophage CSF, is altered in some animal leukaemias.

Normal differentiation can be regulated by low-molecular-weight signalling molecules such as retinoic acid. This pathway can be altered in some cancers; an example is acute promyelocytic leukaemia (see Figures 5.7 and 10.20), in which the retinoic acid receptor α gene is disrupted such that it does not function at normal ligand concentrations. Differentiation is arrested at the stage where the myeloid cells continue to proliferate. Another case of altered differentiation due to uncoupled signal transduction is chronic myeloid leukaemia (see Figure 2.10). Chromosome translocation results in a constitutively active mitogenic signal from the *c-abl* tyrosine kinase oncogene (see Figure 10.8), which stimulates proliferation at the expense of further differentiation.

It is not known how the signals described here contribute to differentiation. Both the cytokines and retinoic acids influence the activity of proteins that regulate gene transcription (see Chapter 10), and so part of the answer must lie in this area of biology. Many transcription factors have been identified at various stages of myeloid differentiation. Current evidence suggests that multiple selective interactions between these factors determine which genes are activated or repressed (Figure 9.20). At an early stage of myeloid differentiation, the model proposes that transcription factors A, B and C are present and form a complex that activates gene 1 and suppresses gene 2. A consequence of gene 1 activation is that C is switched off and D is switched on. The new complex can activate gene 2 and suppress gene 1. This chain reaction would continue until the fully differentiated state was reached; interference with specific transcription would block differentiation at the stage requiring that factor. This model accounts for many features associated with differentiation but identifies neither the genes nor the transcription factors involved; the retinoic acid receptor α (see above) is one of many candidates.

Figure 9.20

Transcription factor rearrangements during differentiation. Each shape is a different transcription factor. (Source: Based on data from Sieweke, M.H. and Graff, T. (1998) *Current Opinion in Genetics and Development*, 8, 545–51. Copyright © 1998. Reproduced with permission of Elsevier.)

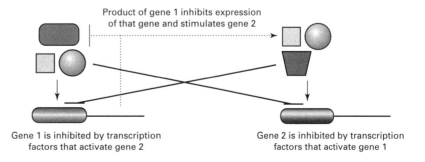

Gene 1 is inhibited by transcription factors that activate gene 2

Product of gene 1 inhibits expression of that gene and stimulates gene 2

Gene 2 is inhibited by transcription factors that activate gene 1

DNA methylation and differentiation

Differentiation involves the coordinated switching on and off of genes specific to the cell type concerned. These changes in gene activity require altered regulation of transcription involving DNA–protein interactions. As commitment to differentiation also necessitates proliferation, those transcriptional alterations must be passed on to the daughter cells. DNA methylation is involved in the process.

Cytosine–guanine (CpG) dinucleotide sequences in DNA can be enzymically methylated at the 5-position of cytosine. Transcription factors will not bind to such methylated sites, and transcription of the gene is therefore diminished. Such methylations on one strand of DNA are passed on to the daughter strand because DNA methylases preferentially act on hemi-methylated DNA (one strand). This method of inheritance is called epigenetic, although it is functionally equivalent to an inactivating mutation. DNA can be demethylated by drugs such as 5-azacytidine, which is incorporated during DNA synthesis, blocks methylase activity and induces differentiation in some cells. Cytosine methylation is inherently mutagenic, because thymine, the product of 5-methylcytosine deamination, is repaired less readily than deaminated cytosine (uracil) (see Chapter 7).

Although DNA methylation provides a mechanism to account for the three requirements of differentiation, altered transcription and inheritance, it is not certain whether its importance is as a causal event or whether it has a secondary role in maintaining the changed phenotype.

If hypermethylation is linked with differentiation, then hypomethylation should be associated with the dedifferentiation occurring during carcinogenesis and progression. The promoter region of the *MAGE* tumour antigen gene is hypomethylated and there is a six-fold decrease in methylation of the α *globin* gene in colorectal cancer as compared with adjacent normal colon. Hypomethylation has also been noted in metastases as compared with primary tumours, suggestive of increased activity of certain genes. Mice in which both **c**ytosine **m**ethyl **t**ransferase (*CMT*) alleles have been lost die during foetal life, and so DNA methylation is required for tissue remodelling and differentiation of individual cell types during that period. Other mice strains have been bred with diminished CMT activity, and they have proved useful in determining biological factors influenced by CMT, particularly in relation to colorectal carcinogenesis. The Min mouse has a germline inactivating mutation in the equivalent of the human *APC* gene that is inactivated in human colorectal carcinogenesis. Min mice mimic humans in that they spontaneously develop multiple intestinal cancers. When Min mice are cross-bred with CMT-deficient animals, the offspring get no intestinal cancers; decreased cytosine methylation switches off carcinogenesis.

Further reading

Proliferation

Bell, S.P. and Dutta, A. (2002) DNA replication in eukaryote cells. *Ann Rev Biochem* **71**, 333–374.
Blagosklonny, M.V. and Pardee, A.B. (2002) The restriction point of the cell cycle. *Cell Cycle* **1**, 103–110.

Bunz, F., Dutriaux, A., Lengauer, C., *et al.* (1998) Requirement for p53 and p21 to sustain G2 arrest after DNA damage. *Science* **282**, 1497–1501.

Chin, L., Pomerantz, J. and DePinho, R.A. (1998) The INK4a/ARF tumour suppressor: one gene–two products–two pathways. *Trends Biochem Sci* **23**, 291–296.

Den Elzen, N. and Pines, J. (2001) Cyclin A is destroyed in prometaphase and can delay chromosome alignment and anaphase. *J Cell Biol* **153**, 121–136.

Jackman, M.R. and Pines, J.N. (1997) Cyclins and the G2/M transition. *Cancer Surv* **29**, 47–73.

Norbury, C.J. (2005) The cancer cell cycle. In *Introduction to the Cellular and Molecular Biology of Cancer*, ed. M. Knowles and P. Selby. Oxford: Oxford University Press.

Apoptosis

Brown, J.M. and Attardi, L.D. (2005) The role of apoptosis in cancer development and treatment response. *Nat Rev Cancer* **5**, 231–237.

Chipuk, J.E., Kuwana, T., Bouchier-Hayes, *et al.* (2004) Direct activation of Bax by p53 mediates mitochondrial membrane permeabilization and apoptosis. *Science* **303**, 1010–1014.

Fennell, D.A. (2005) Apoptosis: molecular physiology and significance for cancer therapeutics. In *Introduction to the Cellular and Molecular Biology of Cancer*, ed. M. Knowles and P. Selby. Oxford: Oxford University Press.

Marsden, V.S., O'Connor, L., O'Reilly, L.A., *et al.* (2002) Apoptosis initiated by Bcl-2-regulated caspase activation of the cytochrome c/Apaf-1/caspase apoptosome. *Nature* **419**, 634–637.

Slee, E.A., O'Connor, D.J. and Lu, X. (2004) To die or not to die: how does p53 decide? *Oncogene* **23**, 2809–2818.

Differentiation

Das, P.M. and Singal, R. (2004) DNA methylation and cancer. *J Clin Oncol* **22**, 4632–4642.

Reya, T., Morrison, S.J., Clarke, M.F. and Weissman, I.L. (2001) Stem cells, cancer and cancer stem cells. *Nature* **414**, 105–111.

Tennen, D.G. (2003) Disruption of differentiation in human cancer: AML shows the way. *Nat Rev Cancer* **3**, 89–101.

Telomerase

Blasco, M.A., Lee, H.W., Hands, M.P., *et al.* (1997) Telomere shortening and tumour formation by mouse cells lacking telomerase RNA. *Cell* **91**, 25–34.

Drayton, S. and Peters, G. (2002) Immortalisation and transformation revisited. *Curr Opin Genet Dev* **12**, 98–104.

Gordon, K.E., Ireland, H., Roberts, M., *et al.* (2003) High levels of telomere dysfunction bestow a selective disadvantage during the progression of human oral squamous cell carcinoma. *Cancer Res* **63**, 458–467.

Newbold, R.F. (2005) Cellular immortalization and telomerase activation in cancer. In *Introduction to the Cellular and Molecular Biology of Cancer*, ed. M. Knowles and P. Selby. Oxford: Oxford University Press.

10 Responding to the environment: growth regulation and signal transduction

KEY POINTS

- Extracellular influences alter cell function via receptor binding and signal transduction to the cell nucleus. The efficiency of this machinery is altered in cancer cells.

- Extracellular signals can be stimulatory (growth factors, hormones) or inhibitory (other cells, extracellular matrix, growth factors, hormones).

- Cancers escape from control by their environment through having (i) decreased sensitivity to inhibitory signals from adjacent cells and the extracellular matrix and (ii) decreased requirement for growth stimulatory factors.

- Endocrine, autocrine and paracrine stimuli are important.

- Polypeptide growth factors have local, autocrine and paracrine effects on multiple cell types.

- Hormones and related low-molecular-weight hydrophobic molecules have endocrine and autocrine actions.

- Cancers can either produce more ligand or become independent of the ligand.

- Signalling pathways use multifunctional proteins at several points to regulate diverse (pleiotropic) functions.

- Cancer cells often alter the functions of these pleiotropic molecules in order to gain a growth advantage.

- Transmembrane receptors alter their conformation in response to extracellular ligands and relay signals to within the cell.

- Membrane receptors can be altered qualitatively or quantitatively in cancer cells.

- Membrane receptors use enzymic (tyrosine kinase, serine/threonine kinase, adenyl cyclase) and non-enzymic methods to transduce signals.

- Protein phosphorylation is used widely to alter protein function.

- Membrane receptors whose intrinsic tyrosine kinase activity is activated by ligands are especially important for growth control.

- Proteins with tyrosine phosphates bind to other proteins with SH domains. This mechanism is used to pass information between proteins.

- Protein phosphatases reverse the effects of protein phosphorylation.

- A cascade of serine/threonine phosphorylations, involving several cellular oncogenes, carries signals to the cell nucleus.

- There is extensive cross-talk between signalling pathways.

- Alterations in *ras* oncogene activity, either by mutation of *ras* or a protein that regulates its function, are common in cancer cells.

- Extracellular low-molecular-weight lipophilic molecules bind and activate intracellular receptors that are gene transcription factors. These receptors can be altered in cancer cells.

- Signals from cell–cell and cell–ECM interactions are transduced by four classes of cell adhesion molecules: integrins, cadherins, selectins and members of the immunoglobulin superfamily. The transmembrane receptors relay signals to the cytoskeleton and the cell nucleus.

- Cell-recognition receptors are altered in cancers.

- Activation of genes coding for growth-regulatory proteins results from all these signalling events. Activation is achieved by altering the phosphorylation status or amount of transcription factor.

General features

Cancer cells attain a degree of autonomy from external regulatory signals that renders them less subject to such signals than normal cells. This autonomy is reflected in a lower requirement for growth-stimulatory molecules such as growth factors and a diminished sensitivity to inhibitory signals provided by adjacent cells and the extracellular matrix (ECM). These stimulatory and inhibitory extracellular stimuli are recognised by receptors and conveyed to the nucleus by complex, multiple pathways with communication (cross-talk) between individual pathways (Figure 10.1). The altered transcriptional activity is directed at obtaining a growth advantage over adjacent cells and is achieved by increasing the efficiency of the intracellular machinery directed at proliferation and by production of secreted growth factors. Additionally, proteases are produced that facilitate invasion (see Chapter 11). The growth factors can modulate functions of the producing cells and functions in the immediate vicinity. This chapter will mainly discuss extranuclear events, nuclear changes having been dealt with in Chapters 5 and 9.

Figure 10.1

Interactions between a cancer cell and its environment.

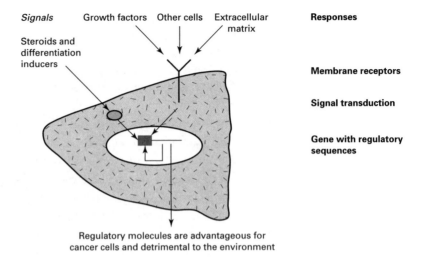

Regulatory molecules are advantageous for cancer cells and detrimental to the environment

Versatility of response pathways

In normal cells, there is a need for versatility and specificity of responses such that different cell types can perform their own specialist functions while utilising common signalling pathways. This is achieved by having key intermediary regulators, usually proteins, common to all cells (Figure 10.2). These *pleiotropic* (multiple-function) proteins receive upstream signals by reaction with one set of proteins and relay the signal by influencing the function of another set of downstream effectors. Specificity is provided by the presence or absence of different upstream and down stream molecules in different cells. This cascade of response pathways between upstream regulators and downstream effectors generates the versatility and specificity required.

Pleiotropic regulation is used at a number of points in the signalling pathway. The *ras* oncogene is one such key intermediate, receiving input signals from extra-cellular molecules via their receptors and transmitting signals to a variety of pathways,

Figure 10.2

Regulation of different functions by one protein (pleiotropic effect).

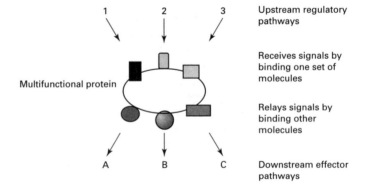

determined by the differentiation status of the particular cell type. Another example is the membrane receptor for epidermal growth factor (EGF). The gene *ErbB1*, also known as an oncogene, codes for a protein that binds either EGF or transforming growth factor alpha (TGF-α) as its upstream regulator, while downstream effectors determine responses via the cytoplasmic tail of the receptor. As some of these effectors are upstream regulators of the ras pathway with its multiplicity of effectors, the potential complexity of responses from a limited number of extracellular signals becomes apparent. In this way, one growth factor can elicit multiple effects in one cell type and different responses in different cell types.

The versatility of response pathways exhibits itself in another way: extensive cross-talk between signalling pathways. In simplistic terms, this means there are many routes by which a single extracellular signal can elicit a given response and whereby different signals synergise to generate a response. Anchorage-dependent growth of normal cells (see Chapter 2) illustrates the latter point, because growth factors will function only if adhesion receptors are also operational; this synergy is lost in many cancer cells.

Oncogenes and protein phosphorylation

The complexity of the signalling pathways makes it difficult to generalise about changes involved in carcinogenesis, but two principles can be identified: (i) the key regulatory proteins are coded for by oncogenes rather than suppressors and (ii) protein phosphorylation is a common method whereby function is altered without requiring *de novo* protein synthesis. Different cancer types use different ways to become autonomous, so that no single change in a gene or signalling pathway predominates. Of the oncogenes involved in signal transduction, *ras* is the one most frequently altered in cancers, but many others are also changed. Examples of proteins involved in both signal transduction and carcinogenesis are given in Table 10.1. They are described in greater detail below, but the point to note here is that several cell compartments are implicated.

Extracellular signals that influence cell growth

Signalling molecules can be large or small and charged or uncharged; to a large extent, their chemical characteristics determine the choice of signal transduction pathway (see Figure 10.1). The large molecules are polypeptides (growth factors) or proteins (membranes of other cells, extracellular matrix), with polysaccharides providing important post-translational modifications, such as extracellular matrix proteins, in some cases. Extracellular polypeptides and proteins act via cell-membrane receptors whose signals must be transduced to the nucleus by intermediary events involving processes as diverse as protein–protein interactions, cytoskeletal changes and movement of macromolecules within intracellular compartments.

Low-molecular-weight lipid-soluble regulators such as steroid hormones and retinoic acid readily traverse the cell membrane and bind to intracellular receptors that are gene transcription factors.

Table 10.1 Signal transduction molecules that are influential in cancers.

Type of molecule	Function
Growth factor	
EGF, IGF	Mitogenic
TGF-β	Inhibits proliferation
	Chemotaxis
	Promotes differentiation
Growth factor receptor	
EGF and IGF receptors	Tyrosine kinase
TGF-β receptor	Serine kinase
Cell recognition	
Integrins	Cytoskeleton
Cadherins	Cell contacts
Signal transduction	
ras	GTP binding
raf	Serine kinase
Transcription factor	
fos, jun, myc	Early replication genes
Oestrogen receptor	Mitogenic
Retinoic acid receptors	Differentiation

EGF, epidermal growth factor; IGF, insulin-like growth factor; TGF-β, transforming growth factor β.

Endocrine, autocrine and paracrine regulation

Extracellular signals can be categorised according to the source of the signal (Figure 10.3). *Endocrine* control involves hormones transported in the bloodstream from producing glands, whereas the other two processes refer to molecules produced locally, either from the same cell (*autocrine*) or from different cells (*paracrine*).

Figure 10.3

Types of extracellular signal.

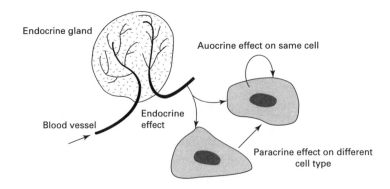

Endocrine gland

Auocrine effect on same cell

Blood vessel

Endocrine effect

Paracrine effect on different cell type

Some transmembrane proteins interact with receptors on adjacent cells; this is called *juxtacrine* regulation. Each type of signal is important in carcinogenesis.

Three categories of extracellular signal will be described: the polypeptide growth factors, the larger glycoproteins involved in cell interactions with other components of the cell's immediate environment such as the extracellular matrix, and low-molecular-weight hydrophobic molecules.

Growth factors

Tissue-culture work provided the first evidence of the existence of factors specifically affecting cell proliferation. It was found that to foster vigorous cell growth, it was necessary to add serum to the basic medium; serum obviously contained a stimulatory agent. Additionally, it was found that the medium in which either normal or malignant cells had been cultured could contain stimulatory or transforming factors. This led to a search concerned with the isolation and purification of growth factors in serum, conditioned media, body fluids and tissue extracts. The names of the growth factors often reflect details of the historical events associated with their discovery. Thus, **p**latelet-**d**erived **g**rowth **f**actor (PDGF) was first isolated from platelets, although it is now known to be produced by a variety of cell types. Transforming growth factor was first isolated from the medium in which virally transformed cells were grown. Later, this was found to be composed of two components, which became known as **t**ransforming **g**rowth **f**actor **α** (TGF-α) and **t**ransforming **g**rowth **f**actor **β** (TGF-β).

The peptide growth factors are grouped into several families on the basis of similarities in structure and amino acid sequence homology. These are the epidermal growth factor family, the platelet-derived growth factor family, the fibroblast growth factor family, the transforming growth factor β family and the insulin-like growth factor family.

Additionally, there are the haemopoietic growth factors. However, as these are structurally diverse, they do not constitute a family in the sense of the groups given above.

Most growth factors stimulate cell proliferation; additionally, several act as angiogenic factors (see Chapter 11). However, in the case of the TGF-β family, there is a wide variety of responses, including inhibition of proliferation and promotion of differentiation. In the body, growth factors are normally concerned with the regulation of proliferation in tissues and responses of cell populations to environmental change. It follows that disturbance of growth factor function is likely to be important in cancer biology.

Local actions on many cell types

Growth factors are most commonly synthesised and act locally within a tumour, although external endocrine routes are also used by insulin in the pancreas and **i**nsulin-like **g**rowth **f**actor **I** (IGF-I) in the liver. The multiple effects of TGF-β just described indicate that within a tumour, growth factor synthesis and effects are not confined to cancer cells and growth of solid cell collections involves interaction between multiple cell types and with the extracellular matrix. Other examples of multiple effects are provided by PDGF and fibroblast growth factor (FGF). Many tumour cells produce these growth factors, both of which are mitogenic for endothelial cells of blood vessels and for normal stromal cells either surrounding or within a tumour mass. Tumour-stimulated angiogenesis at early stages of growth facilitates transition from the avascular state to the vascular state (see Chapter 2) and is also important during metastatic growth (see Chapter 11). Stromal growth is a common feature of epithelial tumours, due partly to paracrine effects of tumour-produced factors. Thus, breast cancer cells can produce PDGF but they do not have PDGF receptors, whereas the stromal cells are receptor-positive and can respond. The converse situation also occurs, in which stromal cells produce the growth factor (ligand) that binds to a receptor on the neoplastic epithelial cells; a good example is IGF and the IGF2 receptor.

Synthesis

Polypeptide growth factors are synthesised as large precursors, which are cleaved by proteases to give final products whose monomer size varies from 6 kDa (TGF-α) to 12 kDa (PDGF, TGF-β). Each growth factor represents a family of molecules, individual members of which can be produced in a tissue-specific way. Thus, for the insulin family, insulin is synthesised in the pancreas and IGF-I is synthesised in the liver (endocrine action) or locally (autocrine or paracrine action) by many cells. IGF-II on the other hand is produced predominantly by foetal cells, although it has been identified in some cancers (Wilms' tumour, sarcomas).

Cancer

Abnormal production of growth factors by tumours has been identified in several situations. The monkey viral oncogene *v-sis* codes for the B subunit of PDGF, the factor responsible for sarcoma production. People with pituitary tumours that secrete growth hormone have increased serum IGF-I due to the effect of growth hormone on the liver, but other cancers generate local IGF-I changes. Small-cell lung cancers produce the autocrine mitogenic polypeptide **g**astrin-**r**eleasing **p**eptide (GRP), also known as bombesin. Blockading bombesin disrupts tumour growth. Indeed, various agents that block growth factor receptors are being tested as potential treatments for advanced cancer (see Chapter 12). In cancers such as lung and ovary, increased production of the mitogenic growth factor TGF-α is associated with poor survival of the patient.

Increased production of normal growth factor by cancer cells commonly results from altered signal transduction consequent to carcinogenic events (see below). This establishes an autonomous loop between the growth factor and gene transcription that contributes to unregulated growth.

Growth factor receptors

General features

Membrane receptors recognise the growth factor at the external face of the cell membrane and relay the signal to the intracellular side; this is how cells recognise and react to these types of external signal. Ligand binding induces conformational changes in the transmembrane protein, which activate its cytoplasmic tail; the consequences depend on the receptor concerned. Different cell types display characteristic profiles of receptors that determine the response potential of the cell concerned. As receptors recognise only specific types of growth factor, this provides an extra degree of specificity as to which cells will respond to a given signal.

For events as important as proliferation, fine control of on/off signals is essential; this is achieved by ensuring that small changes in ligand concentration maximise signal response. Growth factor receptors have dissociation constants in the 10^{-10} M range, which means that they can respond to concentrations of growth factor in the same low range. Magnitude of response is determined by the law of mass action, such that both ligand and receptor levels determine the end result and are manipulated by cancers to achieve a growth advantage.

Cancers have adopted several stratagems to influence receptor activity, ranging from gene amplification (EGF receptor) to mutations that generate constitutively active molecules (*neu* oncogene). Receptor numbers can also be increased by normal events, as is the case with breast cells in which IGF-I receptors are increased by oestrogens and the cells are therefore more sensitive to a given concentration of ligand. Receptors for inhibitory pathways, such as those for TGF-β, can be inactivated by mutations; this occurs in colorectal cancers and lymphoma.

A receptor is a molecule that binds a ligand and generates a biological response. Other ligand-binding proteins exist that do not directly generate a response and are therefore not receptors. In most cases, such binding proteins provide a means of reversibly inactivating the growth factor. This second category of binding protein usually inactivates the ligand but because of the reversibility of the interaction, the protein-bound ligand can act as a pool of readily available ligand. Several IGF-binding proteins in serum and tissues fall into this category. Sometimes, such protein interaction is important for biological activity of the ligand. Thus, TGF-β is synthesised and secreted in a latent form from which the active polypeptide can be released by low pH or proteases. FGFs bind avidly to heparin-containing proteoglycans of the extracellular matrix, which therefore provide a reservoir of the polypeptide, but additional proteins in the cell membrane may function as a means of recruiting growth factors such as TGF-β and FGF to their receptors. Proteins that do not directly transduce signals but contribute to the overall response are called *type II receptors*; *type I receptors* transduce the signal across the plasma membrane.

Growth factor receptors can be divided into two groups depending on whether tyrosine kinases or serine/threonine kinases mediate immediate post-ligand binding events.

Figure 10.4

Transmembrane
receptors involved in
growth regulation.
The receptors are
dimers in reality.

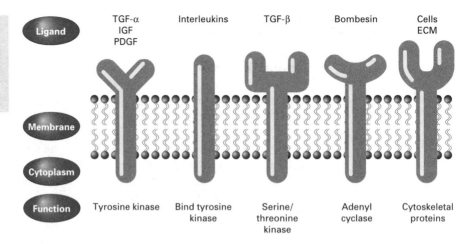

Tyrosine kinase receptors

Proteins modified by phosphorylation of tyrosine residues represent less than 1% of those modified by serine/threonine phosphorylation. The former are involved predominantly in early growth-related events, with subsequent changes in the transduction pathway being dominated by serine/threonine phosphorylations. Although typically involved with membrane events, intracellular tyrosine kinases are also important.

Kinase receptors are divided here into those that contain a tyrosine kinase activity as an integral part of the receptor molecule and those that are inactive in this respect but that can recruit a kinase as a result of ligand binding. The EGF receptor is an example of the first kind and cytokine receptors predominate among the second kind (Figure 10.4).

Receptors with integral kinase activity

Receptors with integral kinase activity have an extracellular ligand-binding domain, a transmembrane region and a multifunctional cytoplasmic tail. The tail has an ATP-binding site plus tyrosine kinase activity capable of phosphorylating itself (autophosphorylation) as well as other proteins. Autophosphorylation of the cytoplasmic face of the receptor generates a docking site for intracellular proteins that provide the next step in the signal transduction route.

The receptors must be in a dimeric form to be active, because the kinase on one chain cannot phosphorylate itself and an interchain phosphorylation is required (Figure 10.5). Different members of the tyrosine kinase receptor family use different methods of achieving dimerisation. TGF-α binds to the EGF receptor in a 1 : 1 ratio; this then dimerises. On the other hand, the IGF-I receptor pre-exists as a dimer and the ligand alters the conformation of the dimer. The PDGF receptor is ligand-dimerised by virtue of the ligand itself being a dimer, each monomer binding to one receptor chain. Members of the EGF receptor family can form functionally important heterodimers with each other. The family contains four subgroups, erbB1

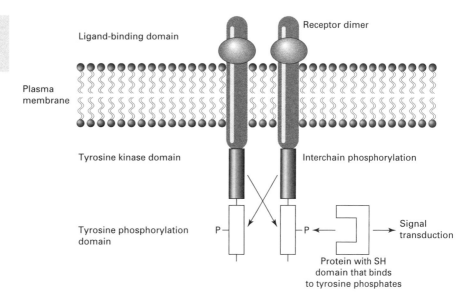

Figure 10.5

Tyrosine kinase receptor signalling.

to erbB4 (**er**ythro**b**lastosis virus protein **B**), each with a distinct ligand specificity. Thus, the EGF receptor (erbB1, HER-1) will bind EGF, TGF-α and amphiregulin polypeptides, whereas erbB2 (HER-2, neu) has no obvious ligands. As ligands activate conformational changes in the receptors, it is important to identify the activating mechanism for erbB2. The EGF receptor achieves this, as growth factor (ligand) binding to the EGF receptor can activate the erbB2 tyrosine kinase pathway by a process called *transmodulation*. A monomer of EGF receptor plus ligand will hetero-dimerise and tyrosine phosphorylate an erbB2 monomer. Tyrosine phosphoryla-tion generates a docking signal for proteins having an **s**rc **h**omology (SH) domain (see below).

Receptors that recruit tyrosine kinases

Transmembrane receptors for cytokines such as interleukins, haematopoietic growth factors (e.g. colony-stimulating factor) and interferons activate tyrosine kinases indir-ectly by ligand–dependent dimerisation and binding of cytoplasmic kinases (Figure 10.6). These **Ja**nus **k**inases (JAKs) – 'Janus' means 'two-faced' – phosphorylate nuclear tran-scription factors called STATs. Additionally, the JAK can phosphorylate the adja-cent chain of the dimerised receptor and activate other mitogenic pathways via ras (see Figure 10.12) and phosphoinositols (see Figure 10.14). This class of receptor is critically important in haemopoiesis, disruption of which can result in leukaemia. This requires coordinate changes in differentiation plus proliferation (see Chapters 2 and 9), each of which is regulated by different regions of the cytoplasmic domain of the cytokine receptor.

Integrins are a second class of receptor that recruit tyrosine kinases. Integrins medi-ate cell–cell and cell–ECM interactions (see below); they activate a **f**ocal **a**dhesion **k**inase (FAK) localised to such points of contact (see Figure 10.17). FAK can be autophosphorylated and bind other proteins, including the tyrosine kinase from the *src* oncogene.

Figure 10.6

Cytokine receptor:
recruitment of a
tyrosine kinase.
Janus kinase (JAK)
phosphorylates
tyrosines on an
adjacent subunit
of the STAT
transcription factor.

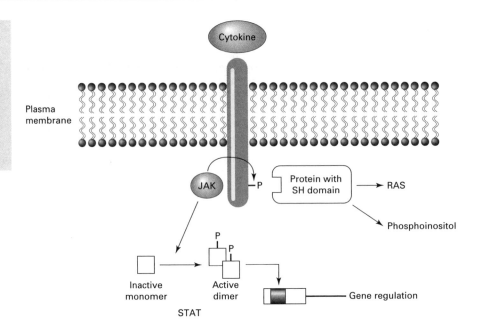

Proteins with domains that bind to tyrosine phosphates

Phosphorylated tyrosines are recognised by amino-acid motifs on other proteins called SH domains. This type of interaction mediates the next step in ligand-induced signal transduction. The amino acids on the C-terminal side of the phosphorylated tyrosine determine the type of SH domain to be recognised, although the whole domain involves a sequence of about 100 amino acids. The type and number of SH domains determine which proteins will bind to the receptor and thereby influence specificity of effect, the other determinant being the presence or absence of the binding protein itself (Figure 10.7). Thus, the PDGF receptor has several autophosphorylation sites capable of binding SH domains of proteins such as src, **p**hosphatidyl **i**nositol **k**inase (PIK), **p**hospho**li**pase **C** (PLC), **GT**Pase-**a**ctivating **p**rotein (GAP) and tyrosine **p**hosphat**ase** (Pase). Depending on the availability of these proteins, several signalling pathways can be activated. PIK is a heterodimer of an 85 kDa adaptor protein that binds to the receptor and a 110 kDa catalytic subunit. PIK contributes to the phosphoinositol pathway and PLC releases diacylglycerol, the natural ligand for protein kinase C (see below). GAP is a bifunctional regulator of ras (see below) and Pase provides a mechanism for inactivating the whole process by hydrolysing the tyrosine phosphates.

The EGF receptor follows a similar pattern, with some SH domains binding similar proteins (PLC) to that of the PDGF receptor and others binding different proteins. The EGF receptor activates ras by a different pathway involving **g**rowth factor-**r**elated **b**inding protein (GRB) (Figure 10.7).

Some SH-containing proteins have their own tyrosine residues capable of phosphorylation by the receptor. GRB becomes tyrosine-phosphorylated and is recognised by the next SH-containing protein in the reaction sequence. Hence, the initial autophosphorylation of the receptor activates a sequence of protein–protein interactions.

Figure 10.7

Signalling events at the cytoplasmic face of tyrosine kinase receptors. Multiple SH domains can dock with tyrosine phosphates on the receptors and activate alternative pathways. The receptors are dimers in reality.

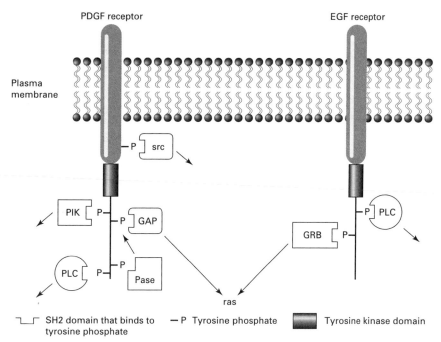

GAP, GTPase-activating protein; GRB, intermediary protein; Pase, protein phosphatase; PLC, phospholipase C; PIK, phosphatidyl inositol 3 kinase; src, tyrosine kinase oncogene.

Protein tyrosine phosphatases

Several tyrosine phosphatases have been characterised that reverse the biological effects of tyrosine phosphorylations. Some of these phosphatases have SH domains; they can therefore bind to tyrosine-phosphorylated sites on receptors and dephosphorylate adjacent sites (Figure 10.7).

Cancer

Tyrosine kinases are altered in many cancers (Table 10.2). Several viral oncogenes code for tyrosine kinases – for example, rat neuroblastoma results from a point mutation in the *neu* oncogene that generates a constitutively active kinase. This mutation changes a valine to a glutamate in the transmembrane domain, which causes the kinase to dimerise in the absence of ligand. In human cancers, tyrosine kinase alterations have been identified at several stages of tumour development. A translocation between chromosomes 5 and 12 activates the PDGF receptor B chain, which is an early event in the development of chronic myelomonocytic leukaemia; this is a different leukaemia from the chronic myeloid leukaemia (CML) described in Chapter 2. Kinase involvement in later stages of carcinogenesis has been identified in several epithelial cancers, although the relationship between kinase activity and stage of carcinogenesis is not always simple. In cervical cancer, EGF receptor activity increases with tumour aggressiveness and mitotic activity; the same is true for lung and ovarian cancers. With each of these examples, increased receptor activity is associated with

Table 10.2 Tyrosine kinases altered in cancers.

Kinase	Function	Cancer
Animal		
neu	Membrane receptor	Rat neuroblastoma
v–kit (virus)	Cytokine receptor	Cat sarcoma
v–src (virus)	Membrane protein	Chicken sarcoma
Human		
EGF receptor	Growth factor receptor	Epithelia
TRK	Growth factor receptor	Thyroid
PDGF receptor	Growth factor receptor	Myeloid leukaemia

EGF, epidermal growth factor; PDGF, platelet-derived growth factor.

decreased likelihood of prolonged survival, which is to be expected given the involvement of these receptors in mitogenic pathways (see below). The picture with breast cancer is more complex; ErbB2 activity increases at early stages of carcinogenesis (well-differentiated *in situ* carcinomas) and then declines and rises again in poorly differentiated invasive cancers. Gene amplification accounts for some but not all cases of higher expression. A chromosome rearrangement in CML results in the production of a fusion protein in which a tyrosine phosphate in one partner (bcr, chromosome 22) binds an SH domain of the other partner (abl, chromosome 9), thereby activating the abl kinase (Figure 10.8). The bcr tyrosine phosphate also spontaneously binds the SH domain of GRB, resulting in ras activation. An additional feature of the bcr–abl fusion is that it alters the intracellular location (nucleus to cytoplasm) of the kinase, which brings it in contact with novel substrates.

Tyrosine kinase inhibitors have been developed and are being used therapeutically in some cancers (see Chapter 12).

Figure 10.8

CML: combined SH domain and tyrosine kinase activation. The chromosome translocation t(9;22) leads to the production of a protein with functions derived from both chromosomes.

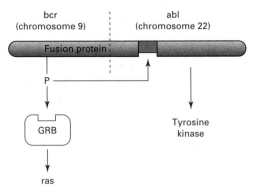

SH domain that binds tyrosine phosphate residues
P Tyrosine phosphate residue
GRB Intermediate docking protein

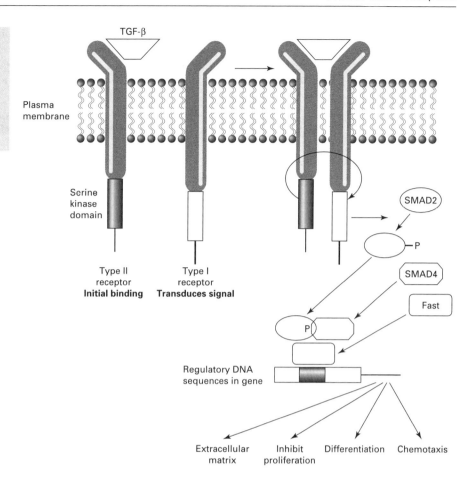

Figure 10.9

TGF-β signalling by serine/threonine phosphorylation. The type II receptor and SMADs 2 and 4 are altered in some cancers.

Receptors that act via serine/threonine kinases

Both stimulatory (phorbol ester) and inhibitory (TGF-β) proliferation signals can be relayed by serine/threonine kinase receptors. The principles are similar to those used by tyrosine kinases, except that the SH domains do not provide the docking mechanism with other proteins.

TGF-β receptor is present in all cells except retinoblastoma cells and thus has widespread functions. These functions can be as varied as inhibition of proliferation, induction of extracellular matrix proteins, chemotaxis and stimulation of another growth factor, such as PDGF. TGF-β initially binds to a type II receptor, which then dimerises with a type I receptor (Figure 10.9). The type II kinase domain phosphorylates and activates the type I kinase domain, which transduces the signal by phosphorylating intracellular proteins of the SMAD family (originally called MAD – **m**others **a**gainst **d**ecapentaplegic). All these phosphorylations are on serine/threonine. Phosphorylation of cytoplasmic SMAD1 or SMAD2 promotes nuclear entry and heterodimerisation with another family member, SMAD4. This oligomeric complex will not bind to specific DNA sequences in regulatory regions of genes until joined by a third protein, Fast. Genes activated directly via this pathway are involved in extracellular matrix production (collagen), inhibition of proliferation (the cyclin-dependent kinase inhibitor p21, transcription factor jun), metastasis (plasminogen activator inhibitor) and differentiation (bone formation). Indirectly, genes requiring the **CREB-b**inding **p**rotein (CBP) coactivator are also inhibited because CBP binds with SMAD2 and SMAD4, and so it is not available to activate those other genes (see below).

The membrane-bound protein kinase C is normally activated by diacylglycerol, but the tumour promotor phorbol ester is also an effective ligand.

Serine/threonine phosphatases

Serine/threonine phosphatases reverse the phosphorylation effects. Several have been identified, with different substrate specificities.

Cancer

Various components of the TGF-β signalling pathway can be altered in different cancers. The gene coding for the type II receptor contains dinucleotide repeats analogous to those occuring in microsatellites and that are therefore sensitive to DNA mismatch repair defects (see Chapters 7 and 8). Hence, colorectal cancers with such defects sometimes contain truncated inactive type II receptors. Missense mutations in type II receptors have also been detected in T-cell lymphomas and head and neck cancers. SMAD mutations are more frequent, with SMAD4 being inactivated in some cancers of the pancreas, colon, breast, ovary and lung; SMAD2 function is lost in colorectal cancers. The net result of these changes is loss of differentiation, increased proliferation and altered cell adhesion. In mice, type I and type II receptors are normally expressed in the luminal (upper) region of colon crypts, where differentiation occurs. Mice with homozygous knock-out deletions of SMAD3 have a high incidence of invasive colorectal cancers, but up to now no SMAD3 mutations have been detected in humans. These facts about SMADs provide an interesting example of how changes in our understanding of molecular events can alter previously held concepts. In colorectal carcinogenesis, the DCC suppressor gene was originally detected as a deletion by its **l**oss **of h**eterozygocity (LOH) and was said to code for a cell-adhesion molecule. It was later identified as a receptor (semaphorin) for extracellular chemotactic peptides (netrins) involved in cell migration. It is now known that the LOH at chromosome 18q (see Table 2.1) also applied to the SMAD4 gene adjacent to the gene for the netrin receptor. SMAD was identified as the relevant gene for colorectal carcinogenesis by experiments with knock-out mice; homozygous deletions of the SMAD gene resulted in colorectal cancers whereas DCC-deleted mice remained cancer-free.

Adenyl cyclase-linked receptors

Adenyl cyclase-linked receptors have a single protein chain that loops across the membrane seven times and a cytoplasmic domain that interacts with two regulatory proteins to form the active adenyl cyclase complex (Figure 10.10). Ligand binding activates the adenyl cyclase and increases intracellular cyclic AMP formation from ATP. This type of receptor is used by polypeptides such as hypothalamic **go**nadotrophin-**r**eleasing **h**ormone (GnRH), whose normal function is to regulate pituitary secretion of

Figure 10.10

Pathways activated by adenyl cyclase-linked receptors.

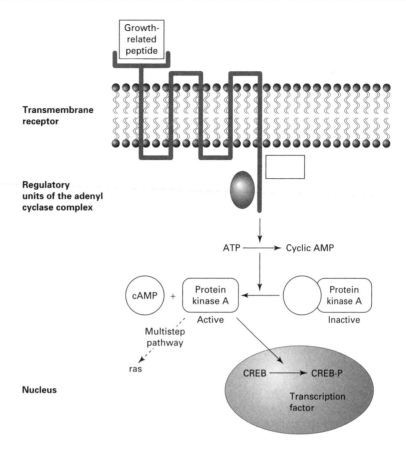

gonadotrophins, which modulate ovarian and testicular steroid hormone production. These hormones have major causal influences on the development of breast and prostate cancer. Additionally, GnRH receptors have been identified on tumour cells, and their growth is influenced by the appropriate ligands. Synthetic ligands of this type are used in the treatment of hormone-sensitive cancers (see Chapter 12). GRP, a growth-related mitogen secreted by certain lung tumours, also uses an adenyl cyclase receptor.

Cyclic AMP binds to and dissociates a dimeric cytoplasmic complex made up of a cyclic AMP-binding protein and serine/threonine **p**rotein **k**inase **A** (PKA). On translocation to the nucleus, PKA phosphorylates and activates the transcription factor **c**yclic AMP **r**esponse **e**lement **b**inding protein (CREB) (Figure 10.10).

Growth factors: from membrane to nucleus

General features

The multiple pathways used by tyrosine and serine kinase receptors to convey their signals are dominated by one feature: a cascade of serine/threonine phosphorylations that alter the functional activities of the proteins involved. These phosphorylations can be reversed by protein phosphatases.

The events involved in this series of reactions are also characterised by a versatility achieved by divergence and convergence of pathways, which goes some way towards explaining how messages from different initial signals converge on a common route and how different cell types can respond in cell-specific ways to a common signal (see Figure 10.2). The *ras* oncogene acts as one of the pleiotropic modulators capable of redirecting input signals from the receptors to alternative pathways.

The end result of this cascade is transcriptional activation achieved by altering either the amount or the functional activity of transcription factors (see Figure 10.1). Several such factors are involved, but *c-fos* and *c-jun* have been particularly well studied. These were originally identified as viral oncogenes that activate growth-related genes. Increasing the amount of protein upregulates c-fos, whereas serine/threonine phosphorylation and dephosphorylation of c-jun are its main activating events. The c-fos and c-jun proteins form a heterodimer that binds to regulatory DNA base sequences (AP1 sites) of genes coding for proliferation-related proteins.

The checkpoints that regulate the cell cycle (see Chapter 9) are the main focus of this sequence of changes, with the G_1 checkpoint being particularly involved. The suppressor activity of Rb is exerted at this focal point and it is inactivated by serine/threonine phosphorylation (see Chapters 5 and 9) resulting from the events described here.

Although regulating proliferation is an important feature of kinase receptor activation, other cell functions such as the cytoskeletal arrangement, apoptosis, invasion and metastasis are also affected.

The ras GTP-binding protein

Normal function

The 21 kDa GTP-binding protein that is attached to the cytoplasmic face of the cell membrane receives input signals from several pathways and relays them to an equally diverse set of effectors (Figure 10.11). Its molecular details were described earlier (see Figure 5.6). Ras is active when bound to GTP and inactive when bound to GDP. The intrinsic GTPase activity of the protein mediates the inactivation step, but an additional protein, GAP, is needed for this process. Activation involves exchanging GDP for GTP, which requires the exchange protein SOS (**s**on **o**f **s**evenless). Input signals from PDGF modulate the activity of GAP in a poorly understood way. GAP is usually described as an inhibitor of ras activation, and so its designation as an activator in conjunction with PDGF is confusing. It is postulated that GAP has two separate functions with opposing effects. IGF and TGF-α/EGF growth factors increase SOS function via an intermediary protein, GRB (see Figure 10.7). The protein–protein complexes required for this set of events involve SH domain interactions.

Ras is synthesised as a precursor with a C-terminal CAAX motif (C = cysteine, A = aliphatic amino acid, X = variable) that loses its three C-terminal amino acids by proteolysis. This leaves a cysteine as the terminal amino acid, which is modified by attachment of a hydrophobic chain (prenylation is the general term), which

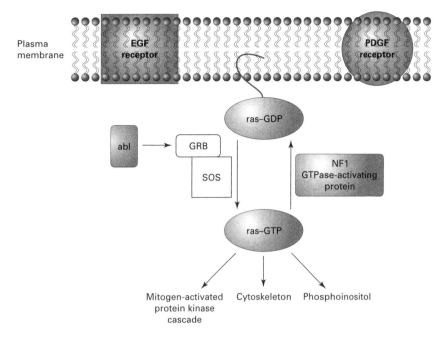

Figure 10.11

Ras regulators and their mutations. Tinted symbols are proteins that can be altered in cancer cells.

abl, tyrosine kinase; GRB, intermediate docking protein; NF1, serves the same function as GAP in some cells; SOS, GTP exchange protein; ⌇, isoprenyl group that links ras to the membrane.

facilitates attachment of ras to the inner wall of the cell membrane (Figure 10.11). Prenylation and membrane insertion are essential for ras activity. The carboxyl of the terminal cysteine is then methylated. The hydrophobic chain is usually a 15-carbon isoprenyl (farnesyl) group, but sometimes a 20-carbon geranylgeranyl chain can be substituted. The main enzyme responsible for farnesyl modification, farnesyl diphosphate protein transferase (farnesyl transferase), is much more active than the equivalent geranylgeranyl transferase, which accounts for the predominance of the farnesyl reaction. These events are discussed in more detail in Chapter 12 as they are targets for new types of drug therapy.

Downstream effectors include phosphoinositols, cytoskeletal proteins and raf, a serine/threonine kinase (Figure 10.11). Two members of the ras superfamily of GTP-binding proteins, rho and rac, modulate actin polymerisation and therefore affect the cytoskeleton (see Figure 10.14). Hence, the ras family of proteins provides a route whereby proliferation and cytoskeletal changes can be coordinately linked.

As far as proliferation is concerned, the most important consequence of ras activation is its attachment to raf, a cytoplasmic serine/threonine kinase, thus recruiting it to the cell membrane, where it effects the next step in the response cascade (see below).

Altered function in cancer cells

The *ras* gene is mutated in about 40% of all human cancers, although mutations can be as high as 90% in pancreatic cancer. In addition to these data, experimental

Table 10.3 Mutations in human myeloid leukaemia (ML) that activate ras.

Gene	Type of change	Function	Leukaemia
Ras	Point mutations	GTPase lost	Acute ML
PDGF receptor	Chromosome translocation t(5;12)	GTP binding prolonged	Chronic mono-ML
Abl	Chromosome translocation t(9;22)	GTP binding prolonged	Chronic ML
NF1	Inactivation	GTPase lost	Childhood chronic ML

(Source: Based on data from Sawyers, C.L. and Denny, C.T. (1994) *Cell*, 77, 171–73. Copyright © 1994. Reproduced with permission of Elsevier.)

evidence from transfection studies, transgenic mice and site-directed mutagenesis indicate that the carcinogenic mutations destroy the GTPase activity of ras and it is therefore maintained in an active GTP-bound form. Molecular details of the *ras* mutations are detailed elsewhere (see Figure 5.5 and Table 5.4). Different *ras* alleles are activated in different cancers – *K-ras* in most cancers, *H-ras* in colorectal and head and neck cancers. Some cancers have normal ras but alterations in other molecules that influence its function. Genes that are mutated in human cancers and that code for proteins that influence ras function have been designated in Figure 10.11. In addition to the tyrosine kinase receptor mutations described above, some cells contain NF1, a protein that has similar actions to those of GAP. Defects in NF1 increase the risk of sarcomas and childhood chronic myeloid leukaemia (CML) due to loss of its GTPase-activating potential. This effectively maintains ras in a GTP-bound state. NF1 therefore has the properties of a suppressor protein.

The varied ways in which cancers can alter one regulatory pathway are illustrated by changes in ras in myeloid leukaermias (Table 10.3). Blocked differentiation of myeloid cells in these leukaemias can result from the disruption of ras itself or indirectly by altering ancillary proteins. NF1 inactivation decreases GTP hydrolysis, while PDGF receptor activation prolongs GTP binding. In CML, increased GTP–ras results from elevated GTP exchange (see Figures 10.8 and 10.11). It is not clear why ras activation by different mechanisms should generate different types of myeloid leukaemia.

Raf and the MAP kinase cascade

GTP–ras will bind raf and translocate it from the cytoplasm to the plasma membrane (Figure 10.12). The serine kinase activity of raf is normally inhibited by sequences at the N-terminal of the protein. When GTP–ras binds to this N-terminal sequence, inhibition is lost and the raf kinase becomes functional. Raf was originally identified as a viral oncogene in which the inhibitory sequences were lost and the serine kinase was constitutively active.

Raf is the first of a series of kinases that activate subsequent members of a cascade, culminating in the phosphorylation of transcription factor c-jun. The general term for these kinases is **m**itogen-**a**ctivated **p**rotein kinase (MAP kinase), so named because it is activated (phosphorylated) by many mitogens, such as the polypeptide

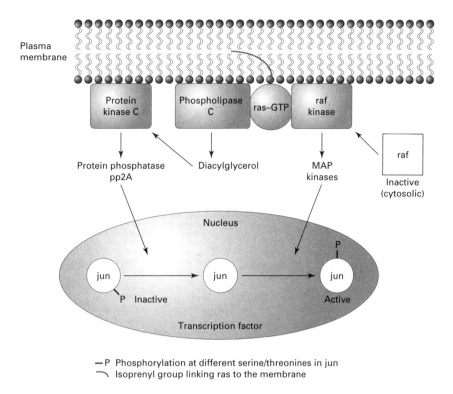

Figure 10.12

Ras activation of jun transcription factor.

—P Phosphorylation at different serine/threonines in jun

⌒ Isoprenyl group linking ras to the membrane

growth factors, serum, phorbol esters and hormones. Individual members of the MAP kinase cascade include, in order of activation, raf (MAP kinase kinase kinase), MEK (MAP kinase kinase) and ERK (**e**xtracellular signal-**r**elated **k**inase, MAP kinase). ERK phosphorylates the ELK transcription factor needed for fos induction (see below). Ionising radiations and free radicals (see Chapter 6) alter serine/threonine protein kinase activity. These **s**tress-**a**ctivated **p**rotein **k**inases (SAPKs) such as JNK are included within the general category of MAP kinases.

Signalling molecules derived from phosphoinositol

Cell membranes contain **p**hospha**t**i**d**yl **in**ositol (PtdIn) lipids made up of inositol linked by a phosphate to glycerol esterified with a long-chain saturated fatty acid and an unsaturated (four double bonds) fatty acid, arachidonic acid (Figure 10.13). Separate **Pt**In **k**inases (PIKs) 3, 4 and 5 add additional phosphate to the inositol moiety. **P**hospho**l**ipase **C** (PLC) releases these phosphoinositols, together with **di**a**c**yl**g**lycerol (DAG), the activator of protein kinase C (see Figure 10.12). Phospholipase A2 can release arachidonic acid from PtdIns to serve as a substrate for prostaglandin and ceramide synthesis (see Figure 10.22). Thus, through these hydrolytic and phosphorylation reactions, phosphatidyl inositol can generate three sets of secondary messengers – DAG, arachidonic acid and phosphoinositols – each of which can influence a spectrum of intracellular pathways.

187

Figure 10.13

Phosphatidyl inositol metabolism.

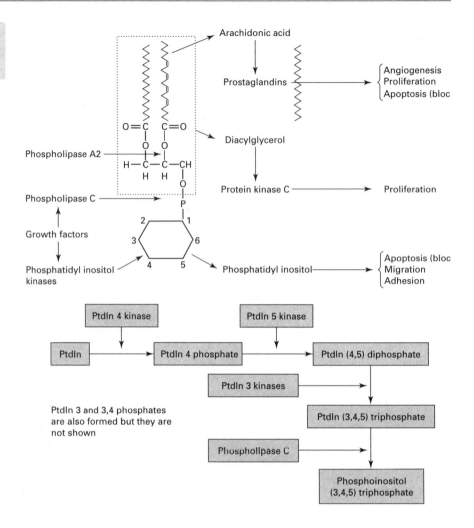

Of the PIKs, the 3-kinase family, referred to here as PIK3, is particularly important in influencing cancer-related events (Figure 10.14). PIK3 is made up of an 85 kDa adaptor subunit with an SH domain and a 100 kDa catalytic subunit. The SH domain binds to tyrosine phosphates on tyrosine kinase receptors (see Figure 10.7). PIK3 can also interact with adenyl cyclase receptors (via GTP-binding adaptors) and possibly with GTP–ras. PIK3 is activated by these interactions and increases the intracellular concentrations of rate-limiting PtdIns; PtdIn (4,5) diphosphate and PtdIn (3,4,5) triphosphate are likely to be the more important compounds that activate downstream events. The PtdIns are inactivated by phosphatases. PtdIns bind to and activate proteins with lipophilic **p**leckstrin **h**omology (PH) domains that include serine/threonine kinases, such as Akt (protein kinase B), p70 and protein kinase C. Akt phosphorylates the pro-apoptotic protein Bad. In its unphosphorylated form, this protein binds and inactivates the anti-apoptotic protein Bcl2 (see Chapter 9), thus activating apoptosis. Phosphorylation of Bad releases Bcl2, thereby inhibiting apoptosis (see Figure 9.16). Phosphorylated Bad is sequestered in the cytoplasm

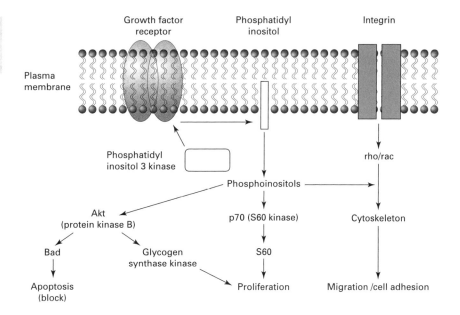

Figure 10.14

Effects of phosphoinositols.

as a heterodimer with the strangely named 14-3-3 protein. Akt also phosphorylates **g**lycogen **s**ynthase **k**inase (GSK), which activates several proteins involved in regulating cell proliferation. p70 phosphorylates a ribosomal protein (S6) that helps regulate the G_1 checkpoint of the cell cycle (see Figure 9.2). The way in which phosphoinositols influence migration is less clear, but they function downstream of integrins and rho/rac (Figure 10.14).

Adhesion of cells to the extracellular matrix also promotes survival by blocking apoptosis via the ras/phosphoinositol/Akt pathway. Activated forms of ras keep this pathway open, which represents a major contribution to the phenomenon of anchorage independence (see Chapter 2).

Nuclear events stimulated by growth factors

The net result of the kinase cascade is altered activity of transcription factors, such as fos and jun, which, in dimeric form, bind to specific DNA base sequences called response elements in the regulatory regions of growth-related genes (see Figure 5.1). A particularly important example of such an element is the AP1 site that binds AP1 protein complexes made up of dimeric complexes of the fos and jun families (Figure 10.15). Each of these oncogenes can be regulated independently by the events described in the preceding section.

Activation of jun involves two ras-related pathways (see Figure 10.12). The activating serine/threonine phosphorylation of jun is mediated by the MAP kinase route, but a different, inhibitory phosphate must be removed first by a protein phosphatase 2A, which is itself activated by a PKC phosphorylation. Thus, activation of jun is accomplished by post-translational phosphorylations but fos is regulated

Figure 10.15

Gene regulation via transcription factors affected by MAP kinases.

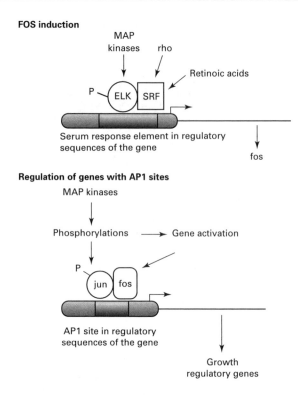

transcriptionally. The promotor region of this gene has several regulatory sites; one is the **s**erum **r**esponse **e**lement (SRE) (Figure 10.15), so called because the growth factors present in serum exert their effects via these DNA base sequences. The SRE binds a dimeric complex made up of one ubiquitous transcription factor, **s**erum **r**esponse **f**actor (SRF), and another, ELK, that is active only when it is serine/threonine-phosphorylated. This activating phosphorylation occurs via the MAP kinase route.

Proteins additional to ELK and SRF are required to form the active transcription complex; these **t**ernary **c**omplex **f**actors (TCFs) include additional serine/threonine kinase such as **j**un **N**-terminal **k**inase (JNK) and the coactivator **CREB**-**b**inding **p**rotein (CBP). Transcription of fos can be altered rapidly by lipophilic factors such as retinoic acid and vitamin D, which induce differentiation; response elements for their nuclear receptors (see below) are present in the regulatory sequences of the *fos* gene. SRF can also be activated indirectly by the GTP-binding proteins rho and rac. Details are sparse, but histone acetylation is important and gene transcription may be stimulated via structural changes in the chromatin. Existence of the rho/rac pathway means that cell adhesions can influence fos transcription (see below). Growth factors that increase proliferation also inhibit apoptosis (see Chapter 9); this inhibition is mediated via phosphoinositol pathways (see Figure 10.14).

There are several MAP kinase signalling pathways, which respond to different external signals. The growth-factor-responsive pathway has been described above; another MAP kinase pathway is activated poorly by growth factors but is sensitive to stress such as low oxygen levels (hypoxia). These kinases, exemplified by JNK,

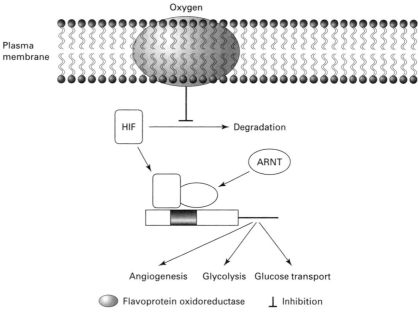

Figure 10.16

Hypoxia and gene transcription.

ARNT, aryl hydrocarbon receptor nuclear transfer factor; HIF, hypoxia-induced factor.

are called **s**tress-**a**ctivated **p**rotein **k**inases (SAPKs). It is not clear how the various kinases are assembled so as to respond to these different stimuli. A multiprotein scaffold may exist to which kinases can be attached and spatially organised so as to confer specificity of response; putative scaffold proteins such as **j**un N-terminal kinase **i**nteracting **p**rotein (JIP) and **MAP** kinase **i**nteracting protein (MPI) have been identified. The oxygen-sensing mechanism involves a flavoprotein oxidoreductase, with the oxygen tension determining whether the flavin cofactor is in an oxidised or reduced state. Another pathway influenced by low oxygen tension is gene activation by **h**ypoxia-**i**nduced transcription **f**actor (HIF) (Figure 10.16). Details are sparse but involve post-transcriptional stabilisation of HIF. This increases HIF concentration and the protein heterodimerises with **ar**yl hydrocarbon **n**uclear **t**ransporter (ARNT), which activates genes with the appropriate enhancer sequences. Additional hypoxia-sensitive HIF-independent mechanisms exist that stabilise mRNAs transcribed from these genes, such as for vascular endothelial growth factor (see Chapter 11). This can activate angiogenesis (see Chapter 11), anaerobic glycolysis and glucose transport. All of these responses help the cell to survive in a low-oxygen environment.

Oncogenic forms of both *fos* and *jun* have been identified in virus-infected cells. They are usually expressed constitutively under the influence of the viral promoter, but additional deletions in the 3′ untranslated region of the mRNA increase its half-life. Although regulation of *fos* and *jun* is important in human cells, gene defects have not been identified in human cancers.

Another set of DNA bases present in regulatory genes bind proteins phosphorylated by the cyclic AMP/PKA pathway (see Figure 10.10). TGF-β signalling via SMAD and Fast transcription factors (see Figure 10.9) was described earlier.

Cell adhesion molecules

Figure 10.17

Cell adhesion molecules and their functions. Homo = same cell type; hetero = different cell types.

Cancers differ from benign growths in their ability to invade surrounding tissues and metastasise to other parts of the body. For epithelial cancers, this involves breaking links with adjacent epithelial cells, migration through the **e**xtra**c**ellular glycoprotein **m**atrix (ECM) and invasion of blood vessels (see Chapter 11). The **c**ell **a**dhesion **m**olecules involved are called CAMs. These varied functions require the recognition of proteins on other cells and the ECM. The changes in recognition patterns that occur during carcinogenesis cannot be defined in simple terms of increased or decreased activity because of the complexity of the processes involved. For example, cell migration as a factor in metastasis requires alternate attachment and detachment of the cell to the ECM so that retention of recognition mechanisms is essential. On the other hand, invasive epithelial cancer cells must lose their attachment to other epithelial cells and to the basement membrane. The one generalisation that can be made is that cancer cells have a different profile of receptors from their normal counterparts.

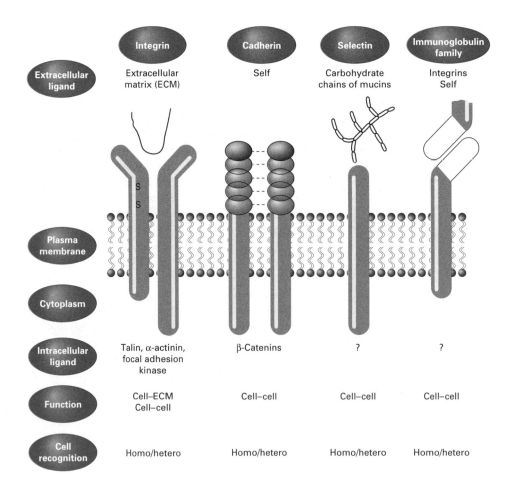

The ability to recognise similar (*homotypic*) or dissimilar (*heterotypic*) cell types or ECM proteins such as collagen, fibronectin and laminin is mediated by four classes of membrane receptor: integrins, cadherins, immunoglobulin family and selectins (Figure 10.17). Additional membrane glycoproteins include syndecans and CD44. These CAMs are, in effect, membrane receptors whose extracellular domains bind ligands that generate conformational changes in the cytoplasmic tail, enabling it to bind specific cytoplasmic proteins. These adaptor molecules link with various signalling pathways that influence cell proliferation, migration, differentiation and apoptosis. Changes in the cytoskeleton (Box 10.1) are of special importance for these events. Anchorage-independent growth in culture is a hallmark of cancer cells (see Chapter 2). This property confers a selective advantage on the cancer cells because they become less dependent on their environment; for a solid tissue, the 'environment' means the surrounding ECM and other cells.

| Box 10.1 | **How a cell interacts with its environment** |

General

Within a tissue, cells interact with other cells of the same (homophilic) or different (heterophilic) types as well as with the glycoproteins and proteoglycans of the ECM. These interactions are mediated by transmembrane glycoprotein CAMs. There are four CAM families: integrins, cadherins, selectins and immunoglobulin-like proteins (see text for details). Additional membrane components include syndecans and the **c**luster of **d**ifferentiation protein CD44. The ECM glycoproteins include several types of collagen, laminin, fibronectin, vitronectin and thrombospondin.

Glycoproteins have various carbohydrate chains covalently attached to the protein through either the −OH of serines and threonines (O-linked) or the −NH$_2$ of asparagine (N-linked). Additional modifications can include sulphations and phosphorylations. Proteoglycans have a core protein with glycosaminoglycan side chains made up of disaccharide repeats of two different sugars (usually hexuronate and hexosamine); tyrosine −OH groups may be sulphated. Important proteoglycans include heparin (heparin sulphate) and chrondroitin sulphate.

CAMs are transmembrane proteins whose external domains function as receptors for ligands that can be ECM proteins or CAMs on other cells. CAMs on other cells can create a terminology problem in deciding which CAM is the receptor and which is the ligand. The term 'counter-receptor' is sometimes used to overcome the problem. The cytoplasmic domain interacts with cytoplasmic proteins that transmit (transduce) the extracellular signals to the cell's interior. This process can also function in reverse, with intracellular signals being transmitted to the exterior.

▶

Intracellular structures

Cells contain networks of polymerised proteins that provide both elasticity and rigidity when required. This cytoskeleton is composed primarily of three such networks, each identified by one of its major proteins: the actin cytoskeleton, the tubulin microfilaments, and intermediate filaments containing cytokeratins (epithelia) or vimentin (other cell types). The actin cytoskeleton, in conjunction with the motor protein myosin and associated proteins, provides contractile structures essential for cell migration and shape. Through ancillary proteins such as talin and α-actinin, the actin cytoskeleton is linked to integrin-containing focal adhesions. Microtubules also polymerise/depolymerise and contribute to the polarity of epithelial cells. Microtubules emanate from a cytoplasmic structure, the centrosome, within which is the centriole. The centriole divides before mitosis and provides an anchorage point in each potential daughter cell for microtubules. These tubulin-containing filaments are linked to individual chromosomes, and so filament contraction retracts each complement of chromosomes into the daughter cells. This retraction requires tubulin depolymerisation; drugs used in cancer treatment can prevent this by stabilising (taxol) or destabilising (vinca alkaloids) the microtubules (see Chapter 12). Intermediate filaments provide the cell with mechanical stability. There are many members of the cytokeratin family: cytokeratins in epithelia, vimentin in other cells and lamin in nuclei. Each type of epithelial cell has a characteristic pattern of cytokeratin expression, which can be used for diagnostic purposes in determining origins of cells in cancers.

Cell junctions

Epithelial cells have several junctional complexes. Those involved in cell–cell contacts include tight (occluding) junctions, gap junctions and desmosomes, all of which can be detected by light microscopy, as well as more diffuse contacts. Cell–ECM interactions are mediated by hemidesmosomes, focal adhesions and other non-junctional contacts. All of these interactions must be perturbed in order that cancerous epithelial cells can escape their immediate environment, invade the surrounding tissue and metastasise to remote parts of the body. Each type of junction contains CAMs characteristic of that junction. Cadherins occur in desmosomes and diffuse contacts; integrins occur in hemidesmosomes, focal contacts and elsewhere; the immunoglobulin family and selectins are linked with non-junctional interactions. Non-epithelial cells have different arrangements of macromolecules, but the CAMs involved have similar mechanistic properties (see text for details). The membrane CAMs interact with the cytoskeleton through adaptor proteins. The nature of these proteins is determined by the CAMs and the cytoskeletal components involved.

Cell migration

Cell migration occurs on the ECM. The front end of the cell extends and attaches to the ECM. This is followed by cell contraction and release at the rear end. The process is then repeated. The intracellular processes are centred on the cytoskeleton, linking through integrins in the plasma membrane (focal adhesions) to the ECM. The on signal for integrin–ECM attachment includes ligand (ECM) interaction, protein phosphorylations and integrin clustering. The off signal involves the internal forces generated by the cytoskeleton and dephosphorylation of focal adhesion proteins. The actin plus myosin cytoskeleton generates the necessary contractile forces. GTP binding proteins such as rho and rac are needed to mediate integrin–actin cytoskeleton linkage.

Extracellular matrix

In this book, the ECM can be considered as two structural entities: the basement membrane and the extracellular stroma. The basement membrane is a distinct structure surrounding collections of epithelial cells and composed of glycoproteins such as collagen IV, laminin, fibronectin, proteoglycans and other proteins. It provides a structural framework on which epithelial cells can function, but it is also involved in bidirectional signalling between epithelium and stroma. The basement membrane is composed of a basal lamina containing the aforementioned components adjacent to the epithelium and a reticular lamina of other collagen types and proteoglycans. The extracellular stroma is a heterogeneous mixture of proteoglycans and glycoproteins.

Some of these properties are due to indirect interactions between growth factor receptors and CAMs. Thus, the effects of liganded growth factor receptors, such as those for EGF or PDGF in normal cells, necessitate the occupancy of CAMs by ECM molecules. In the absence of such occupancy, growth factor binds to its receptor but the mitogenic signal is not transduced to the nucleus; proliferation is blocked at the G_1 checkpoint of the cell cycle (see Chapter 9). Anchorage independence reflects CAM changes that allow the mitogenic signals to reach the nucleus. However, signalling by CAMs is a bidirectional process, and so it can also be viewed as a mechanism that translates genetic information into a three-dimensional pattern of cells in tissues; a major feature of cancer is the disruption of that pattern (see Chapter 3). During normal embryogenesis, considerable cell migration occurs, involving contractile changes in the cytoskeleton directed by components of the ECM. Although cell migration is diminished in adult life, it is regained by cancer cells when they become invasive and metastasise. Again, the migratory property of cancer cells is related to CAM and ECM changes. Cell migration is also important in the formation of new blood capillaries around cancers (see Chapter 11).

Integrins

Integrins promote the assembly of protein complexes containing cytoskeletal elements in response to ligands provided by the ECM or other cells. Tyrosine phosphorylations are required for the formation of those complexes.

This class of receptor is composed of one α and one β protein chain, both of which contribute to ligand binding. At least 15 α and 9 β chains have been identified; it is the combination of different α and β chains that determines ligand specificity, with divalent metal ions such as Ca^{2+} and Mg^{2+} acting as a bridge between the α subunit and the ligand. Table 10.4 provides some examples of ligand specificities of various integrins. Arginine–glycine–aspartate (RGD) motifs commonly but not universally form part of the ECM binding domain. Thus, $\alpha_V\beta_3$ favours an asparagine.proline.any amino acid.tyrosine (NPXY) sequence in its ligands. This ubiquitous integrin interacts with a broad range of ligands, enabling it to signal in many different environments. Although ECM molecules predominate in the list of ligands, other CAMs and extracellular proteins (metalloproteinases) also participate. Functions of those integrins linked with metastasis and angiogenesis are described in Chapter 11.

Ligand binding initially causes clustering of several integrins, which increases the overall strength of cell attachment to the ECM. Structural changes in the cytoplasmic domain of the integrin β subunit, including serine/threonine phosphorylations, facilitate its interaction with proteins such as talin, **f**ocal **a**dhesion **k**inase (FAK) and α-actinin, which transduce signals to intracellular processes (Figure 10.18). In unliganded integrins, the α-subunit blocks the binding sites on the β-subunit for these cytoplasmic proteins; ligand binding relieves that inhibition. FAK can tyrosine phosphorylate some of the attached proteins as well as itself, and these phosphorylations are essential for signal transduction. Those signals promote cell migration, stimulate proliferation and inhibit apoptosis.

Effects on proliferation involve the ras, PLC (see Figure 10.12) and phosphoinositol (see Figure 10.14) pathways. Integrin–ECM interaction recruits FAK, which activates GTP-binding proteins, ras, rho and rac. Ras stimulates cell proliferation via

Table 10.4 Integrin specificity: changes relevant to cancer.

Integrin	Ligand	Function
$\alpha_2\beta_1$	Laminin, collagen	Lost in anchorage-independent cells, lost in breast cancer
$\alpha_3\beta_1$	Laminin, collagen, fibronectin	High in some metastases
$\alpha_4\beta_1$	V-CAM, fibronectin	Arrest of cells in capillaries
$\alpha_5\beta_1$	Fibronectin	Angiogenesis, extravasation of cells from capillaries
$\alpha_6\beta_1$ or $\alpha_6\beta_4$	Laminin	High in cancers of bladder, lung, colon
$\alpha_V\beta_3$	Most ECM proteins Matrix metalloproteinase-2	High in metastatic melanoma, angiogenesis
LFA1 ($\alpha_L\beta_2$)	ICAM	Immune response (see Figure 4.4)

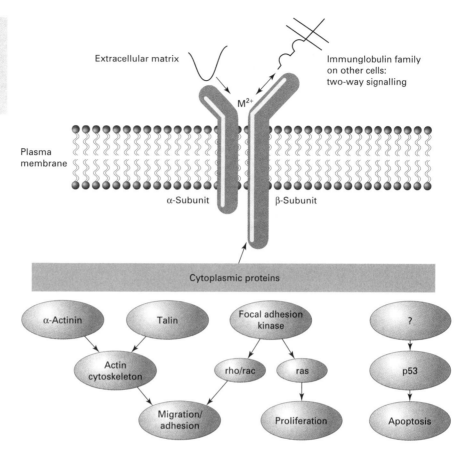

Figure 10.18

Integrin structure and function. Signal transduction involves clustering of multiple integrin dimers.

the MAP kinase pathway (see Figure 10.12), whereas Rho and Rac act via phosphoinositol–mediated steps (see Figure 10.14). Growth factors such as EGF and PDGF also stimulate both of these pathways, but in normal cells they are inactive in the absence of cell adhesion (anchorage dependence). The molecular details involved are unclear, but in the case of PDGF effects on fibroblasts, they are related to concentrations of phosphoinositol intermediates. In the absence of integrin occupancy, PDGF activates (tyrosine phosphorylation) phospholipase C, but the enzyme phosphatidyl inositol-3-kinase is rate-limiting; ECM–integrin interaction activates this enzyme and relieves the block.

Inhibition of apoptosis by integrin-mediated cell adhesion occurs by blocking p53-activated events (see Figure 9.18), but the mechanistic details of this are sparse.

Cancer

The integrin repertoire is altered in cancer cells, but the changes are complex. An approximation would be that integrins involved in tissue organisation are decreased whereas those needed for migration are not. Thus, in breast cancers the $\alpha_5\beta_1$ integrin that recognises fibronectin is decreased, whereas melanomas express increased levels of $\alpha_3\beta_1$ integrin, which binds laminin, fibronectin and collagen. The $\alpha_v\beta_3$ integrin is of special interest because it influences several processes important for carcinogenesis. It binds a wide range of ECM glycoproteins as well as a metallo-proteinase. $\alpha_v\beta_3$ is poorly expressed on normal cells such as capillary endothelial cells and skin melanocytes but is elevated in metastasising cancers such as melanomas. Migration is determined by the ECM on which the cells move and therefore on the cell receptors that recognise the ECM; the wide specificity of $\alpha_v\beta_3$ means that cell migration can proceed over almost any ECM substrate, a property that facilitates invasion and metastasis (see Chapter 11). Its additional property of binding a metalloproteinase to digest a path through the ECM contributes further to invasive potential. Two other processes influenced by $\alpha_v\beta_3$ are apoptosis and angiogenesis. Interaction of this integrin with an ECM ligand promotes cell survival by inhibiting apoptosis (see Figure 10.18). The $\alpha_v\beta_3$ integrin is also elevated in normal capillary endothelial cells participating in angiogenesis. The three properties just described – wide ligand specificity, binding metalloproteinases and inhibition of apoptosis – all facilitate formation of new capillaries (see Chapter 11). Both the anti-apoptotic and angiogenic effects have adverse consequences for the patient and are being targeted as potential forms of treatment. Monoclonal antibodies against $\alpha_v\beta_3$ inhibit its function, thus promoting apoptosis and blocking angiogenesis (see Chapter 12).

Cadherins

Cadherins represent the 'glue' by which adjacent epithelial cells are attached to each other. They are important in determining the pattern of cells in a tissue. The extracellular domain of a cadherin monomer has five repeat sequences that dimerise with similar repeats on the adjacent monomer in the same cell. Ca^{2+} is needed for this interaction (Figure 10.19). The most distal repeat interacts with the analogous repeat of cadherins on the next cell. The names of individual members of this family are frequently prefixed with a letter derived from the cell type in which it was first identified, such as E-cadherin from an **e**pithelial member of the family.

Cadherins transduce the extracellular signals by recruiting β-catenin to their cytoplasmic face. This activates a series of changes centred on changing the pool of available β-catenin in the cytoplasm (Figure 10.19). This pool serves a dual role of regulating both the cytoskeleton and nuclear transcription. The central region of β-catenin contains 13 tandem amino acid repeats (Armadillo repeats from fruit-fly terminology) required for both cadherin and transcription factor interaction. The genes whose transcription is influenced by these events in humans are defined poorly, other than the observation that β-catenin interacts with transcription factors Tcf and Lef. In insects, β-catenin signals to the Wnt pathway involved in wing formation. More information is available about cytoskeletal responses; β-catenin interacts with α-catenin on the actin cytoskeleton and with the normal **a**denomatous **p**olyposis **c**oli (APC) protein, which in turn binds to microtubules. There are two pools of β-catenin, one bound to the actin and microtubule cytoskeletons, the other free and available for downstream effects on gene transcription. APC may play a role in cell movement, but additionally its interaction with β-catenin accelerates ubiquitin-mediated proteolytic destruction of β-catenin. As APC is a key protein in carcinogenesis (see below), its modulation of β-catenin availability indicates an important but indeterminate role for the β-catenin in cell function.

Figure 10.19

E-Cadherin, β-catenin and APC interactions. APC is altered in colorectal cancers, E-cadherin in many cancers and β-catenin in melanomas and prostate cancers.

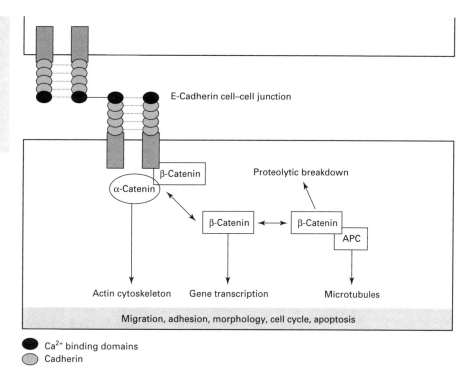

Ca²⁺ binding domains
Cadherin

β-Catenin can be tyrosine-phosphorylated by the *src* oncogene and by growth factor receptors such as EGF (see Figure 10.11). This dissociates APC and alters the cytoskeleton as well as activating gene transcription (Figure 10.19).

Cadherins, APC and cancer

Disruption of tissue organisation associated with carcinogenesis is often accompanied by loss of cadherins, which act as suppressor molecules. Metastases from epithelial cancers often lose E-cadherin expression, thereby facilitating escape of cells from one part of the body to another (see Chapter 11). Loss of E-cadherin expression is sometimes due to hypermethylation of regulatory regions of the gene (see Chapter 9), but in familial stomach cancer there is a germline inactivating mutation in the coding region of the gene.

A defective *APC* gene is inherited in people with adenomatous polyposis coli cancer and both alleles are lost by somatic mutations in sporadic colorectal cancers (see Chapter 8). Loss of APC suppressor function is thus a key (gatekeeper) event in the formation of this type of cancer (see Chapter 2). About 1000 different mutations have been mapped, all of which result in the synthesis of truncated inactive proteins. All of the somatic and most of the germline mutations occur in the middle region of the gene that codes for the β-catenin binding domain. Loss of the β-catenin binding site of APC results in less degradation and higher concentrations of β-catenin in colorectal cancer cells than in normal counterparts. The truncated APC protein will still bind microtubules. The importance of β-catenin in carcinogenesis is emphasised further by the observation that a limited number of melanomas, endometrial cancers and prostate cancers have mutations in its gene, as do a limited number of colorectal cancers with no APC defects. In most cases, these β-catenin mutations stabilise the protein against degradation.

Immunoglobulin superfamily

Immunoglobulin superfamily proteins are single-chain proteins. They have extracellular domains with repeated sequences homologous to those in the recognition domains of immunoglobulins. These repeats recognise similar sequences on adjacent cells. The number of repeats is variable in different members of the family, but the terminal two repeats determine the specificity of interactions. Overlapping terminologies are a problem in that members of this family are called CAMs, which is also the general term for **c**ell **a**dhesion **m**olecules. Individual members of the immunoglobulin CAM family are prefixed with the letter derived from the cell type in which it was first identified. Thus, N-CAM is of **n**eural origin, while V-CAM relates to blood **v**asculature, but their expression is not confined to these cell types.

N-CAM mediates homotypic cell–cell recognition in normal colon epithelium, and its loss represents one of the rate-limiting steps in colorectal carcinogenesis (see Chapter 2). V-CAM is induced by cytokines in vascular endothelia, where its binding to integrins on metastatic cancer cells helps arrest the cells before extravasation (see Chapter 11). ICAM is a third member of this family that has a role in cancer biology. It has similar properties to V-CAM, including its induction by cytokines, but it is also expressed in cancer cells, such as those of the colon, pancreas and kidney. It is not present in the normal progenitor cells in these sites.

Other members of the immunoglobulin family include a membrane receptor (semaphorin) for extracellular chemotactic peptides (netrins) that provide directional stimuli for cell movement, and carcinoembryonic antigen used for diagnostic purposes (see Chapter 12).

Selectins

Selectins are single-chain receptors that recognise carbohydrate side chains of ECM, mucins and cell proteins. They are confined to vascular cells and may play a part in metastasis by arresting cell movement within blood vessels (see Chapter 11).

CD44

Over 20 variants of CD44 are translated from a single mRNA by splicing out different introns. Normal CD44 is a receptor for ECM proteins containing hyaluronic acid. CD44 is expressed widely in normal cells, but it is downregulated in metastatic cancers of the colon, ovary and prostate. Expression of variant CD44s is complex, and no general picture is evident. Thus, variant 6 is not found in normal colon epithelium but increases in amount through the polyp stage until all the cancer cells express it. Variant overexpression also correlates with metastasis in other cases, such as melanoma. It is not known how these effects are achieved.

Syndecans

Syndecans are transmembrane glycoproteins that bind heparin proteoglycans on their extracellular surface and facilitate the function (coreceptor) of other adhesion receptors such as integrins and cadherins. Their cytoplasmic domains can bind enzymes such as protein kinase C and cofactors such as phosphoinositols.

RHO

The RHO gene family includes several members involved in cell migration by regulation of actomyosin-based cytoskeletal filament contraction and the turnover of adhesion sites. Overexpression of RhoC in melanoma cells is alone sufficient to induce a highly metastatic phenotype.

Hydrophobic growth regulatory molecules

Low-molecular-weight hydrophobic molecules such as steroid hormones, retinoic acids and thyroid hormone influence several aspects of tumour development. This section focuses on these compounds but also describes another group, the prostaglandins, which act by different mechanisms. The first group contains compounds of diverse structure (Table 10.5). They are all relatively simple molecules that elicit specific responses in different cell types. This specificity is generated by the presence or absence of individual receptors and by the genes whose transcription they regulate. The ligands include steroid hormones acting by endocrine and autocrine routes, thyroid hormone (endocrine) and derivatives of vitamin D (1,25-dihydroxy vitamin D3) and vitamin A (retinoic acids) obtained either through the diet (vitamins A and D) or by UV-induced reactions in the skin (vitamin D). To circumvent terminology problems, this disparate group are said to be nuclear receptor acting agents.

Nuclear-receptor-mediated events

There are no barriers to cell entry for such compounds, and their physiological effects are mediated by intracellular, mainly nuclear, receptors. The ligand induces conformational changes in the receptor, resulting in dimerisation and exposure of DNA-binding sites, which bind to DNA sequences (hormone-response elements). Transcription from genes containing such elements is altered (Figure 10.20).

Ligands

The structures of three classes of ligand involved with cancers and the nature of this involvement are shown in Table 10.5. They act principally via endocrine routes,

Table 10.5 Hydrophobic molecules involved in cancers and that act by nuclear receptors.

Compound	Involvement	Cancer	Example
Steroids			
Androgens	Tumour promotion, treatment	Prostate	
Oestrogens	Tumour promotion, treatment	Breast, uterus	
Glucocorticoids	Treatment	Leukaemia	
Progestins	Inhibit proliferation, treatment	Uterus, ovary	
Thyroid hormone	Hyperproliferation, differentiation	Chicken erythroblastosis	
Retinoic acids	Differentiation, treatment	Acute promyelocytic leukaemia	

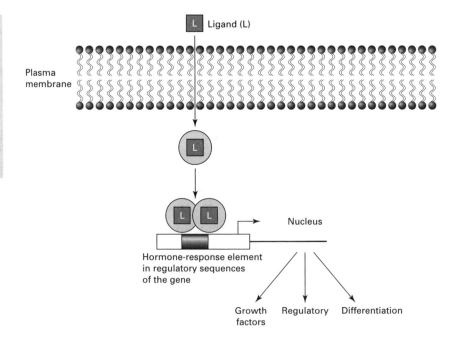

Figure 10.20

Gene regulation by low-molecular-weight hydrophobic molecules. Examples are steroid hormones, retinoic acid and thyroid hormone. The ligand and receptors can be altered in cancer cells.

but autocrine effects may be important in older people (see Figure 12.12). Alteration of ligand types and concentrations is involved at several stages of cancer development. The sex steroids – oestrogens (female) and androgens (male) – are produced endogenously as components of normal development, but they also find widespread use as exogenous agents that regulate contraception (oestrogens and progestins) and muscle development (anabolic androgens). Overexposure to oestrogen from endogenous or exogenous sources increases the risk of endometrial and breast cancer; part of the protective effect of vegetable consumption may be due to antioestrogens in these plants (see Chapter 4). There is speculation that environmental oestrogens (endocrine disrupters) produced as industrial by-products from oils, detergents and pesticides might be responsible for the increased incidence of testicular cancer. Oestrogens are mitogens for cells such as those in endometrium and breast that contain oestrogen receptors; this accounts for the elevated risk of cancer at these sites associated with prolonged oestrogen exposure (see Table 4.3).

Contraceptive pills contain progestins, which, because of their antiproliferative effect, decrease the risk of endometrial and ovarian cancer (see Chapters 4 and 13). Use of anabolic androgens for muscle building is associated with the development of benign liver tumours.

Manipulation of the sex hormone environment is used in the treatment of hormone-sensitive cancers, either by removal of endogenous hormones or by giving antagonists. Glucocorticoids are also used in several treatments (see Chapter 12).

Two isomers of retinoic acid exist with different functions. The *trans* isomer binds to both the **r**etinoic **a**cid **r**eceptor **a**lpha (RARA) and the **r**etinoic acid **X** receptor (RXR), whereas the *cis* isomer binds only to RXR. This specificity has consequences for normal development, because RXR is needed for differentiation responses promoted by vitamin D and thyroid hormone (see below). Altered exposure to vitamin D, thyroid hormone or retinoic acids is not linked with cancer formation, although nuclear accidents such as at Chernobyl (see Chapter 6), increase the incidence of thyroid cancers by a process involving thyroid hormones. These hormones contain iodine (see Table 10.5); the radioactive isotopes iodine-131 and iodine-125 released from the nuclear reaction are incorporated into thyroid hormones and concentrated in the thyroid gland. These isotopes emit ionising γ-radiation, which causes mutational events (see Chapter 6). Retinoic acids, vitamin D and thyroid hormones are all agents that induce differentiation and indirectly block proliferation (see Chapter 9).

Receptors

Receptors are transcription factors whose function is blocked in the absence of ligand due to conformational restraints imposed by other proteins and hypophosphorylation. Details vary with different receptors, but, in general, each receptor protein molecule has a number of overlapping domains, serving different functions (Figure 10.21). Ligand binding to a large C-terminal region dissociates associated proteins such as the **90** kDa **h**eat **s**hock **p**rotein (HSP90), which allows dimerisation and exposure of the DNA-binding domain. With the steroid receptors, homodimers between similar receptors are usually formed, but retinoic acids, thyroid hormone

Figure 10.21

Nuclear receptor protein domains and gene transcription.

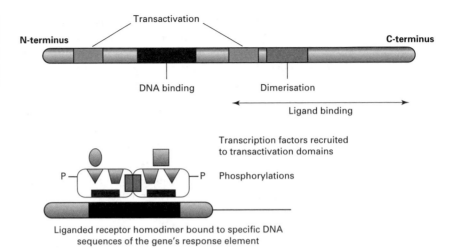

Liganded receptor homodimer bound to specific DNA sequences of the gene's response element

and vitamin D act via heterodimers. These heterodimers comprise an RXR plus its *cis* retinoic acid and the relevant other monomer plus ligand (RARA–*trans*-retinoic acid, thyroid hormone receptor–triiodothyronine, vitamin D receptor–1,25-dihydroxy vitamin D3). Dimerisation also requires serine/threonine phosphorylations. The DNA-binding domain is made up of two separate amino-acid sequences, each containing Zn^{2+}; these *zinc fingers* recognise specific DNA base sequences (hormone-response elements) in regulatory regions of sensitive genes. It is the amino-acid sequence of these fingers plus the base sequence of the response elements that determines which genes are sensitive to which receptors. Other regions of the receptor, known as transactivation domains, bind additional nuclear proteins to form the active transcription complex. The coactivator proteins that form part of the transcription factor complex that activates gene transcription (see Figure 5.1) can be needed for many genes regulated by pathways other than those discussed here. Furthermore, the coactivators can be present in rate-limiting concentrations, so that activation of one gene inactivates others due to competition for coactivators. One such coactivator is **CREB-binding protein** (CBP), needed for growth-related genes regulated by jun, fos (see Figure 10.15), SMAD (see Figure 10.9) and STAT (see Figure 10.6). Retinoic acids and other differentiation-inducing ligands may inhibit proliferation by sequestering these rate-limiting coactivators for their own purposes and thus block transcription from the proliferation-related genes. Figure 5.1, which illustrates general transcriptional regulation, could also be used to describe the hormone-related events.

Hormone antagonists, such as the anti-oestrogen tamoxifen and the anti-androgen flutamide, act by binding to the relevant receptor and exposing the DNA-binding domain but not the transactivation domains (see Figure 13.1). This means that the complex will bind to DNA but will not recruit all the other proteins necessary for initiation of transcription. Plant oestrogens (phyto-oestrogens) occur in seeds and vegetables (see Chapter 4) and act as anti-oestrogens by this mechanism; however, this generalisation should not be pushed too far because phyto-oestrogens can also have agonist properties. Compounds that have both agonist and antagonist effects in a tissue-specific manner are sometimes called selective oestrogen receptor modulators. A second oestrogen receptor, ER-β, has a different ligand specificity and tissue distribution from ER-α (the normal receptor in this book); ER-β may contribute to the selective actions of oestrogens.

Rats have a category of receptors called peroxisome proliferation activating receptors that have been implicated in carcinogenesis, but peroxisome proliferation has not been detected in humans.

The presence or absence of receptors is a major determinant of whether a cell will respond to a ligand, and their concentrations determine the magnitude of response.

Genes influenced by hormone receptors

Proliferation events mediated by these ligands act primarily via the G_1 checkpoint of the cell cycle. Genes that are switched on rapidly include *myc* and *fos*, while those that are activated more slowly include growth factors and their receptors. Oestrogens increase TGF-α production and the number of IGF-I receptors, both events stimulating proliferation. Anti-oestrogens such as tamoxifen block these oestrogen effects but additionally activate genes coding for inhibitory growth factors such as TGF-β. Retinoic acids regulate differentiation-related genes such as osteopontin in bone osteoblasts and lung surfactant protein, but the targets are uncertain in myeloid cells, where defects occur. Retinoic acid activated receptors can block jun N-terminal kinase and thus antagonise genes containing AP1 regulatory sites (see Figure 10.15); many of these are involved in cell proliferation.

Cancer

Changes in receptor type and magnitude occur in cancers. During breast and endometrial carcinogenesis, normal oestrogen receptors are upregulated at the transcriptional level but are then lost in some tumours as they dedifferentiate and become more aggressive. These changes decrease the likelihood of the tumour responding to endocrine treatment (see Chapter 12). However, some oestrogen-receptor-positive breast cancers are resistant to endocrine treatment (see Chapter 12); one possible reason is that there are other pathways of receptor activation. MAP kinases can phosphorylate and dimerise the receptor in the absence of ligand, and so polypeptide growth factors produced by cancer cells could provoke hormone-independent growth. Changes in receptor type have been identified in acute promyelocytic leukaemia in which a t(15;17) chromosome translocation disrupts the retinoic acid receptor in its transactivation domain, thereby blocking differentiation (see Figure 5.7). A rare type of acute myeloid leukaemia has a translocation between chromosomes 8 and 16 that disrupts CBP coactivator function. This prevents normal retinoic-acid-induced differentiation of myeloid cells. In chickens, the erythroblastosis virus carries the oncogene *v-erbA*, which codes for a thyroid receptor homologue and is responsible for generating erythroblastosis, a premalignant condition due to blocked differentiation. The *v-erbA* has deletions and substitutions in the ligand-binding domain such that the oncogene product blocks normal thyroid receptor binding to its response element.

Prostaglandins

This family of bioactive lipids, formed from a 20-carbon fatty acid, arachidonic acid (Figures 10.13 and 10.22), have multiple cellular effects with important clinical effects, as judged from the fact that long-term inhibition of prostaglandin production halves the mortality from colorectal cancer. This serendipitous observation came to light from clinical trials on the use of **n**on-**s**teroidal **a**nti-**i**nflammatory **d**rugs (NSAIDs) such as aspirin to protect against heart problems and to treat arthritis. NSAIDs work by inhibiting two enzymes, **c**ycl**o**o**x**ygenases (COX-1 and COX-2), required for the oxidation of arachidonic acid to produce prostaglandins. Aspirin acetylates a serine −OH at the active site of COX-1 and COX-2, thus preventing prostaglandin synthesis. More selective agents acting by different mechanisms have now been developed (see Chapter 13).

COX-1 is constitutively expressed by many cells, whereas COX-2 can be induced selectively by many mitogens. COX-2 is upregulated at early stages of colorectal carcinogenesis, whereas COX-2 inhibitors block both adenoma and carcinoma formation in the colon. Prostaglandins have autocrine and paracrine effects on cell proliferation, apoptosis and angiogenesis via adenyl cyclase-coupled receptors (see Figure 10.10) and by nuclear receptors of the peroxisome proliferator family. The

Figure 10.22

Prostaglandins: synthesis, function and NSAID inhibition.

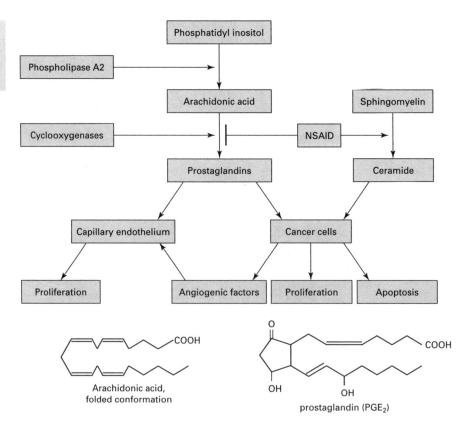

Arachidonic acid, folded conformation

prostaglandin (PGE$_2$)

mechanisms involved are not well understood, but they include stimulation of the production of angiogenic growth factors by cancer cells and promotion of proliferation of capillary endothelial cells. NSAIDs promote apoptosis by a ceramide pathway and block angiogenesis by inhibiting the COX enzymes (Figure 10.22). The COX enzymes may have additional functions relevant to carcinogenesis. Aspirin inhibits acetylaminofluorene binding to DNA, suggesting a role for the cyclooxygenases in carcinogen activation (see Chapter 6). NSAIDs are being tested as agents for preventing or treating colorectal cancer, but they may also be effective in breast and head and neck cancers (see Chapter 13).

Cross-talk between signalling pathways

Normal cells have a network of cross-linked signalling pathways, but it is impossible to do this justice without losing the simple format used here. The interplay between tyrosine and serine/threonine kinase pathways is illustrated in Figure 10.11, and kinase signalling, phosphoinositol and CAMs are illustrated in Figure 10.14; the nuclear receptor and MAP kinase interaction was discussed above.

Under normal circumstances, such cross-communications synergise to give fine control of the processes involved. In cancers, this means that loss of control of one pathway can result in loss of other regulatory mechanisms to the detriment of the normal cells. It can also result in increased adaptability when it comes to cancer treatments based on manipulation of individual pathways; cancer cells are adept at circumventing the actions of inhibitory drugs by switching to alternative pathways (see Chapter 12).

Further reading

Signalling from kinase receptors

Blume-Jensen, P. and Hunter, T. (2001) Oncogenic kinase signalling. *Nature* **411**, 355–365.

Grunwald, V. and Hidalgo, M. (2003) Developing inhibitors of the epidermal growth factor receptor for cancer treatment. *J Natl Cancer Inst* **95**, 851–861.

Leu, T.H. and Maa, M.C. (2003) Functional implication of the interaction between EGR receptor and c-Src. *Front Biosci* **8**, s28–38.

Prigent, S.A. (2005) Growth factors and their signalling pathways in cancer. In *Introduction to the Cellular and Molecular Biology of Cancer*, ed. M. Knowles and P. Selby. Oxford: Oxford University Press.

Cell adhesion

Cavallaro, H. and Christofori, G. (2004) Cell adhesion and signalling by cadherins and Ig-cams in cancer. *Nat Rev Cancer* **4**, 118–132.

Hood, J.D. and Cheresh, D.A. (2002) Role of integrins in cell invasion and signalling. *Nat Rev Cancer* **2**, 91–100.

Liotta, L.A. and Kohn, E.C. (2001) The microenvironment of the tumour–host interface. *Nature* **411**, 375–379.

Signalling by hydrophobic molecules

Claessens, F., Verrijdt, G., Schoenmakers, E., *et al.* (2001) Selective DNA binding by the androgen receptor as a mechanism for hormone-specific gene regulation. *J Steroid Biochem Mol Biol* **76**, 23–30.

Freedman, L.P. (1999) Increasing the complexity of coactivation in nuclear receptor signalling. *Cell* **97**, 5–8.

Gupta, R.A. and DuBois, R.N. (2001) Colorectal cancer prevention and treatment by inhibition of cyclooxygenase-2. *Nat Rev Cancer* **1**, 11–21.

Hansen L.A., Sigman, C.C., Andreola, F., *et al.* (2000) Retinoids in chemoprevention and differentiation therapy. *Carcinogen* **21**, 1271–1279.

Sommer, S. and Fuqua, S.A.W. (2001) Estrogen receptor and breast cancer. *Semin Cancer Biol* **11**, 339–352.

11 Invasion and metastasis

- As malignant tumours grow, they invade adjacent normal tissues.
- Metastasis is the escape of cancer cells from a primary site and their re-establishment at distant secondary locations.
- Metastasis is inefficient because most cells are destroyed in transit, but it is efficient in other ways as most human cancers metastasise successfully.
- Metastasis requires the disruption of local cell–cell interactions, invasion, penetration of blood or lymphatic vessels (intravasation), escape from those vessels (extravasation), migration and growth.
- Metastasis can occur via blood vessels, lymphatics or movement within the body cavities.
- The organ through which the transporting vessels first pass (first-pass organ) is a common site of new growth.
- Tumours can also metastasise to specific sites. The sites are determined by the anatomy of the transporting vessels and by specific features of the cancer cells (the seed) and of the new environment in which they grow (the soil).
- Adhesion molecules help determine sites of metastasis. Local properties such as endothelial function, extracellular matrix composition and growth factor production also contribute.
- Metastases can be dormant for long periods.
- Individual metastases can be of clonal origin.
- Metastasis is a late event in the natural history of carcinogenesis, although early gene changes can influence later events.
- Oncogenes and tumour suppressor genes are important. Metastasis inhibitor genes have been identified.
- Invasion and migration require proteolytic enzymes and polypeptide motility factors.
- Two types of protease are required, both of which are generated from inactive proenzymes by the actions of other proteases. Activators and inhibitors of these events exist.

- Arrest of cancer cells within a vessel is a result of passive entrapment or requires the cooperation of lymphocytes, platelets and endothelial cells.

- Extravasation requires attachment to endothelium, dissolution of the basement membrane and migration.

- Growth at both the new primary and any new site requires the formation of new blood vessels (angiogenesis).

- Angiogenesis is activated by a change in the balance of inhibitory and stimulatory polypeptide factors in favour of stimulation. These factors are produced by cancers and normal cells. It can also be stimulated by hypoxia.

Introduction

As malignant tumours grow, they invade adjacent normal tissues. This expansion is not even; tumours appear to force themselves along lines of least resistance (vessels, fascia) in the surrounding tissues, so that extensions radiate outward from the central mass. Invasion is facilitated by the formation of proteolytic enzymes and an increase in the mobility of the malignant cells. The physical expansion of a tumour can cause occlusion of adjacent blood vessels, which in turn can result in necrosis of surrounding tissues. Metastasis is the process by which cancer cells escape from the primary tumour, penetrate blood or lymphatic vessels, and are transported to distant sites where they establish secondary tumours. By the time a primary tumour is detected, it usually has metastasised and secondary tumours have already established themselves at distant sites. This is taken into consideration in cancer therapy, which usually includes an element of systemic therapy to destroy metastases.

The process of dissemination of tumour cells from the primary tumour is an efficient process. However, the establishment of secondary tumours appears to be relatively inefficient. When a known number of melanoma cells are injected into the bloodstream of a mouse, most are destroyed rapidly in the circulation and very few survive to form secondary tumours. In the clinical context, metastases create major clinical problems, although these can take a long time to become apparent. Even 10 years after apparently successful breast surgery, some women die from metastatic disease. Residual cancer cells can remain dormant for long periods. It should also be understood that secondary tumours can themselves metastasise.

In terms of the natural history of cancer development, invasion and metastasis are considered as late stages of progression, which is not to say that contributory changes have not occurred earlier. Thus, *ras* mutations can increase metastatic potential but are an early gene change in colorectal carcinogenesis (see Chapter 2). The first detected gene alteration in people with familial adenomatous polyposis coli is in the *APC* gene that codes for a protein involved in cell–cell adhesion (see Chapters 2 and 10), disruption of which is a prerequisite for escape from local control. Hence, very early gene changes can contribute to late events in progression.

Both oncogene and tumour suppressor gene products are involved in metastatic spread. The examples of *ras* and *APC* illustrate this point, although a specific metastasis gene has not been identified.

General features

Heterogeneity of metastatic potential

Primary tumours are known to be heterogeneous in several ways, such as drug resistance, growth rates and response to radiation, the presence or absence of hormone receptors (breast and prostate cancers) and melanin (melanomas). This heterogeneity also applies to metastatic ability.

A series of cell lines were derived from a single melanoma cell. Cells from the separate lines were then injected into the bloodstream of normal mice to establish their metastatic efficiency (by counting pigmented metastases on the surface of the lungs after a period of time). It was found that there was a greater variability in metastatic efficiency between the lines than within the lines. As all the cell lines were derived from a single cell, it is clear that this variability in metastatic efficiency arose from the progeny of a single cancer cell. Variations on this procedure were used to study the rapid evolution of differences in metastatic behaviour in an experimental fibrosarcoma. This cancer could be maintained either by subcutaneous transplantation in syngeneic mice or in tissue culture. Starting with transplanted material, lines with high and low metastatic characteristics were established *in vitro* and maintained in culture for about 2 months. Then their metastatic efficiency was compared with that of the parental strain, which had been maintained by transplantation in syngeneic mice. It was found that the low metastatic line remained very similar to the parental strain, while the highly metastatic line had diverged considerably from the parental strain. The two lines were tested for mutability using a common mutagen. The highly metastatic line was nearly five times as mutable as the low metastatic line. Such experiments show that the metastatic characteristics of cells in a tumour vary and that such characteristics are genetically unstable in some cells.

Escape from the primary site and establishment at a new site

The common cancers in humans arise from epithelial cells, which must break contacts with their neighbours, traverse the basement membrane and migrate through the stroma (invasion) in order to reach the blood or lymphatic vessels that will carry them to other parts of the body (Figure 11.1). Invasion distinguishes *in situ* carcinoma from more advanced cancers and is also one of the properties that differentiates benign and malignant lesions (see Chapter 3). Progression to the invasive state also has clinical implications, in that invasive cancers are more life-threatening. A person with breast cancer who has only *in situ* carcinoma can be cured by its excision, but this outcome is not as likely with invasive cancer. When the cells reach

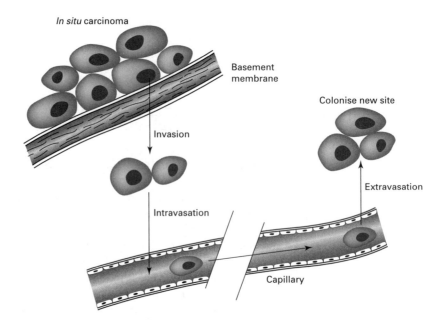

Figure 11.1

Escape of cancer cells to a metastatic site. Within the capillary, cancer cells move as aggregates with other cells (not shown).

the vessels, they have to penetrate them (intravasation), avoid destruction during transit to remote sites, and then repeat the process at the new site (extravasation). Having reached the metastatic site, the cancers must proliferate in the new environment. Again, there are clinical implications regarding cells that successfully complete this series of events. About one-quarter of women whose breast cancer has metastasised to multiple lymph nodes will be alive 10 years after first diagnosis, compared with three-quarters of women with no nodal involvement.

Mesenchymal cancers, such as those arising from bone, have to accomplish a similar set of events, with the exception that the cell–cell contacts are different from those seen in epithelia. Leukaemias are exceptional, in that normal proliferation occurs in the bone marrow or spleen, both of which have direct access to blood vessels.

Routes of transport

Three conduits are used in the transfer of cancer cells to distant sites: lymphatic vessels, blood vessels and the peritoneal cavity (Figure 11.2).

Lymphatic vessels

Lymphatic vessels provide a poor barrier to penetration by cancer cells. Their basement membrane is either rudimentary or absent, the endothelial wall is very permeable, and there is a low internal hydraulic pressure. Lymph moves along the vessels by the external compression provided by natural body movements aided by one-way valves, which direct flow towards the final draining points at the subclavian veins and from here into the superior vena cava. The importance of lymphatic dissemination in metastasis was shown in experiments where the induction of extra lymph vessels in implanted breast tumours in mice was found to enhance metastasis.

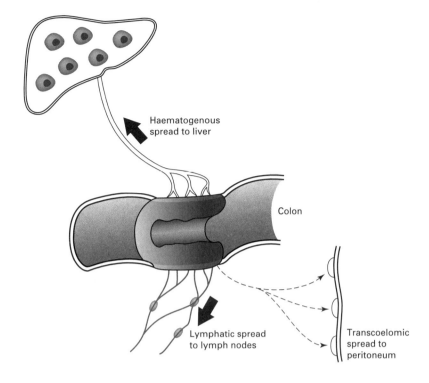

Figure 11.2

Routes of metastasis from a colorectal cancer.

Blood vessels

The capillaries are also favoured routes for dissemination. These vessels consist of a single layer of endothelial cells and a basement membrane, in contrast to veins and arteries, which have additional layers of smooth muscle and supporting cells. It is easier for cancer cells to penetrate capillaries during both intravasation and extravasation. The liver provides a variation of this pattern, in that the main afferent vessel, the hepatic portal vein, breaks down into sinusoids lined by a very thin and incomplete covering of sinusoidal lining cells, giving metastases easy access to hepatocytes (Figure 11.3).

The anatomy of the vascular system partially determines the sites of metastatic growth. Blood from the gut collects in the hepatic portal vein and passes to the liver (Figure 11.3). Blood from the somatic circulation enters the heart by way of the caval vein and passes through the right heart to the lungs. Liver and lungs are therefore common sites for metastatic growth, but other factors also influence sites favoured for the establishment of secondary cancers (see later).

Body cavity

The peritoneal and pleural cavities provide another route for dispersal of metastases between organs within the cavities. In this situation, abdominal and thoracic movements cause movements of the enclosed fluid, which aids the dissemination of cancer cells arising from, say, the ovary or colon.

Figure 11.3

Transport routes of cancer cells around the body. Arrows indicate direction of flow.

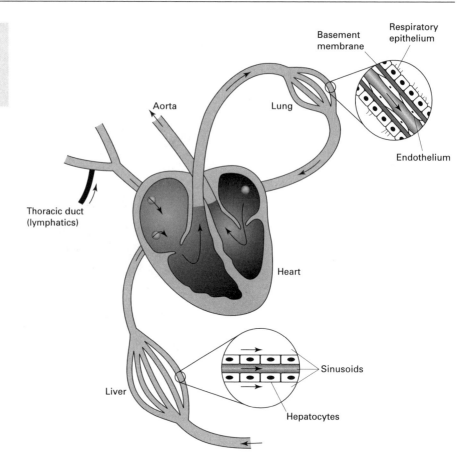

Preferential sites of metastasis

Many primary cancers metastasise to specific secondary sites. Two factors contribute to this selective distribution: the first-pass organ and the growth of cells at favoured sites.

First-pass organ

The organ first encountered by vessels draining areas containing cancers frequently supports secondary tumours. In the abdominal region, the liver is the main first-pass organ for haematogenous cancer cells; therefore, the liver is the common site for metastases from gut cancers (Table 11.1). As normal liver function is essential for life, metastases to this site are a common cause of death. Venous drainage from the head enters the superior vena cava, and so the first-pass organ here is the heart. Attachment and extravasation are clearly difficult in the heart, so cells pass through it to the lungs. The lungs are the main site for the establishment of secondary tumours arising from metastases from sites in the body other than the gastrointestinal tract.

Lymphatic vessels drain into lymph nodes near the affected site. Thus, metastasising breast cancer cells pass to nodes in the axilla (armpits) and establish secondary

Table 11.1 Metastatic sites for human cancers.

Primary site	Metastatic site*	
	First-pass organ	Other sites
Colon	Liver	Lung
Prostate	Liver	Bone
Breast	Liver	Bone, brain
Melanoma	Liver	Brain, bowel
Head and neck	Lung	–

* Blood-borne. Lymph nodes are the first-pass organ for lymphatic spread.

cancers, which can be felt as enlargements. Examination for the presence of axillary node secondaries forms part of the monitoring of people with breast cancer. Lymph-node positivity or negativity is of great importance in determining both the course of treatment and life expectancy in such patients (see Chapter 12). Lymph drains via the left brachycephalic vein into the superior vena cava (see Figure 11.3). Hence, there is a route by which cancer cells in the lymphatic vessels can reach the general bloodstream.

Favoured sites

The distribution of cancer cells to secondary sites cannot always be predicted by the anatomy of the vascular system and simple spread to downstream organs. Cancers from the lung often metastasise to the brain, when it might be expected on anatomical grounds that many other sites might provide equally favoured sites for secondary cancers. Such unexpected distributions were noted by an early physician, Paget, who used the Biblical parable of sown seed (cancer cells) falling on either fertile (favoured) or infertile (unfavoured) soil to explain this situation. In deference to Paget, this is called the 'seed-and-soil concept'. This also implies that the microenvironment at certain sites favours the adhesion and growth of metastasising cancer cells.

Escape from local control and invasion

The first step in metastasis involves cells breaking the bonds between adjacent cells in the tumour before migrating through the stroma to blood or lymphatic vessels. Following dissemination, the cells must then do the reverse, i.e. arrest at some point in the vascular tree and then extravasate and invade adjacent tissues.

These events involve interaction between the cells and the ECM. Many of the molecules involved have been described in Chapter 9. Here, they will be considered only in terms of cell behaviour. Molecules that mediate the action between cells and their immediate environment are collectively called **c**ell **a**dhesion **m**olecules (CAMs) and can be considered as receptors and ligands. CAM is prefixed by a capital letter to designate their original site of identification. Thus, the prefixes N and V refer to **n**erve and (blood) **v**essel, even though their expression is not confined to these cell types.

Three types of recognition process are important: (i) recognition of similar cells (homotypic), (ii) recognition of dissimilar cells (heterotypic) and (iii) cell–ECM interactions.

Cell–cell recognition

Normal cells

In a few tissues such as epithelia, there are distinct structures (desmosomes, adherens junctions, tight junctions, gap junctions) that are concerned with adhesion between adjacent cells. At the molecular level, CAMs are involved through their interaction with similar molecules on the lateral faces of adjacent cells (Figure 11.4). Cell–cell adhesion is mediated mainly by glycoproteins called cadherins. These consist of a single transmembrane chain with four homologous repeats in the extracellular domain; binding specificity resides in the most distal domain. Cadherins work homotypically, that is, they stick to other cadherins extracellularly. Intracellularly, they interact with the cytoskeleton via caterins. Different types of cadherins have tissue-specific distribution, for example E-cadherin is found in epithelia, N-CAM in nervous tissues and colon epithelium, and V-CAM on vascular endothelium binds integrins ($\alpha_4\beta_1$) on lymphocytes (heterotypic interaction). The heterotypic interaction between endothelium and lymphocytes is required for the normal response to inflammation and tissue injury.

Figure 11.4

Changes in adhesion molecules that influence metastasis. (Source: Adapted from Figure 4 in Maemura, M. and Dickson, R.B. (1994) *Breast Cancer Research and Treatment*, 32, 239–60.)

Normal

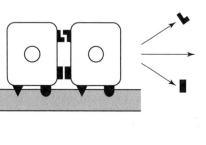
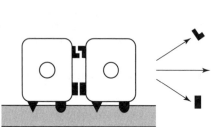

Cancer

P-selectin   L-selectin   E-selectin

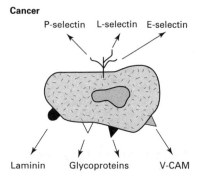

Laminin   Glycoproteins   V-CAM

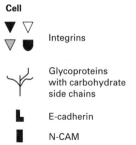

Cell

Integrins

Glycoproteins with carbohydrate side chains

E-cadherin

N-CAM

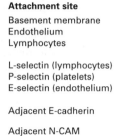

Attachment site

Basement membrane
Endothelium
Lymphocytes

L-selectin (lymphocytes)
P-selectin (platelets)
E-selectin (endothelium)

Adjacent E-cadherin

Adjacent N-CAM

Cancer cells

Breaking of homotypic recognition and changes in heterotypic recognition are characteristic of invasive and metastatic cancers. Proteins such as E-cadherin and N-CAM that promote homotypic recognition function as tumour suppressor proteins in that their loss facilitates escape from local control. This is seen in experimental and clinical settings. Experimentally, antibodies that block cadherin function increase metastatic potential, whereas overexpression of either E-cadherin or N-CAM has the opposite effect. E-cadherin is lost at an early stage of breast carcinogenesis; loss of N-CAM in gliomas is associated with a high probability of metastasis.

Inactivating mutations in the extracellular domain of E-cadherin have been identified in epithelial cancers such as gastric and prostate carcinoma. In keeping with the general principle of cancer cells using multiple mechanisms to achieve the same objective, E-cadherin can also be functionally inactivated by the indirect route, i.e. via mutation of the APC protein that mediates signal transduction from E-cadherin to the cytoskeleton.

Cell–ECM interactions

Normal cells

Integrins provide a major mechanism whereby cells recognise proteins in the extracellular matrix and basement membrane. This family of receptors is formed from a range of α and β subunits, the heterodimer of α and β chains forming the active receptor. Ligands include collagen IV, laminin and fibronectin (basement membrane), and collagen I, laminin and fibronectin (stroma). Specificity as to which ligand is recognised is determined by which α and β subunits make up the receptor (see Table 10.4).

Interaction with the basement membrane provides an important mechanism for regulating cell function. Normal breast epithelium in culture will express differentiated functions such as milk protein production only if grown on an artificial basement membrane. The reason for this is that the gene for one such protein, casein, has regulatory sequences that respond to signals from adhesion molecules. In the absence of these signals, transcription of the gene does not occur. Given the inverse relationship between differentiation and proliferation, loss of basement-membrane interaction in cancers would indirectly generate a more aggressive phenotype. Anchorage-independent growth of cultured cells is a laboratory index of that increased aggressiveness and reflects the altered link between substrate attachment and cell proliferation (see Chapter 10).

Integrins transduce signals from the extracellular matrix and sometimes heterotypic cells to the cytoskeleton. Cells have specialised regions of their membranes called focal adhesions that link the extracellular matrix to the cytoskeleton and other intracellular functions (see Box 10.1). Focal adhesions are sites of integrin accumulation; binding of these receptors to their matrix ligands activates cytoskeletal changes by interaction with a **f**ocal **a**dhesion **k**inase (FAK) capable of phosphorylating its own or other tyrosine residues. Such phosphorylations result from mitogenic signals such as growth factors and are required for the proliferative response (see Figures 10.7 and 10.18).

The $\alpha_3\beta_1$ integrin is localised on the basal surface of normal epithelial cells, where it binds to laminin in the basement membrane (see Figure 11.4).

Cancer cells

Integrin changes resulting from carcinogenesis cannot be defined in simple terms of increase or decrease, but cancers often have different types and membrane distributions of these receptors compared with their normal counterparts. In general, integrins involved in tissue organisation are decreased whereas those needed for migration are not. Several integrin changes relevant to carcinogenesis are listed in Table 10.4, and the increased expression of $\alpha_V\beta_3$ illustrates the influence that integrins can have on invasion and metastasis. $\alpha_V\beta_3$ has a broad ligand specificity, is little expressed on normal cells but is increased on melanoma cells and normal endothelium participating in cancer-directed angiogenesis (see below). The ability of this integrin to recognise virtually any of the glycoproteins of the ECM means that cells expressing $\alpha_V\beta_3$ can migrate over whatever matrices they encounter on their route to distant parts. The integrin's ability to bind metalloproteinases also helps digest a path through the ECM. Upregulation of $\alpha_V\beta_3$ coincides with the appearance of a more aggressive growth pattern. Melanomas initially expand radially, but invasion is heralded by a change in direction to vertical growth. Upregulation of $\alpha_V\beta_3$ integrin occurs at this stage. In contrast to these increased expressions, $\alpha_2\beta_1$ that recognises laminin and collagen is decreased in colorectal and breast cancers.

Laminin receptors (integrins $\alpha_3\beta_1$ and $\alpha_6\beta_1$) are frequently upregulated in epithelial cancers such as those of endometrium and breast; their distribution is altered such that they are found throughout the cell membrane, not only in the basal region.

Upregulation of all types of protease (serine/threonine, cysteine, aspartate and metalloproteinases) is a common event in carcinogenesis, with increased secretion of plasminogen activator, a serine protease, preceding the acquisition of anchorage-independent growth in culture (see Figure 2.6). Activation of these enzymes facilitates invasion, extra- and intravasation, and angiogenesis (see below).

Intravasation

Cancer cells attach to the stromal face of the blood vessel basement membrane, digest that membrane with proteases (see below) and migrate between the endothelial cells into the bloodstream. Entry into lymphatic vessels is easier because there is no basement membrane to circumvent.

Transport in the bloodstream

Cells are carried in the direction of blood flow. While they are in the bloodstream, cells must first avoid destruction and then have their movement arrested at potential sites of new growth. The bloodstream is a hostile environment, with more than 99% of injected cancer cells being destroyed by a combination of mechanical stresses, proteolytic destruction and surveillance by the host immune system. Immune surveillance can also occur outside the vessels; it involves cells of the immune system and **m**ajor **h**istocompatibility **c**omplex (MHC) proteins on the cancer cells.

The contribution of host immune surveillance to metastatic spread is a subject of debate, because, other than viral cancers in which foreign proteins are expressed, cancer cells are composed of host proteins that are unlikely to activate the immune system. Strains of mice that are immunodeficient due to lack of T-cells do not develop increased numbers of metastases when injected with cancer cells, but they do have natural killer cells capable of destroying abnormal cells, so this does not rule out a host contribution. On the other hand, MHC changes are common in cancer cells. MHC-I proteins are required for antigen presentation to cytotoxic T-cells, and so loss of MHC proteins should give the cancer cell a survival advantage. In experimental systems, overexpression of MHC-I proteins decreases metastatic potential, and metastatic potential is correlated inversely with MHC-I expression in a range of melanoma cell lines. Clinically, lymph-node metastases from breast, colorectal and kidney cancers have lower expression of MHC-I proteins than the primaries from which they were derived.

Cancer cells are transported in the blood as single cells or as aggregates (emboli) of several cancer cells, lymphocytes and adhering platelets (Figure 11.5). Formation of emboli may provide protection from mechanical stress and immune attack. The formation of emboli also facilitates attachment to the endothelium and therefore helps arrest the cancer cells at potential metastatic sites.

Extravasation

Escape from the vessel involves three steps: (i) attachment to the endothelial lining; (ii) retraction of the endothelial cells followed by cancer cell attachment to, and destruction of, the basement membrane; and (iii) migration into the surrounding stroma (Figure 11.5).

Arrest within the blood vessel

Arrest within the blood vessel occurs by attachment of cancer cell aggregates, lymphocytes and platelets (emboli) to the capillary endothelial cells, each of the three cell types that constitute the embolus participate in this process. Platelets interact with fibrinogen on the endothelial surface; via their P-selectin, they interact with endothelial proteoglycans. Endothelia from different tissues vary in their properties, which contributes to the site-specificity of metastases. Endothelial cells carry organ-specific cell-membrane determinants, some of which have been identified as CAMs and selectins. Endothelial E-selectins bind to proteoglycans on the tumour cells, the proteoglycans being characterised by sialylated fucosylated lactosamine side chains. $\alpha_4\beta_1$ integrins on both the tumour cell and lymphocytes contribute to this initial braking of the embolus movement and its tethering to the endothelium. This weak heterophylic cell interaction does not achieve complete arrest; stronger cell interactions

Figure 11.5

Stages of extravasation.

Embolus formation

Platelets   Cancer cells   Lymphocytes

Attachment to endothelium

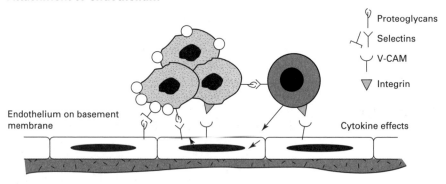

Endothelium on basement membrane

Proteoglycans
Selectins
V-CAM
Integrin

Cytokine effects

Retraction

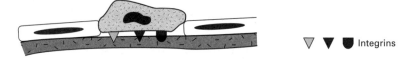

Integrins

Invasion

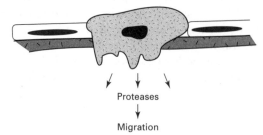

Proteases

Migration

between $\alpha_4\beta_1$ integrins and endothelial V-CAM (see Table 10.4) are required to achieve that. Normal endothelium expresses low levels of V-CAM, but cytokines (interleukin-1, tumour necrosis factor) from both lymphocytes and tumour cells upregulate V-CAM expression. Strong interaction between tumour cell, lymphocytes and endothelium results from clustering of the integrins (affinity modulation) that form multiple interactions with V-CAM (see Chapter 10). This generates a localised stop mechanism. Endothelia from many sites express V-CAM, but L-CAM is present in lung; this provides a degree of selectivity as to which metastatic site is selected ('soil').

The process just described is a normal response to tissue injury, with T-cells accumulating at an inflammation site providing the cytokines. Cancers use this mechanism to stop their movement by interaction of endothelial V-CAM with integrins on the cancer cell. This heterotypic cell interaction is the first phase of extravasation.

An analogous process involving endothelial selectins and carbohydrate side chains on cancer cell-membrane proteins or attached platelets contributes to arrest of movement. Cytokine induction of E- and P-selectins on the endothelial surface are capable of recognising carbohydrate side chains on the cancer cells (E-selectin) or platelets (P-selectin) that form the embolus. Many cancers have ill-defined altered expression of surface glycoproteins that facilitate this heterotypic interaction.

Experimental injection of radioactively labelled tumour cells into the circulation shows rapid clearance from the blood, with most of the radioactivity being sequestered in the lungs. Some experimental evidence indicates that proliferation in arrested cells occurs in the vascular channels before extravasation. This implies that the initial growth of metastases is not absolutely dependent on prior extravasation.

Escape from the blood vessel

Retraction of the endothelial cells exposes the glycoproteins of the basement membrane, to which the cancer cells attach and then digest with proteases and glycosidases. The basement-membrane proteins include laminin, collagen IV and fibronectin, which are ligands for the integrin family of receptors on the cancer cell surface (Figure 11.5). Different cancers display distinct patterns of integrins. Thus, bone cancers (osteosarcomas) have increased $\alpha_1\beta_1$ integrin, whereas colorectal cancers possess $\alpha_6\beta_4$ forms. As $\alpha_1\beta_1$ recognises collagen and laminin whereas $\alpha_6\beta_4$ binds laminin, it follows that glycoprotein composition of basement membrane and extracellular matrix of a target site can contribute to 'soil' specificity. Differential expression of laminin receptor also influences 'soil' specificity. Epithelial cancers, such as those originating from the colon, lung and breast, have high expression of this receptor, but non-epithelial cancers such as of bone and brain do not.

Proteases involved in metastatic spread

Endopeptidases involved in metastatic spread are used at three stages: (i) invasion of the primary growth site, (ii) digestion of the endothelial basement membrane and (iii) invasion of the metastatic site. Two major types of protease are secreted by the cancers, categorised according to whether they require Zn^{2+} or Ca^{2+} (metalloproteinases): those that require the ions are collagenase types I and IV and stromolysin;

Figure 11.6

General features of extracellular protein digestion.

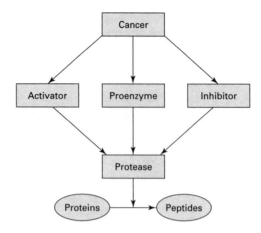

those that do not require the ions have a serine residue at the active site (serine proteases) – plasminogen is an example.

A feature common to both categories is that these proteases are secreted as inactive proenzymes, which must be activated by other proteases (Figure 11.6). Tissue inhibitors of activation also exist, such that invasion can be influenced by any of three components: the amount of proenzyme, the activator (a protease) and the inhibitor (a protease inhibitor). All these components can be produced by normal cells, but their balance is altered in cancers in favour of proteolysis.

The serine protease precursor plasminogen is converted to the active protease plasmin by other proteases called plasminogen activators (Figure 11.7). These activators must themselves be proteolytically converted from inactive proenzyme forms. Plasminogen activators are categorised as tissue-type (tPA) or urokinase-type (uPA). This nomenclature, based on their original characterisation, can be confusing; uPA is most important in tissue proteolysis, but the prime function of tPA is to dissolve blood clots. Antibodies directed against uPA inhibit invasion, whereas overexpression has the opposite effect. Synthetic inhibitors of uPA such as amiloride also decrease the number of metastatic colonies in model systems. Cancer cells have membrane receptors for uPA, which concentrate that enzyme along with associated proteolytic activity at centres of active invasion.

Metalloproteinases fall into three categories, as defined by their substrate specificity. Collagenases such as MMP1 digest collagens I, II, III, VII, VIII and X; gelatinases such as MMP2 digest gelatin, fibronectin, elastin and collagens I, IV, V, VII and X; and stromelysins (MMP3) hydrolyse fibronectin, laminin and collagens IV, V and IX. Thus, the MMPs can digest all the individual components of the ECM and remove physical barriers to metastasis. In addition to these secreted MMPs, a few transmembrane members of the family exist. MMPs are secreted as latent proenzymes, which have their prodomains removed by the extracellular serine protease, plasmin or other MMPs (Figure 11.7). Plasmin can thus serve two functions: digestion of the ECM and activation of MMPs. The active site of MMPs contains a histidine.glutamate.any amino acid.glycine.histidine motif; the two histidines co-ordinate the Zn^{2+} that is essential for activity. **T**issue **i**nhibitors of **m**etallo**p**roteinases

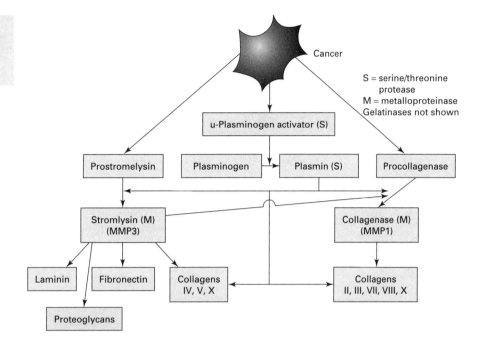

Figure 11.7

Proteases and their precursors involved in metastasis.

(TIMP) can also be secreted by cells; if this occurs, it is associated with decreased metastatic potential. TIMPs are broad-spectrum inhibitor proteins that form complexes with MMPs. They all contain cysteine residues arranged so that six intrachain −S−S− bonds are formed. Synthetic MMP inhibitors are being tested as potential antimetastatic drugs (see Chapter 12).

Digestion products of ECM glycoproteins such as collagen XVIII and plasminogen can influence angiogenesis (see below).

Migration

After extravasation, the cancer cells must migrate to their new site of growth. This requires continued production of proteases to digest the matrix, but additional features are also important. Migration is achieved by alternate attachment of the leading edge of the cell to matrix proteins and detachment of the rear edge. Integrins in the cancer membrane mediate these events by transducing the external signals from the matrix to the actin cytoskeleton of the cell. Movement is achieved by contraction and relaxation of this cytoskeleton (see Box 10.1).

Peptides released during proteolysis of matrix also act as chemotactic agents to attract additional cancer cells to the region. Proteolysis of matrix proteins does not always destroy the peptide sequences that form the binding site of the protein. Such peptides are capable of binding to integrins, thereby blocking cell attachment to the matrix and facilitating movement elsewhere.

Another class of polypeptides called motility factors are also important for migration as they stimulate movement by different mechanisms from those just mentioned.

They can be produced by normal cells and act in a paracrine manner on cancer cells, or they can be produced by cancer cells themselves and have an autocrine action. The names of these factors, such as autocrine motility factor, scatter factor and migration-stimulating factor, reflect their original method of detection.

As with the related growth factors, surface receptors exist that can be altered in cancers. In the case of scatter factor, the receptor is a tyrosine kinase coded by the *c-met* oncogene.

Growth

Proliferation of the cancer cells at their new site is initially confined to a cuff of cells within 1 mm of the blood vessel. This growth occurs under the influence of locally produced growth factors; the distance is determined largely by the diffusion of oxygen from the blood. For further growth, new blood vessels must be formed (angiogenesis) to supply essential nutrients and oxygen and to remove wastes.

Angiogenesis

Angiogenesis (Figure 11.8) is the formation of new blood vessels from pre-existing vascular beds. In many physiological situations, such as in wound healing, angiogenesis is a transient phenomenon and the new vascular bed will regress after it has fulfilled its function. However, in pathological situations, such as the establishment of secondary tumours, the vascular bed persists. In the latter context, angiogenesis is the step that determines whether a cancer remains dormant or develops. Although

Figure 11.8

Phases of angiogenesis.

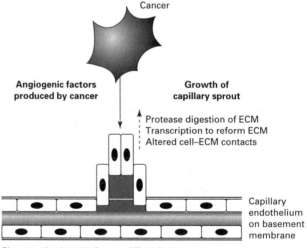

Cancer

Angiogenic factors produced by cancer

Growth of capillary sprout

Protease digestion of ECM
Transcription to reform ECM
Altered cell–ECM contacts

Capillary endothelium on basement membrane

Phase 1 Angiogenic factors diffuse from cancer
Phase 2 Proliferation and invasion of endothelial cells
Phase 3 Maturation: lumen formation, arteriovenous loop formation, recruitment of supporting cells

Figure 11.9

Influence of hypoxia on angiogenesis.

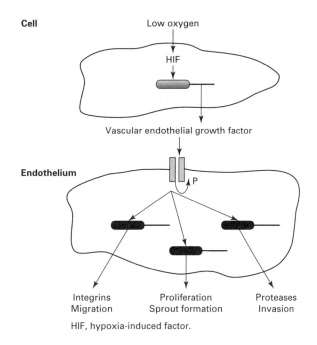

HIF, hypoxia-induced factor.

this section will consider angiogenesis mainly in the context of the establishment of secondary tumours, it should be appreciated that the same process is also essential for the establishment of primary tumours at their site of origin (see Figure 2.3).

The microcirculation is composed of capillaries, which are essentially tubes of endothelial cells with a basement membrane; proliferation rarely occurs in endothelial cells. Angiogenesis initially involves stimulation of endothelial cell proliferation and migration. Later, it commonly involves recruitment of other cells, such as smooth-muscle cells, concerned with the morphogenesis and maintenance of the new vessels.

Angiogenesis is stimulated by angiogenic factors, which are predominantly peptides. Many angiogenic factors are also growth factors (see Chapter 10); among the most important of these are **f**ibroblast **g**rowth **f**actor (FGF) and **v**ascular **e**ndothelial **g**rowth **f**actor (VEGF). Angiogenic factors are produced in very small quantities by many normal tissues. Production is upregulated in a physiological context by low oxygen tension (hypoxia) and in a pathological context by tumours (Figure 11.9). Hypoxia activates a series of serine/threonine protein kinases, the **s**tress-**a**ctivated **p**rotein **k**inases (SAPKs), which stimulate transcription from specific genes via **h**ypoxia-**i**nduced transcription **f**actors (HIFs) (see Chapter 10). The tumour suppressor gene *VHL* (**v**on **H**ippel–**L**indau) codes for a protein pVHL, which forms a complex with other proteins (Cul2, elongin B, elongin C, Rbx1). This complex degrades HIF in an oxygen-dependent manner. Cells lacking pVHL do not degrade HIF in response to oxygen. Because HIF controls the production of angiogenic factors such as VEGF, when it is not degraded the result is uncontrolled proliferation and the formation of a blood-vessel tumour (haemangioblastoma). VEGF is secreted as a large glycoprotein, which can be cleaved to yield a smaller but still active protein. Like FGF, VEGF can be stored as inactive complexes with ECM proteoglycans such as heparan; that active growth factor is released by ECM digestion (Figure 11.10).

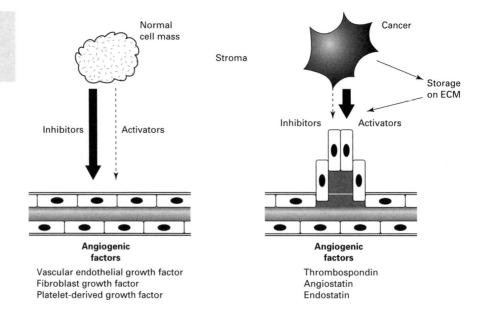

Figure 11.10

Activators and inhibitors of angiogenesis.

The importance of VEGF in angiogenesis is illustrated by knock-out mice; in VEGF$^{+/-}$ embryos blood-vessel formation is abnormal but not abolished, while VEGF$^{-/-}$ embryos die in mid-gestation.

The paracrine effect of VEGF is mediated via transmembrane receptors that are present only on endothelial cells, and so VEGF is mitogenic only at this site. FGF receptors have a wider distribution. VEGF and FGF have synergistic effects on endothelial cells. VEGF receptors are typical tyrosine kinase receptors in that they require dimerisation, tyrosine phosphorylation of the cytoplasmic domain and recruitment of SH domain proteins (see Chapter 10). Recruited proteins include phospholipase C, GAP and phosphatidyl inositol-3-kinase, each capable of transducing the proliferative signal to the endothelial cell nucleus (see Figure 11.9 and Chapter 10). The VEGF receptor gene also contains an HIF response element and is activated by hypoxia. In addition to these proliferative effects, VEGF also promotes the secretion of serine proteinases and metalloproteinases and induces integrins, VCAM and ICAM, all of which facilitate capillary sprout invasion of the ECM.

In a number of experimental situations, it can be demonstrated that there is a marked increase in the number of blood vessels within tumours before the phase of rapid growth. A similar relationship has been shown in collections of preserved human material (gliomas, breast, cervical and prostate cancers), where an increase in capillary density can be related to stage. These findings imply that angiogenesis is essential for tumour growth.

Anti-angiogenesis

In physiological situations, new capillary beds regress at the end of function, and so it could be expected that there are further regulating factors concerned with this degeneration. Indeed, several anti-angiogenic factors, such as angiostatin, endostatin and thrombospondin, have been identified. The thrombospondin gene is activated by p53 (see Figure 5.13), which helps to block angiogenesis; mutant p53 does not have this effect. Angiostatin and endostatin are products of the proteolysis of plasminogen and collagen XVIII; they may act by binding to and blocking growth factor receptors needed for endothelial proliferation. Administration of anti-angiogenic factors could have an indirect anti-cancer effect by causing regression of the blood supply to the tumour. In experimental situations, when endostatin was administered to nude mice carrying human tumours, the tumours shrank to a point where some were barely detectable.

Lymphangiogenesis

Until recently, lymphatic vessels have been difficult to study because they could not be distinguished from capillaries using normal histology. This has changed since the discovery of a specific marker for lymphatic endothelium, LYVE-1 (an antibody). Investigations have shown that the development of lymphatics is under the control of a system similar to the VEGF system regulating angiogenesis. In lymphangiogenesis, two members of the VEGF family, VEGF-C and VEGF-D, act on a specific receptor VEGF-R3, which is limited to lymphatic vessels. When VEGF-C and VEGF-D were experimentally overexpressed in tumours transplanted into mice, there was an increase in lymphangiogenesis and an increase in metastasis.

Now that the basic features of angiogenesis are known, attention is being focused on its manipulation for therapeutic purposes. Avenues of investigation include blocking $\alpha_v\beta_3$ integrins and inhibiting MMPs with synthetic peptides (see Chapter 12). Direct strategies involving angiogenic factors have been less successful for several reasons. For example, tumours can upregulate production of angiogenic factors when challenged with anti-angiogenic agents. Additionally, tumours frequently express multiple angiogenic factors (some pancreatic tumours can express up to eight angiogenic factors), which makes targeting difficult.

Gene changes involved in metastasis

Many gene products that influence metastatic spread have been mentioned in the preceding sections of this chapter. An important point to note is that different pathways are utilised by different cancers, and so there is no gene change that is common to all cancers. A caveat to this generalisation is that the gene products involved in angiogenesis are common to all cancers.

Both oncogenes and tumour suppressor genes are involved in metastasis, some of which have been implicated in other aspects of cancer biology. Thus, *ras* activation is associated with increased proliferation and is an early event in colorectal carcinogenesis. Ras-transfected cells have increased metastatic potential. Other oncogenes such as *v-src* and *v-raf* can also increase proliferation, tumorigenicity (transformation in culture) and invasiveness. Although properties such as transformation and proliferation are essential for metastasis, the following experiment shows how they can be separated. Experimentally, ras transforms some cells without affecting metastasis, while viruses such as adenovirus can block metastatic properties of ras but not its transforming effect. This indicates that transformation and metastasis can be divorced and metastasis is not simply a consequence of early events in carcinogenesis and proliferation. It is not clear how changes in a gene such as *ras* can influence transformation in some situations and metastasis in others. As ras is a focal point for multiple upstream and downstream signal pathways (see Chapter 9), it is possible that different responses are modulated in different cells.

Work investigating differences between cell lines with high and low metastatic potential has indicated that there is a group of 'signature genes' concerned with the metastatic phenotype. One such investigation used cells lines derived from a person with breast cancer with extensive metastases to lungs; 54 candidate genes were identified. Some of these genes were overexpressed and some were underexpressed. The genes included genes for a growth factor, a chemokine, metalloproteinases, an interleukin receptor and a cell adhesion receptor. Several of these candidate genes were also found in biopsy material derived from a group of patients with breast cancer; many of these patients developed lung metastases later.

Twist, a transcription factor and morphogenetic regulator, has been found to be strongly upregulated in metastasising clones of mouse mammary tumour. As Twist is a key inducer of mesoderm in embryogenesis, it is implicated in promoting an epithelial–mesenchymal transition and is a good candidate for orchestrating the many changes associated with metastasis.

Further reading

Metastasis

Achen, M.G., McColl, B.K. and Stacker, S.A. (2005) Focus on lymphangiogenesis in tumour metastasis. *Cancer Cell* **7**, 121–127.

Al-Mehdi, A.B., Tozawa, K., Fisher, A.B. *et al.* (2000) Intravascular origin of metastases from the proliferation of endothelium-attached tumour cells: a new model for metastasis. *Nat Med* **6**, 100–102.

Chang, C. and Werb, Z. (2001) The many faces of metalloproteases: cell growth, invasion angiogenesis and metastasis. *Trends Cell Biol* **11**, S37–S43.

Hart, I. (2005) The spread of tumours. In *Introduction to the Cellular and Molecular Biology of Cancer*, ed. M. Knowles and P. Selby. Oxford: Oxford University Press.

Minn, A.J., Gupta, G.P., Siegel, P.M., *et al.* (2005) Genes that mediate breast cancer metastasis to lungs. *Nature* **436**, 518–524.

Yang, J., Mani, S.A., Donaher, J.L., *et al.* (2004) Twist, a master regulator of morphogenesis, plays an essential role in tumour metastasis. *Cell* **127**, 927–939.

Angiogenesis

Burke, N.A. and DeNardo, S.J. (2001) Antiangiogenic agents and their promising potential in combined therapy. *Crit Rev Oncol Haematol* **39**, 155–171.

Reynolds, L.E., Wyder, L., Lively, J.C., *et al.* (2002) Enhanced pathological angiogenesis in mice lacking β3 integrin or β3 and β5 integrins. *Nat Med* **8**, 27–34.

Skobe, M., Hawighorst, T., Jackson, D.G., *et al.* (2001) Induction of tumour lymphangiogenesis by VEGF-C promotes breast cancer metastasis. *Nat Med* **7**, 192–198.

Tahtis, K. and Bicknell, R. (2005) Tumour angiogenesis. In *Introduction to the Cellular and Molecular Biology of Cancer*, ed. M. Knowles and P. Selby. Oxford: Oxford University Press.

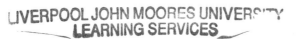

Principles of cancer treatment

- Different types of treatment are required first when the cancer is detected and later when the cancer has spread.
- It is important initially that the primary cancer is either removed or reduced in volume.
- The fewer cells there are when treatment begins, the greater the probability of achieving a cure.
- If a cancer has metastasised, drugs or radiotherapy are used.
- The objective of treatment is to prevent proliferation (cytostatic effect) and to kill the cancer cells (cytotoxic effect).
- Cell sensitivity to therapeutic agents varies at different times of the cell cycle.
- Future behaviour of a cancer can be predicted from its characteristics at the time of first treatment. The useful characteristics are tumour size, degree of spread from the original site, histological appearance and biochemical markers of growth and aggressiveness.
- Chemotherapy disrupts DNA synthesis and cell division by mechanisms common to all cells. This causes side effects.
- Optimal drug treatment reflects a compromise between effects on the cancer and toxicity to normal tissues.
- Drugs used in chemotherapy include alkylating agents that damage DNA, antimetabolites that inhibit nucleic acid synthesis, and natural products that have several effects.
- Combinations of drugs are more effective than single agents.
- Chemotherapy is used as a primary (neoadjuvant) therapy or as an adjuvant to other types of treatment. It is the main method for treating advanced cancer.
- Cancers arising from hormone-sensitive cells regress if deprived of hormone. This receptor-mediated process is not common to all cells, and so hormone treatment has fewer side effects than chemotherapy.
- Radiotherapy generates DNA strand breaks through free-radical formation.

- Photodynamic therapy involves laser activation of sensitive compounds that generate free radicals.
- Cells with DNA damaged by chemotherapy or radiotherapy die by the apoptotic pathway.
- New forms of treatment are being investigated based on interference with signal transduction, gene function, angiogenesis and cytokine action. Improved immunotherapy is also a goal.
- Cells within a cancer have heterogeneous sensitivities to drugs. This can be due to the properties of the cells, their place in the cell cycle or their distance from blood vessels.
- Resistance to drugs is acquired as a result of treatment. This can be due to altered cell permeability, altered metabolism, increased number of targets or more efficient DNA repair.

Introduction

It is possible to screen vulnerable populations for the pre-malignant signs or early stages of some cancers. In order to be effective, such screening must be applied to all the population at risk; it is useful only in cancers where there is a reasonable chance of a cure. Screening is expensive, and so it is used only for a few cancers and only in countries that can afford it. Breast cancer is screened for using specialised X-ray imaging (mammography) to image small lesions. Screening for cervical cancer employs cytological examination of a smear of cells, which are obtained by gently scraping the cervix and then stained with a specialised stain (Papanicolaou's stain). In colorectal cancers, the primary test is the detection of occult blood in the faeces; if positive, this is followed by direct visual inspection using endoscopy. Other cancers have less distinct diagnostic features and are screened less commonly. One example of this group is prostate cancer, which can be screened using a combination of a blood test for prostate-specific antigen (PSA) and digital rectal examination for prostate enlargement. Similarly, screening for stomach cancer can be carried out using indirect radiography and measurement of serum pepsinogen I and II levels. When pre-malignant or early malignant stages are detected by screening, prompt treatment can halt the progress of the disease.

It is more usual that the patient detects symptoms and reports these to a doctor, who then makes a preliminary diagnosis and refers the patient to a hospital with specialised staff and better diagnostic tools. Hospital examination may include imaging, biopsy to provide material for histopathology and clinical biochemistry. If the diagnosis is confirmed, then the state of development of the cancer (staging) is established, because the type of treatment is determined by the stage.

As cancer therapy is radical and involves several types of treatment, it is delivered by teams of specialists working in large hospitals. The principal therapeutic modalities are surgery, radiotherapy and chemotherapy, although other disciplines such as imaging, nursing and psychology provide important components in the whole treatment. In the case of solid tumours, the first step is usually surgical removal of the primary cancer together with a margin of normal tissue, as such cancers are commonly irregular in shape. Then the area around the site may be irradiated to destroy any possible remnants of the tumour. At the same time, cytotoxic drugs can be given to kill residual cancer cells and possible metastases. In such circumstances, the secondary treatments are referred to as adjuvant therapy; they are not the major modality, but they are an essential supplement to back it up. This is the usual pattern of treatment, but there are some situations where alternative approaches are used. In regions of anatomical complexity, such as the head and neck, and in regions of vital biological function, such as the brain and spine, surgery would cause many problems, and so radiotherapy is sometimes the preferred modality. In disseminated cancers such as leukaemia, the only modality that can be used is chemotherapy (Figure 12.1).

Chemotherapy almost inevitably causes depression of the haemopoietic system. This means a reduced output of blood cells, which results in reduced resistance to disease, anaemia and thrombocytopenia (reduced number of platelets). To combat these potentially dangerous side effects, supportive therapy in the form of antibiotic cover, GM-CSF, erythropoietin and thrombopoietin may be given.

If the primary tumour is detected at an early stage and the therapy is prompt, then the patient can be cured. However, if all the original cancer has not been removed or destroyed, then after a period any remaining tumour cells will start to grow again. Should secondary cancers develop, the therapeutic cycle is repeated. However, metastases are less frequently cured and will commonly cause death. The period of time from the first detection to death is called the overall survival time.

In some cancers, it is possible to constrain proliferation using cytostatic agents without eliminating the tumour. The breast is sensitive to oestrogens, and anti-oestrogens can provide a means of checking the growth of breast cancers. This type of

Figure 12.1

Clinical events in the treatment of cancer.

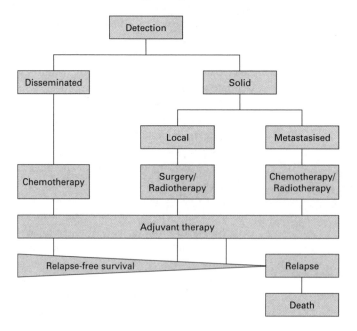

therapy is reasonably tissue-specific and non-toxic, thus offering some advantages over chemotherapy using cytotoxic agents, but it does not result in a cure.

The ideal treatment would be one that removed all the cancer cells without affecting normal cells; such a treatment does not exist and may be unattainable. Chemotherapy and radiotherapy will destroy not only proliferating cancer cells but also proliferating normal cells; it follows that side effects are almost inevitable.

Principles behind the treatment of cancer

Definition of response

It is important to have agreed criteria as to what constitutes a response so that effectiveness of regimens can be compared and patients informed as to the likely outcome of their treatments.

Relapse-free or overall survival times are good ways of covering both objectives. As people relapse at different rates, it is usual to plot a graph showing the proportion of patients with no detectable cancer or the proportion who are still alive at different times after treatment. Figure 12.2 shows such a graph of overall survival for people with breast cancer, whose cancers had (node-positive) or had not (node-negative) metastasised to the lymph nodes at the time of initial surgery. In the node-negative group, about one-quarter of the patients had died within 10 years, with little change thereafter, whereas three-quarters of the node-positive patients had died within the same time period and the group continued to do badly. It is bad news if cancer has spread at the time of first treatment. In order to compare different subgroups of patients, treatments or cancer types, it is inconvenient to present many such graphs; however, information can be presented in a simpler format as the proportion of patients being relapse-free 5 years after treatment. Table 12.1 presents these data for different cancers. In all cases, metastasis is accompanied by worse

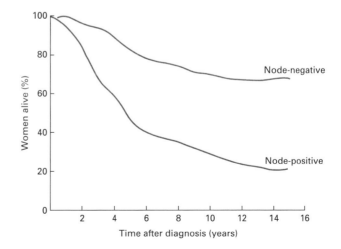

Figure 12.2

Overall survival for people with breast cancer. Node status was determined at the time of first treatment. (Source: Adapted from Figure 1 in Galea, M.H., *et al.* (1992) *Breast Cancer Research and Treatment*, **22**, 207–19.)

Table 12.1 Mean survival rates for various cancers after treatment.

Cancer	Percentage alive at 5 years*
Prostate	99
Breast	86
Bladder	82
Colorectal	63
Non-Hodgkin's lymphoma	58
Ovary	55
Leukaemias	43
Stomach	24
Lung	15
Pancreas	4

* Note that these values are averages and that they have a wide variation due to stage at diagnosis and effectiveness of therapy.
(Source: Adapted from Brenner, H. (2002) *The Lancet*, 360, 1131–35. Reprinted with permission from Elsevier.)

outcome; pancreatic and lung cancers have a poorer prognosis than prostate cancer, with colorectal and ovary cancers showing intermediate characteristics. The data for people with non-metastatic testicular cancer indicate that they are cured by the primary treatment.

Another set of definitions applied to advanced cancers classifies responses according to whether a cancer disappears completely (complete response), disappears partially (partial response), remains static (no change) or continues to grow (progressive disease). Partial and complete responses are often combined. A response period of 6 months is usually specified.

Using these criteria, chemotherapy can achieve response rates of 50%, although this figure covers wide variations depending on the type of cancer and the treatment used.

Patient criteria: stage and grade

When comparing different patients or treatments, like must be compared with like, such that the patients in the comparison groups begin with similar stages of cancer. Two types of criteria are used for this: one based on tumour size and degree of spread, i.e. stage of disease, and the other based on the cellular characteristics of the cancer, i.e. grade. Thus, a large cancer that has invaded its surroundings and metastasised to other parts of the body is at an advanced stage compared with a cancer that is confined to one site. Staging is done by the TNM system, based on the three criteria of **t**umour size, spread to the lymph **n**odes and **m**etastasis to distant sites. A stage 1 cancer is one of small size that has not progressed outside its original site, whereas a stage 4 growth is large and has spread widely. Figure 12.3 shows the influence of tumour stage on overall survival of women with breast cancer; one-quarter of stage 1 patients are alive at 10 years compared with none of the stage 4 group even at 5 years.

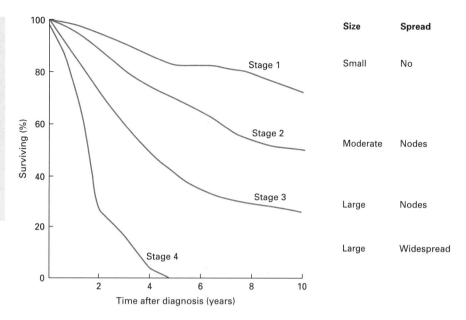

Figure 12.3

Overall survival for people with breast cancer. Staged at diagnosis.
(Source: Jordan, V. Craig (1987) *Estrogen/ Antiestrogen Action and Breast Cancer Therapy.* Madison, WI: University of Wisconsin Press. Copyright © 1987. Reprinted by permission.)

A low-grade tumour has a histological resemblance to the tissue of origin, whereas a high-grade cancer has undergone so many changes that it resembles the tissue of origin only marginally. Criteria for grading include number of mitoses, irregularities in nuclear shape (nuclear pleiomorphism) and architectural resemblance to normal tissue.

Both stage and grade are important because they measure different parameters of the cancer and can be used to predict the likely course of the cancer.

Early detection means better results

It was pointed out in Chapter 2 that if a cancer can be physically detected, then it has been developing for a long time, such that a 1 cm tumour has passed through three-quarters of its lifespan (see Figure 2.9). As time equates with increased cellular change towards aggressiveness, it follows that the earlier a cancer can be detected, the fewer changes it will have undergone and the more likelihood there will be of getting a good response to treatment. Animal experiments have indicated the increased likelihood of achieving a cure when small numbers of cancer cells are present at the start of therapy (Table 12.2). If a drug treatment kills 99.999% of the cells, then the fraction left alive is 0.001%. This is referred to as a 5 log kill, because 1×10^{-5} of the starting cells remain. Injection of 10^4 cells followed by the same degree of kill would leave no cells alive and all the animals would be cured. Injection of 10^9 cells followed by a 5 log kill would leave 10^4 viable cells, which are capable of killing all the animals. An intermediate number of remaining cells would result in the cure of some but not all animals. Achieving a 5 log kill is just possible in animals but virtually unattainable in patients because of toxic side effects. To put this in perspective, a cancer comprising 10^9 cells is only just detectable by physical

Table 12.2 Influence of cell number on response to a 5 log (99.999%) cell kill by a chemotherapeutic agent.

Cell number		Percentage of animals with tumours
Before treatment	**After treatment**	
10^4 (0.01 mg)	0	0
10^6 (1 mg)	10	50
10^9 (1 g)	10^4	100

examination of patients (see Figure 2.9), and so it is problematic to achieve a cure by anything other than surgical removal of all the cells.

These types of data indicate that early detection of very small or pre-malignant growths should result in more cures. Screening large numbers of people for early signs of cancer should, therefore, be beneficial, provided that a suitable test is available. Abnormal cells can be detected in smears taken from the cervix, and this form of cervical screening does save lives (Figure 12.4). Cervical smear tests were introduced widely into Denmark and Finland in the late 1960s, and death rates from cervical cancer have fallen since then. In contrast, tests were not introduced widely into Norway until the 1980s and deaths did not fall there until after this date. Screening for breast cancer by imaging the internal features of the breast using weak X-rays (mammography) can also be beneficial. Deaths from breast cancer are falling in some countries, reflecting partly the widespread use of mammography and partly the added benefits of more efficient treatments.

Figure 12.4

Effect of screening on deaths from cervical cancer. Widespread screening programmes were available in Denmark and Finland but not in Norway. (Source: Läärä, E., Day, N.E., and Hakama, M. (1987) Trends in mortality from cervical cancer in the Nordic countries: association with organised screening programmes. *Lancet* i 1247–9.)

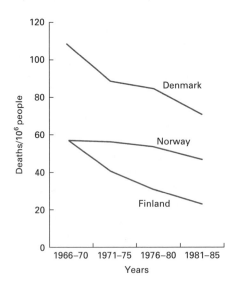

Surgery

The primary aim of surgery is to remove the entire tumour and, when appropriate, any metastases in regional lymphatics. This is the cornerstone of treatment for solid tumours, and it can, in some cases, result in a complete cure. In earlier times, cancer surgery often resulted in undesirable loss of function and deformities; more recently, there has been a trend to minimise surgery and to retain as much form and function as possible. A good example of this conservative trend is provided by the current therapy for breast cancer. In the past, radical mastectomy provided an adequate means of local control; however, the consequent effects could involve other organs and were often psychologically traumatic. Currently, partial mastectomy (lumpectomy) with adjuvant therapy is favoured because it provides a means of control that is as good as that provided by radical mastectomy, without the mutilating effects. The use of imaging techniques to define the size and position of deep-seated tumours and their surrounding organs can provide important information before surgery and radiotherapy. Such advances have led to an improvement in outcome of cancers such as that of the stomach, where surgery is essentially the only possible curative treatment.

In a few rare cancers with a strong familial basis, it is possible to prevent the disease using pre-emptive surgery. Such procedures include colectomy for young asymptomatic patients with familial adenomatous polypitis, and mastectomy for double homozygous carriers of the *BRCA1* and *BRCA2* genes.

Radiotherapy

Most therapeutic radiography uses specialised apparatus that delivers a narrow beam of high-energy X-rays to a well-defined area of the body. This allows treatment of both superficial and deep-seated tumours without surgical trauma. Damage to the adjacent and overlying tissues is minimised by selective shielding and by varying the direction of the beam so that the total dose occurs only at the site of the tumour. Such precision requires prior imaging in order to define the position of the tumour and adjacent organs, together with the use of stereotactic apparatus and computer-aided planning of irradiation. This is important because some organs, such as the lens of the eye, the spinal cord, the lung, the kidney and the small intestine, have a poor capacity to repair radiation damage.

The intended outcome of radiotherapy is to kill malignant cells by causing irreparable damage to their DNA. Cycling cells are radiosensitive, but tumour stem cells or quiescent G_0 cells are relatively resistant. Because of this, radiation doses are fractionated, so that the total dose is delivered over a period of days. This allows any damaged normal tissues to repair themselves while the tumour stem cells become reoxygenated and start proliferating. Subsequent doses will then destroy the reactivated tumour cells. Reoxygenation is also important, as oxygen is required for the generation of the free radicals necessary to produce full effectiveness (oxygen effect).

Less commonly, radiotherapy involves the use of radioactive sources. In units that do not have a therapeutic X-ray unit, radio-cobalt sources can be used to provide a beam of gamma rays for external radiotherapy. Another application is brachytherapy, which uses radiation from radioactive sources either placed close to or inserted in the tumour. Plastic-covered flexible iridium-131 wires can be inserted into tumours of the tongue, breast, brain and buccal mucosa to produce effects similar to those produced by external radiotherapy systems.

Chemotherapy

The term 'chemotherapy' is conventionally confined to the use of cytotoxic or cytostatic drugs that respectively kill malignant cells or prevent them from proliferating. The efficacy of such drugs depends on the concentration of the drugs reaching the tumour, the duration of exposure, and the proportion of the population that is proliferating. The latter point is important, as the drugs act mainly on proliferating cells, and tumours commonly include subpopulations of cells that are not dividing. This action is not limited to malignant cells; it affects proliferating cells throughout the body, resulting in numerous untoward effects. Cytotoxic drugs can also be specifically toxic to vital organs such as the heart and the kidney, and so they must be used with utmost caution. To some degree, the side effects can be minimised by careful dosing, by using combinations of drugs with different toxicities (combination or polychemotherapy) and by using supportive procedures. During the course of treatment, the target cells may become resistant to the drugs used, and so many chemotherapists prefer to use high doses initially in the hope of killing all the malignant cells before resistance develops.

Cellular heterogeneity

By the time a cancer reaches the stage of requiring treatment, molecular changes associated with progression have taken place to a variable extent, and so the constituent cells behave in a heterogeneous manner. This is reflected in the fact that some cells respond to treatment while others remain unresponsive. This heterogeneity is due to the individual characteristics of the cells and to their location within the cancer (Figure 12.5). Unfortunately, individual cells can develop resistance against drugs to which they are exposed (intrinsic resistance). The mechanisms underlying that resistance are discussed later on. Some potentially sensitive cells are resistant because of external factors (extrinsic resistance). This can be due to their stage in the cell cycle or their location relative to blood vessels. Cells that are in G_1 are refractory to most treatments, compared with those in S or M. Thus, if DNA synthesis takes up 1% of the cycle time, then only 1% of cells will be in the S phase at any moment and only 1% of cells will be sensitive to S-phase-specific drugs. In some cancers, such as of the colon and skin, where stem cells are present, a cure will not be achieved unless they are destroyed; killing the other cells will help but will not eliminate the cancer.

Location of the cells within a cancer can also influence response because drugs must reach those cells from the general circulation. The further a cancer cell is from a blood vessel, the less likely the cancer cell is to receive enough drug to kill it. Likewise, radiotherapy relies on the generation of reactive oxygen species from

Figure 12.5

Cells within a cancer have different sensitivities.

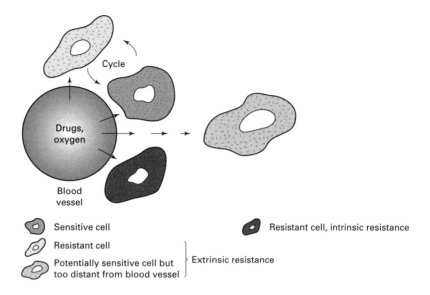

molecular oxygen to damage the DNA (see Chapter 6), and this oxygen is delivered by the blood. Hypoxia increases with distance from a blood vessel, and so radiation sensitivity decreases with distance. Some areas of a tumour are well vascularised whereas others are not; poorly vascularised cells will be hardly affected by drugs. For example, it would take an antibody several months to travel from the outside to the centre of a 1 cm tumour by diffusion alone. Blood vessels within the cancer are essential if this time period is to be reduced.

Cytostatic and cytotoxic effects: cell death and proliferation

The best results are obtained if cancer cells are killed (cytotoxic effect) rather than their growth arrested but left viable (cytostatic effect). This is not to suggest that cytostatic effects are not beneficial. Definitions of whether a response has occurred include a 'no change' category, which is considered to be a partial success rather than a partial failure because cancer expansion has been stopped. It is also worth remembering that growth is a balance of proliferation and death and that relatively small changes in either property can tip the balance in favour of increased or decreased size (Table 12.3). It has been estimated that during active growth, for every 100 cells that divide to give 200 daughter cells, 80 die, thus leaving 120 to continue the expansion process. The dying cells do not necessarily come from the proliferating pool; however, if the number dying can be increased to more than 100, then there would be a net cell loss and the tumour would shrink. This type of argument is used in favour of maximising the doses of chemotherapeutic drugs that a patient can stand in order to optimise cell kill at a time of low tumour cell burden.

With the realisation that cell death can be actively induced via the apoptosis pathway, attention is being directed at its manipulation as a form of treatment. Indeed,

Table 12.3 Influence of cell death and proliferation on tumour growth.

	Regression	Growth	
Cell death	← Stasis	⇌ Proliferation	

Number of cells dying per 100 proliferating★	Net change	Result
80	+120	Growth
100	0	Stasis
120	−20	Regression

★ To generate 200 daughter cells.

DNA damage, be it drug- or radiation-induced, activates the apoptosis pathway (see Chapters 6 and 9). The other form of cell death, necrosis, can also be increased by preventing angiogenesis. In the absence of new blood-vessel formation, oxygen and essential nutrients are not available to maintain cell functions and necrotic death ensues. Death sets in at about 150 μm either side of a blood vessel, which limits tumour size to 300 μm around individual vessels.

Cell-cycle-specific effects

The majority of drugs used for treating cancer are based on preventing DNA synthesis or mitosis. Actions of individual drugs are discussed later, but some general points will be described here.

Most of the agents mentioned in Figure 12.6 act at specific phases (phase-specific drugs) of the cell cycle, whereas others, such as cyclophosphamide, function at several phases and are referred to as cycle-specific. This distinction is a relative one in that most drugs act at several phases of the cycle but are especially effective at certain points. Thus, cultured cells are four times more sensitive to ionising radiation during mitosis than during DNA synthesis, with intermediate effects being seen in G_1. Likewise, vincristine blocks cells in mitosis but the effective interaction between it and its target, tubulin, occurs earlier.

It is also evident from Figure 12.6 that treatment regimens are aimed at several molecules, although effects on DNA predominate. Again, these specificities should be taken only as guidelines, because **5-fluorouracil** (5FU) inhibits DNA synthesis as well as RNA transcription (see below).

Two of the agents mentioned in Figure 12.6, hormones and retinoic acid, are more specific because they affect only cells that contain specific intracellular receptors for these ligands. Retinoic acid induces differentiation in one form of leukaemia, acute promyelocytic leukaemia (see Chapter 5), and thus blocks their proliferation, whereas steroid hormone antagonists block receptor-positive cells in G_1 (see Chapter 10).

Figure 12.6

Drug effects related to
the cell cycle.

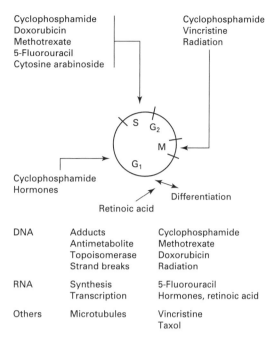

Cyclophosphamide
Doxorubicin
Methotrexate
5-Fluorouracil
Cytosine arabinoside

Cyclophosphamide
Vincristine
Radiation

Cyclophosphamide
Hormones

Retinoic acid

Differentiation

DNA	Adducts	Cyclophosphamide
	Antimetabolite	Methotrexate
	Topoisomerase	Doxorubicin
	Strand breaks	Radiation
RNA	Synthesis	5-Fluorouracil
	Transcription	Hormones, retinoic acid
Others	Microtubules	Vincristine
		Taxol

Apoptosis as a conduit for cell killing

Cells damaged during therapy must be removed; apoptotic death can achieve this
objective. Ionising radiation and genotoxic drugs, which include many used in
chemotherapy, switch on the repressor gene *p53* that stops proliferation and activates apoptosis (see Chapters 6 and 9). Cells with defective p53 are resistant to some
chemotherapeutic agents and to radiation damage. An attractive hypothesis is that
resistance to apoptosis may contribute to drug resistance. Oncogene-transformed mouse
cells are sensitive to apoptosis induced by 5FU, doxorubicin and radiation only if
normal p53 is present; loss of function of p53 results in resistance to each of these
agents.

Side effects

Minimising the side effects of treatments is a major consideration in deciding therapeutic options. In breast cancer, hormone therapy has fewer side effects than
chemotherapy and is the preferred method for certain patients (see below). Agents
that are relatively non-specific because they modulate general functions such as proliferation present special problems. Because cancer cells can have increased levels
of signal transduction molecules such as growth factor receptors, they can respond
to lower doses of some drugs, but side effects will still occur. Treatments under
development are directed at increasing specificity by targeting drugs preferentially
to cancer cells (see below).

Haemopoietic cells are particularly sensitive to cytotoxic drugs, and treatment commonly results in anaemia and reduced white blood cell numbers, with resulting decreased resistance to infection. The former can be treated either with blood transfusions or erythropoietin, and the latter with either antibiotics or G-CSF/GM-CSF treatment. Alternatively, protection can be achieved by removing bone marrow before therapy and returning it after the completion of treatment (autologous bone-marrow transplantation).

Germ cells in the ovary and testis are chemosensitive, and so young patients may become sterile as a result of treatment. Although this cannot be prevented, storage of ova and semen is possible so that parenthood need not be denied to people receiving such treatment.

Nausea and vomiting are common side effects of chemotherapy because the drugs involved activate vomiting centres in the brain stem; these effects can be alleviated by 5-hydroxytryptamine receptor antagonists or corticosteroids.

Drug resistance

Some cells have an intrinsic resistance to chemotherapeutic agents, but almost all cells have mechanisms by which they can acquire resistance when exposed to a drug. The various ways by which this resistance is acquired are listed in Table 12.4, together with the drugs involved. Development of resistance is the main cause of treatment failure following an initial good response. Mechanisms involved with drug resistance are described here, and additional points about specific drugs are given later.

Membrane transport and the P-glycoprotein

When cells are exposed to a single drug such as vincristine, they develop cross-resistance to other drugs derived from natural products that are of dissimilar structure and function, such as doxorubicin and etoposide, as well as to vincristine itself. Their only common feature is that they are lipophilic. This insensitivity is caused

Table 12.4 Mechanisms of resistance to chemotherapeutic drugs.

Process	Cause	Drugs affected
Decreased influx	Folate transporters	Methotrexate
Increased efflux	P-glycoprotein	Vincristine, doxorubicin
Increased inactivation	Glutathione–S–transferase	Alkylating agents
Decreased activation	Kinases	5-Fluorouracil, cytosine arabinoside
	Polyglutamation	Methotrexate
Increased targets	Dihydrofolate reductase	Methotrexate
Increased DNA repair	Repair proteins	Doxorubicin, alkylating agents
Poor blood supply	Inadequate drug	All drugs
Sanctuary sites	Blood–brain barrier	All drugs

by an approximately 1000-fold increase in the level of P-glycoprotein, a 170 kDa transmembrane protein that functions as an ATP-dependent efflux pump for the drugs. Increased expression can result from either gene amplification or increased transcription from the normal gene. This is called the **m**ulti**d**rug **r**esistance (MDR) phenotype; the responsible genes are the *MDR* genes. Compared with cells that have normal levels of P-glycoprotein, MDR cells can be 100 times more resistant to drugs such as doxorubicin. The normal function of P-glycoprotein is as a Cl⁻ ion efflux pump. Its ability to pump out such diverse chemicals is due to multiple binding sites on its cytoplasmic face. The drug can reach the internal plasma membrane but it is then transferred to the exterior before reaching the cytoplasm. Ca^{2+} ion channel blockers such as verapamil will compete with vincristine for binding sites; thus, verapamil can reduce the degree of resistance to vincristine.

The cross-resistance does not apply to all drugs, because alkylating agents and antimetabolites are unaffected by levels of P-glycoprotein. There is a good general correlation between P-glycoprotein expression and degree of drug insensitivity.

Resistance mechanisms for alkylating agents and antimetabolites are more specific than MDR, causing cross-resistance to other drugs only if they use the same enzyme-transport mechanisms or if they are subject to the same repair mechanisms. Cells can become resistant to methotrexate by loss of reduced folate carrier, the membrane protein required to transport it into the cell. These cells would be cross-resistant to other antifolates, such as raltitrexed, which use the same transporter.

Drug metabolism

All drugs are inactivated by metabolism, but some require a metabolic activation step before they are active. Changes to both processes can result in resistance. Alkylating agents are conjugated to glutathione by glutathione–*S*-transferase, and upregulation of this enzyme increases the rate of drug inactivation. Antimetabolites such as 5FU and cytarabine are activated by phosphorylations, and the kinases involved (see below) are downregulated by prolonged drug exposure. A different type of drug-induced change to an activation step occurs with methotrexate. Methotrexate inactivates its target protein dihydrofolate reductase on its own, but that activity is enhanced once it penetrates the cell by addition of four to six glutamate residues (see below). This process does not alter the ability of methotrexate to inactivate dihydrofolate reductase, but it does reduce efflux, meaning that methotrexate remains active for a longer period. Loss of the polyglutamation process reduces this activity.

Altered targets

Prolonged exposure to methotrexate also causes amplification of the gene for its target protein dihydrofolate reductase. The amplified genes are expressed so that insufficient drug is available to inhibit all the dihydrofolate reductase. The same end result, increased enzyme activity, can also be achieved by gene mutations.

DNA repair

Cells contain efficient mechanisms for repairing damaged DNA (see Chapter 7). Increased activity of this complex series of processes therefore minimises the biological effect of DNA damage caused by alkylating agents and natural products such as doxorubicin.

Blood supply and sanctuary sites

Poor blood supply results in inadequate drug delivery (see above), while the blood–brain barrier prevents drugs carried in the blood from reaching cancer cells growing in the brain. These are called sanctuary sites.

Tumour markers

The ability to predict how a cancer might behave is useful in deciding what treatment to give or in monitoring whether a treatment is working. This can be achieved by looking at the physical characteristics of the cancer and of tissue and serum from the patient. Patient characteristics such as nodal status and TNM stage are used to decide whether adjuvant therapy is required at first diagnosis (see above). Serum or tissue analysis can refine the decision-making by providing additional information. The main questions that can be answered in this way are: How fast is the cancer growing? Is it likely to metastasise? Which is the best drug to use, and is the drug effective? The majority of chemicals that provide such information are proteins detected by specific antibodies, so the term 'antigen' will be used to describe them. They are known as tumour markers. The term 'prognostic factor' is sometimes used, but this can include features such as nodal status and histological tumour grade. The availability of **p**olymerase **c**hain **r**eaction (PCR) kits to amplify and detect altered DNA base sequences in minute samples of cells has identified additional uses for tumour markers, such as the detection of tumour cells in blood or lymph nodes and the diagnosis of cancer types that are difficult to categorise by conventional pathology. Indeed, this methodology, plus the ability to detect antigens in tissue sections by immunohistochemical means, makes the dividing line between chemical pathology and histopathology (see Chapter 3) somewhat artificial.

Blood

A few cancers produce antigens that enter the general circulation; these can be assayed in a serum sample. Such assays are useful in two contexts: screening undetected cancer and monitoring the behaviour of an established cancer, since the amount of antigen present is related to the number of cancer cells present. **P**rostate-**s**pecific **a**ntigen (PSA) can be used in screening for prostate cancer; however, this test can yield both false negatives and false positives, as PSA is elevated in benign prostate hyperplasia. The glycoprotein CA-125 is raised in about 80% of women with ovarian cancer and can be used as a marker for ovarian cancer; however, CA-125 may also be elevated in a smaller proportion of people with cancers of the breast, colon and pancreas, and it is elevated in pregnancy. The CA-125 level can be used to determine how much cancer may be present (tumour burden) and to monitor how much of the cancer is destroyed by chemotherapy.

In healthy people, the only nucleated (DNA-containing) cells in the blood are leucocytes; people with cancer have additional blood-borne metastatic cells. These cells are too sparse to be detected by conventional means but they can be identified through the remarkable sensitivity of the PCR. Amplification of specific DNA sequences by this method means the cells can be assayed in samples containing fewer than ten nucleated cells. All cells in an individual contain essentially the same DNA, and so directly detecting specific sequences would not achieve the desired objective of distinguishing cancer cells from normal leucocytes. However, expression of those sequences in the form of mRNA is relatively cell-specific, and so specificity can be achieved by first converting the mRNA sequences to their DNA homologues with a **r**everse **t**ranscriptase enzyme followed by PCR (RTPCR). The choice of which mRNA to monitor depends on the cell of interest, but cytokeratins are particularly useful for detecting epithelial cancer cells; epithelia express different cytokeratins from those in leucocytes (see Box 10.1).

Tissue

Tissue is available at the time of surgery or as a result of biopsy at other times. Expression of a wide range of antigens can be assayed either biochemically or immunohisto-chemically. Cell-sorting devices can identify the number of proliferating cells or ploidy status of the nuclear DNA.

The biological properties of a cancer for which assays are useful are cell proliferation, aggressiveness and treatment sensitivity. A rapidly growing aggressive tumour will recur quickly and requires treatment immediately. Proliferation can be assayed by incorporation of bromodeoxyuridine into DNA followed by its quantitation with an antibody raised against the nucleoside. A simpler assay is immunohistochemical detection of nuclear antigens related to DNA synthesis. Two antigens of proven use are **p**roliferating **c**ell **n**uclear **a**ntigen (PCNA) and Ki-67. PCNA is required for DNA polymerase function (see Chapter 9); the action of Ki-67 is less clear. Flow cytometry can also be used to assess the proportion of S-phase cells in a population: DNA in tumour nuclei is stained with a fluorescent dye and fractionated according to the DNA content per nucleus. The number of cells with double DNA content indicates the cells in S+G_2 of the cell cycle before mitosis.

Aggressiveness is a vague term covering many functions, and a multitude of antigens has been proposed for its prognosis. Two groups are worth mentioning: adhesion molecules and growth factor receptors. Invasion and metastasis require loss and gain of various cell adhesion molecules (see Chapter 11). E-cadherin is lost in many metastatic epithelial cells, whereas integrins can increase or decrease depending on the type of integrin and the type of cell. Growth factor receptors such as epidermal growth factor and erbB2 (see Chapter 10) are elevated in malignant tumours, and increased expression of either of these antigens indicates a poor prognosis. An aneuploid DNA profile detected by flow cytometry also points to an aggressive cancer.

There are few antigens available to predict responses to treatment. There is no totally reliable marker for response to chemotherapy. However, the presence of oestrogen and progestogen receptors in endometrial and breast cancers indicates a high probability of response to hormone therapy.

Chemotherapy

Chemotherapy uses cytotoxic drugs that disrupt the cell cycle, thus causing the death of proliferating cells. The ways in which these work, and the processes affected, are given in outline in Figure 12.6 above and in Table 12.5. The agents used are

Table 12.5 Processes affected by chemotherapeutic drugs.

Agent	Process affected	Cancers treated
Alkylating agents		
Cyclophosphamide	DNA synthesis	Breast, leukaemia
Cisplatin	DNA synthesis	Ovary, testis
Antimetabolites		
Methotrexate	Dihydrofolate reductase	Breast, placenta
5-Fluorouracil	Thymidylate synthase, RNA synthesis	Stomach, breast, colorectal
Cytosine arabinoside	DNA polymerase	Leukaemia, lymphoma
Natural products		
Doxorubicin	DNA and RNA synthesis	Lung, breast, leukaemia
Vincristine	Tubulin polymerisation	Lymphoma, testis
Taxol	Tubulin depolymerisation	Ovary, breast

divided into several different categories based in part on the manner in which they work and in part on their chemical nature.

Regimens using single drugs can be effective; for example, methotrexate alone is effective in the treatment of early choriocarcinoma (cancer of the placenta). However, it is more usual to use several drugs. The beneficial effect of this approach is illustrated in Figure 12.7, which shows that with increasing numbers of drugs used the remission rate is improved in patients with Hodgkin's lymphoma. Different combinations are used for different cancers; each combination is given an acronym. There are

Figure 12.7

Number of drugs in a combination. The graph shows remission of Hodgkin's lymphoma for drug combinations containing one, two and four drugs. (Source: Reproduced from Fig. 17.2 in Franks, L.M. and Teich, N.M. (eds) (1991) *Introduction to the Cellular and Molecular Biology of Cancer*, Second Edition. Oxford: Oxford University Press. Copyright © 1991. Reprinted with permission of Oxford University Press.)

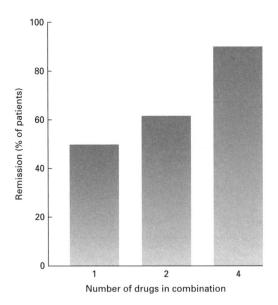

many of these (CHOPP, VAD, MOPP, etc.), but it is sufficient here to give one example, CMF, which contains cyclophosphamide, methotrexate and 5FU. Cyclophosphamide is an alkylating agent, while the methotrexate and 5FU are antimetabolites. Cells develop different types of resistance to each of these compounds (see above), and so combination increases the likelihood that one of the drugs will be effective on the cells. Each drug has its own toxicity profile, and thus individual toxicities can be minimised without diminishing the overall cytotoxic effect. Many cytotoxic drugs are themselves carcinogens (see Chapter 6) and, in rare cases, dissimilar cancers may appear several years after successful chemotherapy.

The potential benefits of primary (neoadjuvant) chemotherapy are being investigated, but its worth in both the adjuvant and metastatic settings is established. Adjuvant chemotherapy after surgery plus radiotherapy for Wilms' tumour (kidney) in children can double the survival rate. Beneficial but less dramatic effects are seen with adult tumours. Chemotherapy is often the only treatment option for metastatic cancers.

Most chemotherapeutic agents in current use were discovered years ago, but treatment responses have improved because the agents can now be delivered to the cancer more efficiently. Maintaining an effective concentration of the drug over a long period of time is more effective than giving one large dose; it also produces fewer side effects. For cycle-specific drugs, prolonged delivery also has the benefit of targeting cells at different cycle phases because the cells eventually reach a phase at which the drug is most effective.

Drugs can sometimes be perfused through the affected area without entering the general circulation.

Not all cancers respond well to cytotoxic drugs. The leukaemias and lymphomas, germ-cell cancers and choriocarcinomas generally respond well, but melanomas and cancers of the liver, pancreas, brain, kidney and thyroid do not.

Alkylating agents

Alkylating agents form adducts with DNA bases, which disrupts DNA synthesis (see Chapter 6). Most alkylating agents have two functional groups, each of which can react with a DNA base and form interstrand and intrastrand cross-links within the DNA double helix. These links can be formed at any stage of the cell cycle, and thus alkylating agents are not phase-specific.

Cyclophosphamide

The structure of cyclophosphamide is shown in Figure 12.8, together with the guanine adducts resulting from its metabolic activation and through which its effects are mediated. Cyclophosphamide metabolites block proliferation at several stages of the cycle (see Figure 12.6) and are used in combination with methotrexate and 5FU for treatment of many cancers, such as those of the breast. The side effects of cyclophosphamide include immunosuppression, hair loss and sterility. Resistance to its actions occurs through changes in cellular transport and increased DNA repair. Alkylating agents such as nitrosoureas methylate DNA guanines (see Figure 6.7), which are repaired by alkyl transferase (see Figure 7.4). There is increased activity of alkyl transferase in brain tumours, which renders them less sensitive to methylating drugs.

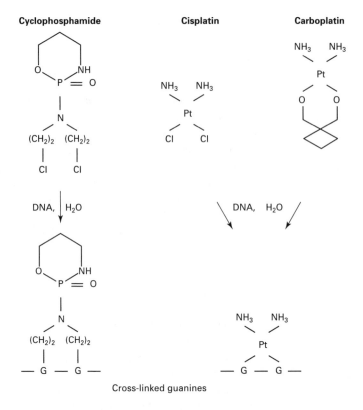

Figure 12.8

Alkylating agents that cross-link DNA guanines.

A related compound, ifosfamide, is as effective as cyclophosphamide but has a different toxicity profile.

Cisplatin

Cisplatin and its analogue carboplatin are converted to alkylating species in the body (Figure 12.8), preferentially forming adducts at the N-7 position of guanine and adenine. These adducts can interact with adjacent bases on the same strand (intrastrand adducts) or on separate strands (interstrand adducts). The order of preference for adduct formation is G : G > A : G > others. Intrastrand adducts distort the DNA helix, while interstrand links prevent strand separation, so that replication is inhibited or abnormal.

Cisplatin is particularly effective against ovarian and testicular cancers. Cisplatin has an advantage over other chemotherapeutic agents in that it has minimal effect on the bone marrow. Its main toxicities are nausea, renal dysfunction (nephrotoxicity) and neural effects. Carboplatin has a similar anti-tumour profile to cisplatin but it has greatly reduced side effects, especially with regard to nephrotoxicity.

Resistance to cisplatin can result from its altered cellular transport, enhanced repair of damaged DNA or inactivating reactions of the cisplatin with sulphydryl groups in proteins and glutathione. Cisplatin derivatives are not influenced by MDR mechanisms, but they are substrates for glutathione-*S*-tranferase, the detoxifying enzyme that conjugates the drug with reduced glutathione (Figure 12.9); cisplatin-resistant

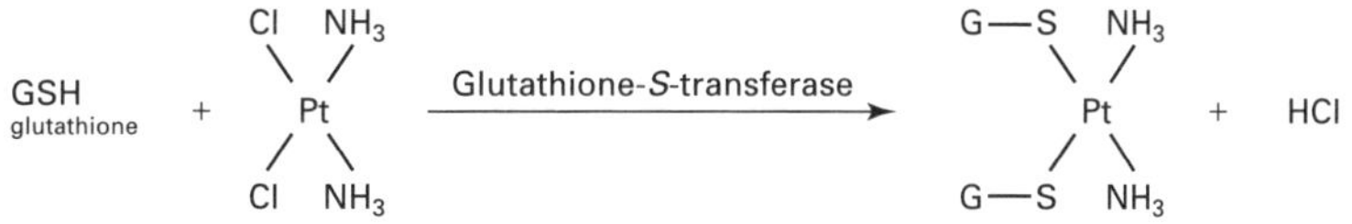

Figure 12.9

Cisplatin resistance may be due to glutathione-*S*-transferase.

cancers can overexpress this enzyme. Cisplatin also upregulates metallothionine, whose sulphydryl groups interact with the drug by a reaction analogous to that of glutathione. Decreased efficiency of apoptosis may play a role in cisplatin resistance. In experimental systems, increased expression of the anti-apoptosis protein Bcl2 (see Chapter 9) correlates with decreased drug sensitivity of ovarian and breast cancers, but the correlation is not good enough to use Bcl2 as a predictive test for chemoresistance in patients.

Antimetabolites

Antimetabolites inhibit nucleic acid synthesis. The mechanism by which this occurs depends on the compound.

Methotrexate

Methotrexate is one of the few drugs capable of curing a cancer, choriocarcinoma, on its own, although it is more commonly used in combination with other agents. Methotrexate is a derivative of folic acid and competitively inhibits the enzyme **dihydrofolate reductase** (DHFR), essential for purine and pyrimidine production and therefore DNA synthesis (Figure 12.10). Folic acid is reduced to tetrahydrofolic acid (FH_4), which accepts a one-carbon fragment from serine to form either N^5,N^{10}-methylene-FH_4 or N^{10}-formyl-FH_4. The methylene group in N^5,N^{10}-methylene-FH_4 can be donated to phosphoribosyl glycinamide in the purine biosynthetic pathway, while the formyl group of N^{10}-formyl-FH_4 methylates dUMP under the action of thymidylate synthase, thus forming dTMP. In the process of carbon donation, FH_4 is converted to FH_2 and must be reconverted to FH_4 by DHFR. Methotrexate, which has a methyl group on the N-10 position of folic acid plus a 4-amino group, inhibits this hydrogenation, which depletes the pool of reduced folate.

If high doses of methotrexate are used, its toxic effect on the bone marrow cells can be considerable. However, this can be counteracted by providing reduced folate in the form of leucovorin (folinic acid, N^5-formyl-FH_4).

Methotrexate enters the cell by active transport. Drug resistance can result from decreased activity of this transport process. Two other types of resistance are encountered: amplification of the *DHFR* gene and decreased polyglutamate formation within the cell. Exposure to methotrexate can generate a several-thousand-fold amplification of the *DHFR* gene plus DNA regions on either side, to the extent that the changes can be seen in stained chromosomes. This can take the form of homogeneous staining regions within the chromosome due to the amplified DNA, or it can take the form of double minute chromosomes that are separate from the standard chromosome. Amplification of the *DHFR* gene results in overexpression of the enzyme; methotrexate will not inhibit all the available enzyme. Folic acid

Figure 12.10

Folic acid: structure and derivatives. Methotrexate inhibition of nucleic acid synthesis.

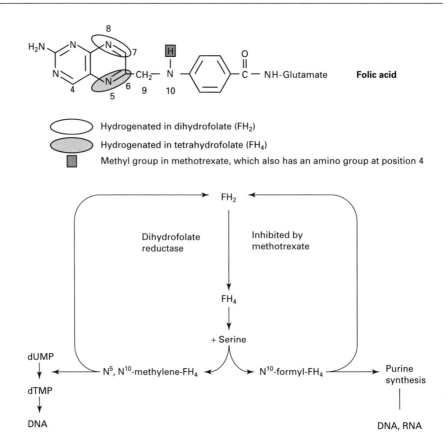

Hydrogenated in dihydrofolate (FH_2)

Hydrogenated in tetrahydrofolate (FH_4)

Methyl group in methotrexate, which also has an amino group at position 4

can have four to six glutamate residues added within the cell; this biologically active derivative is retained within the cell to a greater extent than the parent compound. The enzymes involved in glutamate addition become less active in cancers, and so the inhibitory activity of the methotrexate is diminished.

5-Fluorouracil

5FU is a derivative of uracil that can be phosphorylated and incorporated into RNA, which is thus not functional (Figure 12.11). Additionally, 5FU produces 5–fluoro–dUMP, which forms an inactive ternary complex with the N^5,N^{10}-methylene-FH_4 and thymidylate synthase, thereby inhibiting DNA synthesis. 5FU is used to treat breast and stomach cancers. Its main toxicity is to bone marrow cells. Resistance results from increased catabolism and downregulation of its activating enzymes.

Cytarabine (Ara-C)

When deoxyribose in cytidine is replaced by arabinose, another five-carbon sugar, the product is Ara-C. This can be phosphorylated to form Ara-CTP, which is an inhibitor of DNA polymerase α. Some Ara-C is also incorporated into DNA. Both processes block DNA synthesis, and so Ara-C is an S-phase inhibitor. It is effective against leukaemia. Its main toxicity is on bone marrow. Resistance results from loss of activating kinases and increased catabolism.

Figure 12.11

5-Fluorouracil: structure and actions.

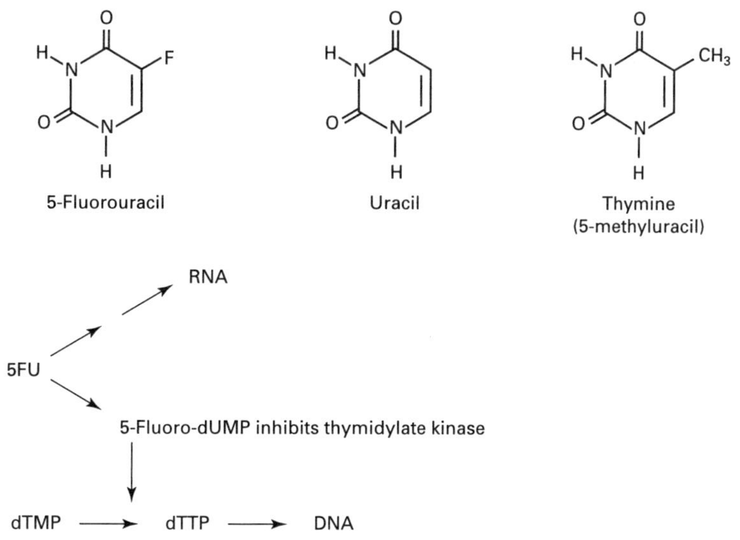

5-Fluorouracil   Uracil   Thymine (5-methyluracil)

5FU → RNA

5FU → 5-Fluoro-dUMP inhibits thymidylate kinase

dTMP → dTTP → DNA

Natural products

Topoisomerase inhibitors

The topoisomerases are enzymes concerned with uncoiling of hypercoiled DNA during and after replication. There are inhibitors for the two major types of topoisomerase – topoisomerase I (inhibited by the camptothecins, e.g. topotecan) and topoisomerase II (inhibited the epipodophyllotoxins, e.g. etoposide). Both types of inhibitor cause the formation of double-strand breaks and the death of the cell. At a cellular level, they induce G_2 arrest and apoptosis.

Microtubule poisons

These drugs disrupt the function of the spindle during mitosis. Consequently, the chromosomes do not separate, the dividing cell becomes blocked at metaphase and apoptosis ensues. The vinca alkaloids (vincristin, vinblastine, vinorelbine) prevent the polymerisation of tubulin, while the taxanes (Paclitaxel, docetaxel) stabilise the microtubule and prevent depolymerisation; this leads to the formation of abnormal spindles and apoptosis. These compounds are effective against a wide spectrum of cancers such as the leukaemias and lymphomas and ovarian, breast and testicular cancers.

Anthracyclin antibiotics

These antibiotics (doxorubicin, epirubicin) have several effects on DNA. They intercalate and cause partial unwinding of the double helix. They also generate free radicals, cause single- and double-strand breaks and bind to topoisomerase II, the enzyme concerned with untangling DNA, which induces cleavage, unwinding and rejoining of the DNA strands. These agents are used mainly in breast cancers and leukaemias.

Hormone therapy

Breast cancer and prostate cancer are the most common cancers in women and men, respectively, in the Western world (see Figure 1.3). The normal progenitor cells require oestrogens (women) or androgens (men) for their proliferation. This mitogenic effect of the sex steroids is mediated by specific intracellular receptors, which are gene transcription factors (see Chapter 10) that overcome a block in the G_1 phase of the cycle. Antagonising this effect generates a cytostatic response, although additional cytotoxic effects may occur. Because relatively few cell types contain these receptors, drugs aimed at their disruption have a degree of specificity that is missing from chemotherapeutic agents. As breast and prostate cancers occur predominantly in older people, disruption of reproductive function, the main side effect of hormone therapy, is not considered a problem. This is not true for younger women, however, in whom the menstrual cycle can be disrupted.

Treatment of hormone-sensitive cancers is based on the principle of depriving the cancer of the mitogenic hormone, which can be achieved either by preventing steroid synthesis or by blocking their effects at the target cell level via the receptor machinery (Figure 12.12).

Figure 12.12

Depriving breast cancers of hormone.

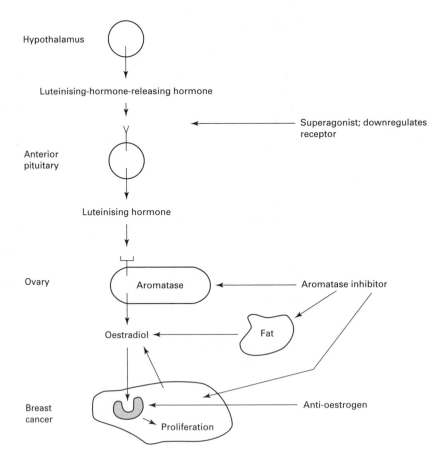

Disruption of steroid synthesis

Depletion of sex steroids was originally achieved by surgical removal of the relevant gland – ovary, testis, adrenal or pituitary. However, currently, pharmacological manipulation is the method of choice, except for ovarian destruction by radiotherapy without recourse to surgery. Inactivation of ovarian function is effective only in premenopausal women, as the postmenopausal ovary has already stopped producing oestradiol. As far as breast cancer is concerned, oestradiol (Figure 12.12) is the main oestrogen in humans and is synthesised mostly in the ovary, and so the function of the ovary is central to treatments based on removing oestradiol. Ovarian function is regulated by polypeptide hormones produced by the anterior pituitary gland – **l**uteinising **h**ormone (LH) and **f**ollicle-**s**timulating **h**ormone (FSH). These hormones are collectively known as gonadotrophins. The release of LH and FSH is modulated by polypeptides synthesised in hypothalamic centres of the brain. **LH-r**eleasing **h**ormone (LHRH), synthesised in the hypothalamus, is especially important, because its effect can be blocked by antagonists. In postmenopausal women, the ovary becomes refractory to pituitary hormones and ovarian oestradiol synthesis stops, but synthesis continues at a low level in extraglandular sites such as fat cells and breast cancer cells. This represents a change from an endocrine effect (in premenopausal women) to an autocrine response (in postmenopausal women) of oestradiol.

LHRH superagonists

The hypothalamic decapeptide LHRH stimulates membrane receptors in the pituitary gland to release LH. Synthetic analogues of LHRH bind so avidly to the LHRH receptors that the analogues downregulate the receptors. These LHRH superagonists thus desensitise the pituitary gland, causing decreased oestradiol production in the ovary. These agonists are also effective against prostate cancer because the same hypothalamic-pituitary regulation process occurs in both sexes. Additionally, the LHRH agonists may have direct antiproliferative effects on the cancer cells.

Inhibitors of steroid synthesis

Another way to decrease oestradiol production is via drugs that block steroid biosynthesis. The last step in this pathway requires an aromatase enzyme that converts testosterone to oestradiol. Aromatase inhibitors such as formestane (4-hydroxy-androstenedione) are clinically effective, with the advantage over LHRH agonists that aromatase inhibitors also block extraglandular oestrogen synthesis. These steroidal aromatase inhibitors irreversibly inactivate the enzyme (type I or suicide inhibitors). Non-steroidal triazols such as anastrozole (type II inhibitors) are reversible.

Steroid receptor antagonists

Anti-oestrogens bind to oestrogen receptors but do not activate gene transcription (see Chapter 10). Receptor binding by the antagonist prevents oestradiol binding and blocks its mitogenic effect (see Figures 12.12). A few oestrogen-sensitive genes, such as the gene for TGF-β, act in reverse, such that they are activated by anti-oestrogens and inactivated by oestrogens. Anti-oestrogen blockade of oestradiol

Figure 12.13

Structure of oestradiol and its antagonist tamoxifen.

Figure 12.13

Structure of oestradiol and its antagonist tamoxifen.

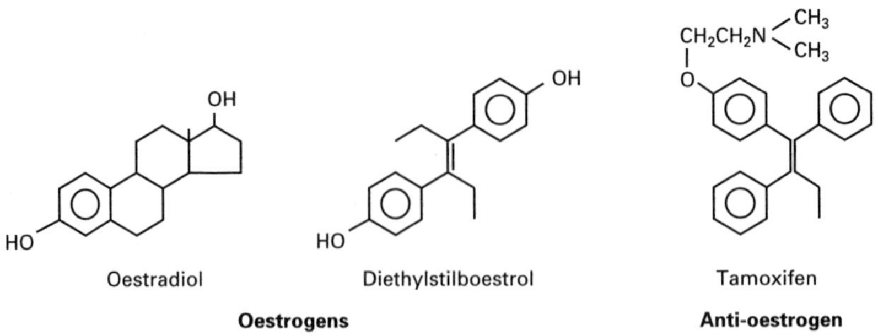

binding to its receptor synergises with the induction of growth-inhibitory polypeptides to stop proliferation.

The most widely used anti-oestrogen in the past was tamoxifen, a derivative of the non-steroidal oestrogen diethylstilboestrol (Figure 12.13). Interference with the action of other classes of steroid hormone, such as progestogens, glucocorticoids and androgens, is also effective in treating advanced breast cancer. Interestingly, male breast cancer responds to the same hormone treatments as does the female disease. An analogous situation occurs with prostate cancer in men; its growth is driven by androgens from the testis. Anti-androgens such as flutamide induce remission.

The main side effect of tamoxifen is interference with sexual functions such as ovulation. However, it also causes secondary cancers of the endometrium. Because of this, tamoxifen will probably be phased out and replaced by selective aromatase inhibitors such as anastrozole, which do not increase the incidence of endometrial cancer. Aromatase inhibitors work by preventing the conversion of adrenal androgens to oestrogens in adipose tissue (fat). In postmenopausal women, this aromatase action provides the only source of oestrogens. Resistance to tamoxifen can result from loss of receptors, but many receptor-positive breast cancers are hormone-insensitive, and thus other mechanisms must exist. One possibility is hormone-independent up-regulation of locally produced growth factors. Another route to hormone insensitivity is ligand-independent activation of steroid receptors via the MAP kinase signalling pathway (see Chapter 10).

Immunotherapy/biological response modifier therapy

Although progress in this area has been substantial, these forms of therapy cannot yet be considered as significant as surgery, radiotherapy and chemotherapy. With regard to immunotherapy, there are two basic approaches. Active immunotherapy involves the use of vaccines or bacterial products, while passive immunotherapy involves administration of antibodies or lymphoreticular cells. The major problem appears to be that cancer antigens found on the cell surface of affected cells are also found in normal tissues, although at different levels or developmental stages. This lack of a distinct difference has meant that immunisation against tumours is difficult. Additional problems arise in the way in which the antigen is presented to the immune system. T-cells can be seen to become tolerant of tumour antigens rather than responsive to them. Cancer vaccines either treat existing cancers (therapeutic vaccines) or prevent the development of cancer (prophylactic vaccines). Therapeutic vaccines against melanomas have been developed, and some have undergone extensive clinical trials. One of these, Melacine, a vaccine prepared from melonoma cell lysates, has been used in trials comparing responses with polychemotherapy. Melacine showed advantages in that it was non-toxic and allowed a better quality of life when compared with chemotherapy alone. Prophylactic vaccines are considered later.

One seemingly unusual agent is used to decrease progression, prevent recurrence and increase survival in bladder cancer. This is BCG, an attenuated strain of the tuberculosis bacterium. BCG probably acts by stimulating a non-specific inflammatory reaction that results in an increase in the production of cytokines and immunoglobulins, which in turn act on the tumour.

Investigations using passive immunotherapy have produced some interesting results. One such trial was undertaken on people with cancer who had not responded to conventional therapy. Blood was removed from the patients and treated with **i**nterleukin-**2** (IL-2) to produce **l**ymphokine-**a**ctivated **k**iller (LAK) cells. These cells were reinfused together with IL-2 and interferon. The LAK cells have the ability to destroy cancer in a non-specific way. Such experimental approaches appear to produce partial responses and unfortunately do not result in complete cures.

The biological response modifiers are a heterogeneous group including **i**nterfer-**on**s (IFNs), **i**nterleukins (ILs) and colony-stimulating factors. The IFNs are produced naturally by cells of the body in response to infection by viruses and fungi. One of this group, IFN-α, is being used to treat several cancers such as melanoma and chronic myeloid leukaemia. The ILs are cytokines that occur naturally in the body. One of this group, IL-2, appears to stimulate the growth and activity of cells of the immune system to constrain the activity of cancer cells. The colony-stimulating factors are concerned with the production of blood cells other than lymphocytes and can be used in supportive therapy to minimise the adverse effects of chemotherapy.

Photodynamic therapy

Visible light on its own does not damage cells, but it can have deleterious effects in the presence of light-sensitive (photosensitive) chemicals such as porphyrins plus oxygen. Naturally occuring porphyrins such as haemoglobin bind and transport oxygen (O_2). In the laboratory, haemoglobin can be modified with acid, so that light in the 630 nm (red) region of the spectrum provides energy to transfer an electron from the photosensitive porphyrin to oxygen and generate the reactive superoxide radical $O_2^{\bullet}$. The porphyrin is thus a prodrug. This free radical has a short half-life (< 0.04 μs) and therefore will damage only those molecules less than 0.02 μm from the site of O_2 formation. Given a cell diameter of about 10 μm, this means that only cells containing porphyrin are directly destroyed, although there are secondary effects such as an inflammatory response with accumulation of leucocytes and an immune reaction. Photodynamic therapy has been adapted such that the porphyrin is given systemically and the target cancer is illuminated with 630 nm light focused on the cancer and not the surrounding tissues.

Multiple processes are activated, such as vascular shutdown, an inflammatory reaction, stress–activated kinase increase (see Chapter 10) and apoptosis. All of these contribute to treatment effectiveness, but apoptosis is particularly relevant. The basis for the selective uptake of the porphyrin by the cancer cells is unclear, but it involves both the high blood-vessel density in cancers and the presence of mitochondrial membrane binding sites for porphyrins. Formation of $O_2^\bullet$ radicals in the mitochondrial membrane activates the apoptosis pathway downstream from the processes requiring RNA and protein synthesis such as p53 formation (see Figure 9.14). Cell death is thus independent of p53 status and stage in the cell cycle, and so the potential causes of intrinsic and extrinsic resistance are circumvented.

The most commonly used photosensitiser is porfimer sodium, a partially purified haematoporphyrin derivative. Photodynamic therapy has been used successfully to treat cancers of the bladder, head and neck, and oesophagus. Side effects include skin photosensitivity and renal problems. Local heating also occurs due to the activating light.

New forms of treatment

The improvement of existing combinations of therapeutic modalities and the development of new therapeutic packages will undoubtedly lead to improved remission times and will, occasionally, result in complete cures for some cancers. However, it is likely that the main development in cancer therapy will occur in the field of molecular medicine. As more is understood about the molecular defects that lead to malignancy, it may well be possible to use these as targets for destruction or rectification. Such an approach is much more specific in action than conventional cytotoxic chemotherapy and should be less prone to development of drug resistance and toxic side effects. The list below and in Table 12.6 is not meant to be comprehensive but is intended to cover major developments to date.

Tyrosine kinase inhibitors

Tyrosine kinases (TKs) are of great importance in signal-transduction pathways, and so it follows that TK inhibitors are potentially important agents to be used to switch off active pathways. One such agent, imatinib, targets the TKs ABL (bcr/abl), c-Kit and PDGFR. Imatinib has been strikingly successful in the treatment of chronic myeloid leukaemia, which expresses bcr-abl, and gastrointestinal stromal tumours, which express c-Kit. Imatinib has also been used in trials with other tumours such as glioblastoma multiforme, which overexpresses PDGFR. Other TK inhibitors, such as gefitinib and eriotinib, are being evaluated in clinical trials involving several cancers (Figure 12.15).

Also included in this group is trastuzumab, a monoclonal antibody against EGFR2/HER2, which is overexpressed in breast cancer cells. Trials comparing

Table 12.6 New forms of cancer treatment either in use or in late clinical trials.

Drug	Type	Target	Diseases
Tyrosine kinase inhibitors			
			Chronic myeloid leukaemia
Imatinib	Small molecule	ABL	Gastrointestinal stromal tumour
		Kit	Chronic myelomonocytic leukaemia
		PDGFR	Dermatofibrosarcoma protuberans
Gefitinib (Iressa)	Small molecule	EGFR	Lung cancer
Trastuzumab	Monoclonal antibody	EGFR2/HER2/neu	Breast cancer
Cetuximab	Monoclonal antibody	EGF	Colorectal cancer
Angiogenesis/metastasis inhibitors			
			Renal cancer
Bevacizumab (Avastin)	Monoclonal antibody	VEGF	Colorectal cancer
Neovastat	Small molecule	MMP	
Vitaxin		Integrins	
Gene silencing			
Oblimersen	siRNA	Bcl2	Lung cancer
			Melanoma
			Non-Hodgkin's lymphoma
			Acute leukaemias
Prophylactic vaccination			
Vaccine		HBV	Hepatocellular cancer
		HPV-16, 18	Cervical cancer

overall survival times in people with breast cancer treated with docetaxol alone and in combination with trastuzumab show the combination results in better survival times. Similar results have been found using cetuximab, another monoclonal antibody, which blocks the EGFR in colorectal cancer. The combination of cetuximab with the topoisomerase inhibitor irinotecan was found to be better than treatment using cetuximab alone.

Angiogenic/metastasis inhibitors

Bevacizumab is a monoclonal antibody against VEGF and is therefore a potent block of angiogenesis. It is being used in combination with conventional chemotherapy to treat colorectal cancer.

Other agents block angiogenesis and metastasis indirectly by inhibiting MMPs (Figure 12.16), which are essential in cell migration through tissues. These include proteinase antagonists such as Neovastat and integrin antagonists such as Vitaxin.

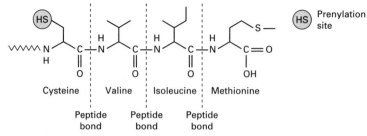

Figure 12.14

Prenylation of ras: a target for therapeutic drugs.
(Source: Based on data in Lobell, R.B. and Kohl, N.E. (1998) *Cancer and Metastasis Reviews*, **17**, 203–210.)

Cysteine | Valine | Isoleucine | Methionine

Peptide bond | Peptide bond | Peptide bond

Natural C-terminal substrate for farnesyl transfersae

Aromatic group

Protease-resistant bonds

Removed within the cell

Competitive inhibitor L739, 749

Gene silencing

It is possible to silence oncogenes using oncogene-specific siRNAs (Figure 12.17). One of these, Oblimersen, has been used to silence *Bcl2* and is being used in clinical trials involving several cancers.

Elimination of causal agents

The major cause of hepatocellular cancer is the **h**epatitis **B** **v**irus (HBV). It is possible to prevent HBV infection with the use of a prophylactic vaccine. By reducing the incidence of HBV infection, it is possible to reduce the incidence of

Figure 12.15

Competitive inhibitors of ATP binding to tyrosine kinases.
(Source: Based on data in Kohls, W.D., Fry, D.W. and Kraker A.J. (1997) *Current Opinion in Oncology*, **9**, 562–68.)

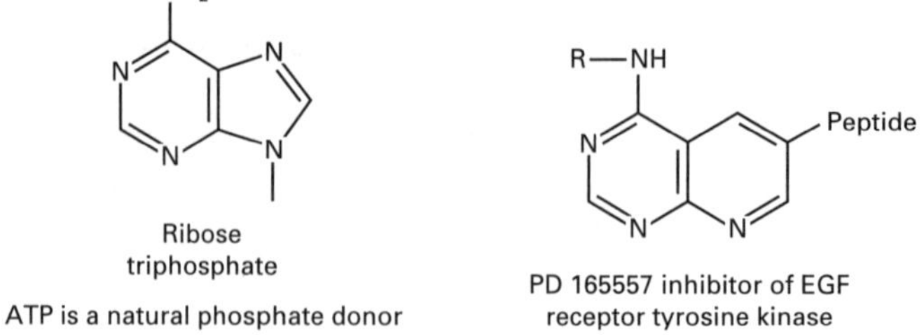

Ribose triphosphate

ATP is a natural phosphate donor

PD 165557 inhibitor of EGF receptor tyrosine kinase

Figure 12.16

Inhibition of metalloproteinases by Zn^{2+}-chelating peptides.

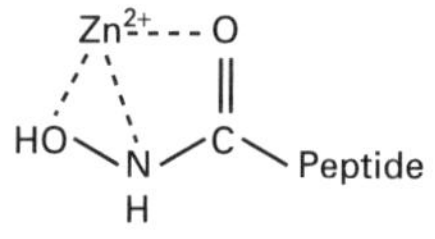

Hydroxamate end group

hepatocellular cancer. Large-scale trials carried out in Taiwan and Korea have yielded convincing evidence to support this approach; now many countries where hepatocellular cancer is common vaccinate children against HBV. Infection with **h**uman **p**apilloma **v**irus types **16** and **18** (HPV16 and 18) is causally associated with cervical cancer. The production of prophylactic vaccines against these viruses is not as advanced as that for HBV. Nevertheless, large-scale trials have shown that vaccination against HPV16 and 18 greatly reduces the incidence of cervical cancer, and it is likely that this vaccination will be deployed in order to reduce the incidence of this cancer. There is also interest in the development of a vaccine to prevent *Helicobacter pylori* infection, which in turn should reduce the incidence of stomach cancer.

Figure 12.17

Antisense oligodeoxynucleotides can destroy specific mRNAs.

Gene therapy

Gene therapy involves insertion of genes into malignant or normal cells in order to modify gene expression for therapeutic benefit. Genes are transfected using either viral or non-viral vectors. When viruses are used, they must be attenuated, i.e. rendered

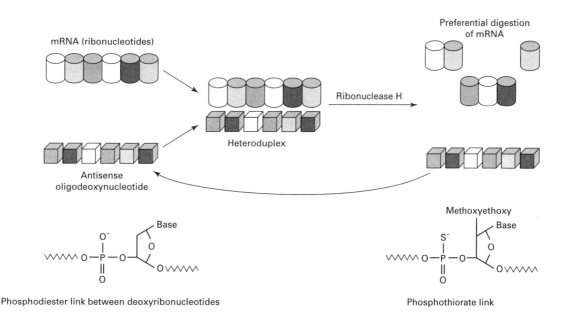

mRNA (ribonucleotides)

Preferential digestion of mRNA

Ribonuclease H

Heteroduplex

Antisense oligodeoxynucleotide

Phosphodiester link between deoxyribonucleotides

Phosphothiorate link

259

Figure 12.18

Identification of tumour antigens and their immunodominant peptides.

1. Transfect recombinant melanoma DNA to express proteins (expression library)

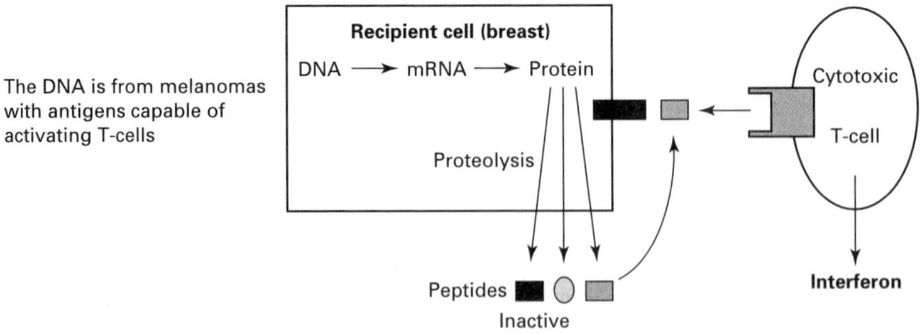

The DNA is from melanomas with antigens capable of activating T-cells

Recipient cell (breast)

DNA ⟶ mRNA ⟶ Protein

Proteolysis

Cytotoxic

T-cell

Peptides ▰ ◯ ▱
Inactive

Interferon

2. Isolate recipient cells that promote interferon production
3. Isolate melanoma DNA coding for protein/peptides
4. Repeat stages 1, 2 and 3 with fragments of DNA from stage 3
5. Sequence DNA to identify responsible genes; predict amino acid sequence of protein/peptides
6. Synthesise immunodominant peptide; test for biological effect (interferon production, lysis of recipient cell)

no longer harmful to the patient. Gene therapy has the potential of very high specificity owing to the ability to pinpoint targets concerned with control of proliferation. Many types of gene therapy have been developed to exploit the many defects that occur in cancer cells. However, such treatments are still in the developmental stage, and in only a few cases have they been developed to the clinical trial stage. These strategies include a group that could be called mutation compensation, which can work in several ways, including restoration of the function of a mutated tumour suppressor gene (e.g. retinoblastoma) by inserting the normal gene or by ablating the function of a dominant oncogene. Another strategy involves a form of molecular chemotherapy in which the transgene is deleterious to the cancer cells, either directly or indirectly. Examples include genes that increase the sensitivity to chemotherapy (e.g. the *P450* gene that sensitises breast cancer to cyclophosphamide), suicide genes that are toxic to cancer cells and genes such as that for GM-CSF, which protects bone marrow cells from the depressing effects of chemotherapy.

Gene–expression profiling

This technique involves obtaining a small quantity of mRNA from the malignant cells. This mRNA is labelled with a fluorescent dye and hybridised on the surface of a robotically spotted array of thousands of cDNAs or oligonucleotides. The display provides a rapid way in which to analyse the expression of thousands of genes simultaneously. Using computer analysis of such data, major subgroups of patients can be established on the basis of occurrence of overexpressed or underexpressed genes. In several types of cancer, subgroups of patients established using these procedures have distinctly different survival times. Therefore, although gene-expression profiling is not therapeutic, it could be used to establish prognostic subgroups, so that clinicians could direct therapy to those who would best benefit from it.

Further reading

Alikhan, M.A., Phooskooru, V. and Kohli, M. (2004) Re: Randomized trial of adjuvant therapy in colon carcinoma: 10-year results of NSABP protocol C-01. *J Natl Cancer Inst* **96**, 1794.

Barnett, F.H., Scharer-Schuksz, M., Wood, M., *et al.* (2004) Intra-arterial delivery of endostatin gene to brain tumours prolongs survival and alters tumour vessel ultrastructure. *Gene Ther* **11**, 1283–1289.

Bartelink, H., Horiot, J.C., Poortmans, P., *et al.* (2001) Recurrence rates after treatment for breast cancer with standard radiotherapy with or without additional radiation. *N Engl J Med* **345**, 1378–1387.

Bykov, V.J. and Wiman, K.G. (2003) Novel cancer therapy by reactivation of p53 apoptosis pathway. *Ann Med* **35**, 458–465.

Camidge, D.R. and Joderell, D.I. (2005) Chemotherapy. In *Introduction to the Cellular and Molecular Biology of Cancer*, ed. M. Knowles and P. Selby. Oxford: Oxford University Press.

Cheater, J.D. (2005) Cancer gene therapy. In *Introduction to the Cellular and Molecular Biology of Cancer*, ed. M. Knowles and P. Selby. Oxford: Oxford University Press.

Cummings, J., Ward, T.H., Ranson, M. and Dive, C. (2004) Apoptosis pathway-targeted drugs from bench to the clinic. *Biochim Biophys Acta* **1705**, 53–66.

Cunningham, D., Humblet, Y., Siena, S. (2004) Cetuximab monotherapy and cetuximab plus irinotecan in irinotecan-refractory metastatic colorectal cancer. *N Engl J Med* **351**, 337–345.

Dolmans, D.E., Fukumura, D. and Jain, R.K. (2003) Photodynamic therapy for cancer. *Nat Rev Cancer* **3**, 380–387.

Fentiman, I.S. (2005) Local treatment of cancer. In *Introduction to the Cellular and Molecular Biology of Cancer*, ed. M. Knowles and P. Selby. Oxford: Oxford University Press.

Fentiman, I.S., van Zijl, J., Karydas, I., *et al.* (2003) Treatment of operable breast cancer in the elderly: a randomised clinical trial EORTC 10850 comparing modified radical mastectomy with tumourectomy plus tamoxifen. *Eur J Cancer* **39**, 300–308.

Geldart, T., Glennie, M.J. and Johnson, P.W.M. (2005) Monoclonal antibodies and therapy. In *Introduction to the Cellular and Molecular Biology of Cancer*, ed. M. Knowles and P. Selby. Oxford: Oxford University Press.

Harper, D.M., Franco, E.L., Wheeler, C., *et al.* (2004) Efficacy of a bivalent L1 virus-like particle vaccine in prevention of infection with human papilloma virus types 16 and 18 in young women: a randomised controlled trial. *Lancet* **364**, 1757–1765.

Hersy, P. (2002) Advances in non-surgical treatment of melanoma. *Expert Opin Investig Drugs* **11**, 75–85.

Jackson, A.M. and Porte, J. (2005) Immunotherapy of cancer. In *Introduction to the Cellular and Molecular Biology of Cancer*, ed. M. Knowles and P. Selby. Oxford: Oxford University Press.

Kerbel, R. and Folkman, J. (2002) Clinical translation of angiogenesis inhibitors. *Nat Rev Cancer* **2**, 727–739.

Kiltie, A. (2005) Radiotherapy and molecular radiotherapy. In *Introduction to the Cellular and Molecular Biology of Cancer*, ed. M. Knowles and P. Selby. Oxford: Oxford University Press.

Krause, D.S. and Van Etten, R.A. (2005) Tyrosine kinases as targets for cancer therapy. *N Engl J Med* **353**, 172–187.

Liu, T.G., Yin, J.Q., Shang, B.Y., *et al.* (2004) Silencing of hdm 2 oncogene by siRNA inhibits p53-dependent human breast cancer. *Cancer Gene Ther* **11**, 748–756.

Michiels, S., Koscielny, S. and Hill, C. (2005) Prediction of cancer outcome with microarray: a multiple random validation strategy. *Lancet* **365**, 488–497.

Oltersdorf, T., Elmore, S.W., Shoemaker, A.R., *et al.* (2005) An inhibitor of Bcl-2 family proteins induces regression of solid tumours. *Nature* **435**, 677–681.

O'Regan, R.M. and Jordan, V.C. (2002) The evolution of tamoxifen therapy: selective oestrogen-receptor modulators and downregulators. *Lancet Oncol* **3**, 207–214.

Overall, C.M. and Lopez-Otin, C. (2002) Strategies for MMP inhibition in cancer: innovations for the post-trial era. *Nat Rev Cancer* **2**, 657–672.

Sasieni, P. and Cuzick, J. (2005) Screening. In *Introduction to the Cellular and Molecular Biology of Cancer*, ed. M. Knowles and P. Selby. Oxford: Oxford University Press.

Thun, M.J., Henley, S.J. and Patrono, C. (2002) Nonsteroidal anti-inflammatory drugs as anticancer agents: mechanistic, pharmacologic, and clinical issues. *J Natl Cancer Inst* **94**, 252–266.

Websites

See the clinical trials page of the National Cancer Institute website:
www.cancer.gov/clinicaltrials

- Some cancers can potentially be prevented.
- Statutory regulation of the use of known carcinogens is used to prevent some cancers.
- Cancers caused by viruses can be prevented by vaccination against the agents concerned.
- Chemoprevention of breast cancer has been achieved with anti-oestrogens such as tamoxifen and with aromatase inhibitors.
- Ovarian and endometrial cancer risk is decreased by use of the combined oral contraceptive pill.
- Non-steroidal anti-inflammatory drugs may reduce the risk of developing colorectal cancer. However, there are serious side effects with this approach.
- There is no strong association between specific components of diet and cancer. However, increasing fruit and vegetable intake and decreasing the intake of fat and red meat probably reduces the risk of getting several cancers.

Introduction

Preventing or limiting exposure to known carcinogens appears to be a logical way to reduce the incidence of cancer. However, in complex societies, this is not always possible or practicable. Nevertheless, as cancer is the second major cause of death in developed countries, governments and individuals should consider steps to reduce the incidence of cancers. In only a few instances is effective regulation of carcinogens possible; what remains are education and enlightened persuasion.

Limitation of exposure to tobacco smoke

The role of tobacco smoke in the development of several cancers is well established. Many governments seek to limit the smoking habit by imposing a high duty on tobacco products, banning advertising of such products and giving health warnings on the packaging of tobacco products. Some authorities also endeavour to reduce tobacco smoke inhalation by non-smokers (passive smoking) by banning smoking in places of work and entertainment.

At a personal level, attempts to stop smoking are aided by skin patches that release nicotine into the body. Nicotine is the major substance that causes tobacco dependency; an exogenous supply of this drug from such patches helps to break the smoking habit.

Statutory regulation of physical and chemical carcinogens

The use of some carcinogens can be regulated by statute. Sources of ionising radiation are controlled at national level, radiation users are registered, and the dose absorbed by such workers is monitored regularly. Building regulations in regions with a high geological seepage of radon require new buildings either to incorporate an impermeable membrane in their foundations or to provide a ventilated sump below the ground floor. In the workplace, there are regulations limiting either the use or the handling of known carcinogens. For example, in the UK, there are regulations concerned with the use of benzene, the scavenging of hardwood sawdust and the removal of asbestos from older insulated installations.

Limitation of exposure to solar radiation

In regions where people with pale skins are exposed to high fluxes of ultraviolet light, children and agricultural workers are encouraged to avoid the midday sun, to wear a brimmed hat when outside and to protect exposed skin with sun-block.

Control of infective agents

In a few cancers, specific infective agents are causal agents (see Chapter 5). If these agents are regulated, then the incidence of the related cancer should be reduced. Currently, there is a major international programme to vaccinate children against the hepatitis B virus in order to prevent hepatocellular cancer in countries with a known high incidence of this disease. Vaccines against the forms of human papilloma virus that cause cervical cancer have been developed and are likely to be deployed shortly (see Chapter 12).

Breast cancer, tamoxifen and anastrozole

The major risk factor for breast cancer is oestrogen overexposure (see Chapter 4), and so opposing oestrogen overexposure should be beneficial. Over several decades,

Figure 13.1

Oestradiol and tamoxifen binding to the oestrogen receptor. Other proteins are involved but are not illustrated here.

Domain structure of oestradiol receptor

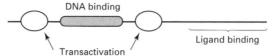

DNA binding

Transactivation

Ligand binding

Inactive receptor in absence of ligand: DNA-binding domain occluded

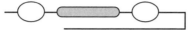

Oestradiol binding: DNA-binding and both transactivation domains exposed

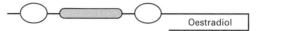

Oestradiol

Tamoxifed binding: DNA-binding and one transactivation domain exposed

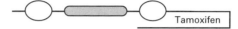

Tamoxifen

the partial oestrogen agonist tamoxifen has been used clinically as an adjuvant in breast cancer therapy in order to reduce recurrence. This approach has been broadly successful, but it also increases the incidence of endometrial cancer. Because of this, it is likely that the use of tamoxifen will be phased out and the aromatase inhibitors will be used instead. These work indirectly by blocking the major source of oestrogen in postmenopausal women, namely by the conversion of androgens from the adrenal gland to oestrodiol (Figure 13.1). Concomitant increase in the incidence of osteoporosis can be regulated by the use of bisphosphonates.

Endometrial/ovarian cancer and the contraceptive pill

Long-term use of combination oral contraceptives approximately halves the risk of endometrial cancer and also reduces the incidence of ovarian cancer (Figure 13.2). However, there is a small increase in the risk of breast cancer. This latter kind of information fuels a dilemma that can be addressed only by a personal decision on the balance of the several risks.

Colon cancer and non-steroidal anti-inflammatory drugs

Non-**s**teroidal **a**nti-**i**nflammatory **d**rugs (NSAIDs) such as aspirin were found to decrease mortality from colon cancer by half when taken for diseases such as arthritis (Figure 13.3). These agents work by inhibiting the COX enzymes and prostaglandin production (see Figure 10.22). Prostaglandins stimulate angiogenesis and cell

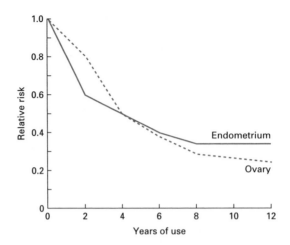

Figure 13.2

Risk of ovarian and endometrial cancers in women taking oral contraceptives. (Source: Based on data from Stanford, J.L. (1991) *Contraception*, 43, 543–46. Copyright © 1991. Reproduced with permission of Elsevier.)

proliferation, and blocking their synthesis also increases apoptosis (see Chapter 10). Inhibiting prostaglandin synthesis production would influence all of these functions and may thus inhibit cancer formation. Laboratory studies have demonstrated the relevance of these effects to colon carcinogenesis. The Min mouse, which lacks the *APC* gene (see Chapter 2), develops colon polyps; deleting the *COX-2* gene decreases both the size and the number of the polyps. COX inhibitors have a similar effect on chemically induced colon cancers. Unfortunately, aspirin used over long periods of time can cause gastrointestinal ulceration and renal toxicity, while COX-2 inhibitors used long-term increase the incidence of serious cardiovascular disorders. Clearly these agents require further refinement before being applied on a wide scale.

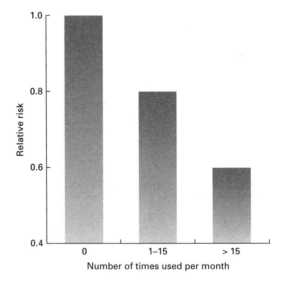

Figure 13.3

Mortality from colorectal cancer in people taking aspirin. (Source: Based on data in Thun, M.J., Namboodri, M.M. and Heath, C.W. (1991) *New England Journal of Medicine*, 325, 1593–96.)

Diet

According to some international bodies, 30−40% of cancers are preventable by dietary means. This encapsulates the potential benefit of dietary manipulation, but it is a best-case scenario; actually achieving changes of such a magnitude is an improbable objective. Table 13.1 indicates that potential benefits would accrue for a range of cancers and points to the major food components involved. When considering these estimates of preventable cancers, we must remember that the data on which they are based were obtained mainly from observational epidemiological investigations in countries with different dietary habits (China versus USA) or in groups with different lifestyles (vegetarians versus meat-eaters) within one country (see Chapter 4). This type of study provides substantial evidence that food intake is an important factor, but it overestimates the magnitude of change that could be achieved in practice. Although the data indicate the food items involved, they do not reveal which components in those foods are the active agents. Nevertheless, any decrease in cancer incidence has to be a good objective.

Food contains both good and bad components, with good items including fruit and vegetables (Table 13.1). It is unknown how a predominantly vegetarian diet reduces the risk of cancer; probably many factors are involved. The lack of clear causal relationships has not deterred national and international bodies from recommending diets containing more fresh fruit and vegetables than have been consumed in the past. Many countries encourage people to eat five to nine portions of fruit and vegetables per day. This good advice is worth following; however, based on previous experience with coronary heart disease, it is unlikely to achieve a maximum response, as people seem to prefer the hamburger to the lettuce. The European Prospective Investigation of Cancer and Nutrition (EPIC), a large prospective study involving a cohort of 520 000 participants that was initiated in 1992, will undoubtedly yield interesting information in this area.

There have also been attempts to reduce cancer incidence by taking antioxidant micronutrient supplements. To date, no clear epidemiological evidence supports this

Table 13.1 Diet and the five major (global) cancers: overall, three to four million cancers are preventable.

Site	Incidence (millions)	Prevent by diet (estimate)	Dietary factor	
			Good	Bad
Lung	1.3	25%*	Fruit and vegetables	
Stomach	1.0	70%	Fruit and vegetables	Salt, salty foods
Breast	0.9	40%†	Fruit and vegetables	Fat, alcohol
Colon	0.9	70%	Fruit and vegetables	Meat, alcohol
Mouth, pharynx, nasopharynx	0.6	40%	Fruit and vegetables	Alcohol, salty fish

* Smokers and non-smokers.
† If started before puberty; 15% if started in adult life.
(Source: Based on data in World Cancer Research Fund/American Institute for Cancer Research (1997) *Food, Nutrition and the Prevention of Cancer: A Global Perspective*. Washington, DC: American Institute for Cancer Research. Reprinted with permission.)

Figure 13.4

Risk of developing lung cancer in smokers taking β-carotene.

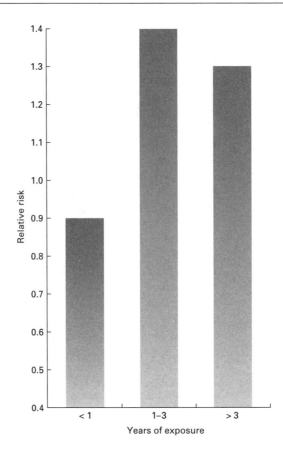

concept. Indeed, one large overview analysis has indicated that supplementary vitamins (A, C and E and beta-carotene) may actually increase all-cause mortality, while selenium may be protective.

The lack of clear evidence linking diet to the incidence of cancer might occur because studies usually depend on subjective recall of the food consumed (via dietary questionnaires) in order to estimate the quantity of the dietary component eaten. Imperfect recall results in a bias, which confounds establishment of clear associations. In a comparative study using a single population, data obtained from a food diary showed a significant association between fat intake and breast cancer, while data obtained using a food-frequency questionnaire did not.

The current weight of opinion favours the concept that dietary fibre may be protective against cancers of the gastrointestinal tract (see Chapter 4) and that the consumption of red and processed meat increases the risk of colorectal cancer.

Further reading

Bange, J., Zwick, E. and Ullrich, A. (2001) Molecular targets for breast cancer therapy and prevention. *Nat Med* **7**, 548–552.

Bingham, S.A., Luben, R., Welch, A., *et al.* (2003) Are imprecise methods obscuring a relationship between fat and breast cancer? *Lancet* **362**, 212–214.

Bjelakovic, G., Nikolova, D., Simonetti, R.G. and Gluud, C. (2004) Antioxidants for prevention of gastrointestinal cancers: a systematic review and meta-analysis. *Lancet* **364**, 1219–1228.

Bueno-de-Mesquita, H.B., Ferrari, P. and Riboli, E., on behalf of EPIC (2002) Plant food and the risk of colorectal cancer in Europe: preliminary findings. In *Nutrition and Lifestyle: Opportunities for Cancer Prevention*, eds E. Riboli and R. Lambert. Lyons: IARC Press.

Chang, M.H., Chen, C.J., Lai, M.S., *et al.* (1997) Universal hepatitis B vaccination in Taiwan and the incidence of hepatocellular carcinoma in children. *N Engl J Med* **336**, 1855–1859.

Collaborative Group on Hormonal Factors in Breast Cancer (1996) Breast cancer and hormonal contraceptives: collaborative reanalysis of individual data on 53 297 women with breast cancer and 100 239 women without breast cancer from 54 epidemiological studies. *Lancet* **347**, 1713–1727.

Green, A., Williams, G., Neale, R., *et al.* (1999) Daily sunscreen application and betacarotene supplementation in prevention of basal-cell and squamous-cell carcinomas of the skin: a randomised controlled trial. *Lancet* **354**, 723–729.

Harper, D.M., Franco, E.L., Wheeler, C., *et al.* (2004) Efficacy of a bivalent L1 virus-like particle vaccine in prevention of infection with human papilloma types 16 and 18 in young women: a randomised controlled trial. *Lancet* **364**, 1757–1765.

Michels, K.B. (2005) The role of nutrition in cancer development and prevention. *Int J Cancer* **114**, 163–165.

Norat, T., Lukanova, A., Ferrari, P. and Riboli, E. (2002) Meat consumption and colorectal cancer risk: dose–response meta-analysis of epidemiological studies. *Int J Cancer* **98**, 241–256.

Rosenbaum Smith, S.M. and Osborne, M.P. (2000) Breast cancer chemoprevention. *Am J Surg* **180**, 249–251.

Solomon, S.D., McMurray, J.J., Pfeffer, M.A., *et al.* (2005) Cardiovascular risk associated with celecoxib in a clinical trial for colorectal adenoma prevention. *N Engl J Med* **352**, 1071–1080.

Surh, Y.-J. (2003) Cancer chemoprevention with dietary phytochemicals. *Nat Rev Cancer* **3**, 768–780.

Appendix: Features of selected cancers

The cancers in this appendix are those whose incidence and mortality are listed in Table 1.1. Data for these cancers relate to European and North American populations. Unless stated otherwise, the factors mentioned increase the risk. Multiple changes in gene structure and function have been identified in every cancer studied; a comprehensive list would not distinguish between genes that play a causative role in carcinogenesis and those that have ancillary effects such as changes relevant to progression. Furthermore, for any one type of cancer, specific gene changes often occur in only a proportion (commonly about one-third) of those cancers; there are multiple routes to a common end point, cancer. Rather than provide a catalogue of genes, only those genes that are *probably* involved in early rather than late responses are considered here. Brief details are given of the major genes involved in early responses. Investigation of cancer-associated genes is advancing rapidly, so for up-to-date information of this area it is probably best to refer to a reliable website such as the Cancer Genetics Web at www.cancerindex.org/geneweb.

Figure A.1

New cases and deaths from the main cancers. USA, 1995, percentage of all cancers at stated site.

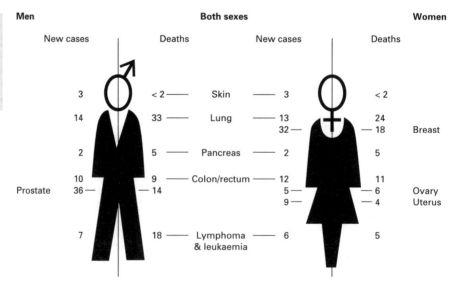

Bladder (Figure A.2)

- More than 90% of bladder cancers are transitional cell carcinomas.

- This is the fourth most common cancer in men and the eleventh most common cancer in women.

- Incidence: greater over the age of 50 years.

- Risk factors: many chemicals used in industrial processes (however, use of these has been banned for about 40 years), sex (twice as common in men than in women), smoking, bladder stones, repeated infections.

- Gene changes: *NAT2*, *GSTM1* (regulating the enzymes concerned with the breakdown of carcinogens), *HRAS*, *ERBB2*, $p16^{INK14A}$.

- Treatment: intravesicular BCG, surgery (radical cystectomy), radiotherapy, chemotherapy. If diagnosis and treatment are prompt, 5-year survival is 65%.

Figure A.2
Urinary bladder.

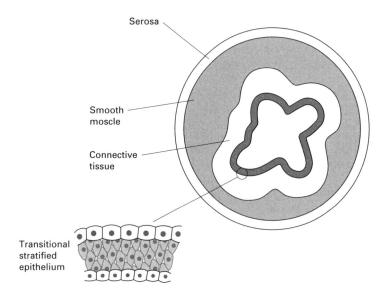

Breast (Figure A.3)

- Adenocarcinomas: mostly of ductal (80%) or lobular (10%) epithelium.

- Lifetime risk of getting breast cancer: women, 1 in 11; men, 1 in 1000.

- Five-year survival rates: 80% (Table 12.1; Figures 4.3, 12.2 and 12.3 for subgroup data).

- Risk factors: age of first pregnancy (< 30 years, lower risk), early menarche, late menopause, family history, breastfeeding (premenopause, lower risk), diet (see Chapter 4).

Figure A.3

Breast. Epithelial cells give rise to cancers. See also Figure 3.3. Blue type indicates cells that give rise to cancers.

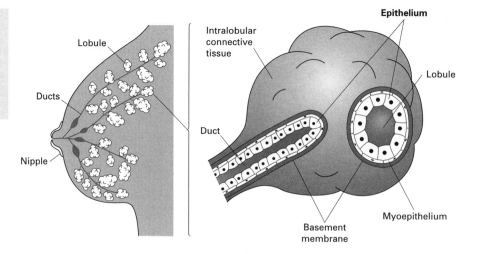

- Metastasis: lymph nodes, bone and locally in the breast.

- Inherited gene changes: *BRCA1* and *BRCA2*, *p53* (see Figures 4.6 and 8.2 and Tables 8.3–8.5).

- Sporadic gene changes: oestrogen receptor (see Table 10.5), cyclin D (see Figure 9.9), EGF/ErbB family (Nathanson, K.I. (2001). *Nat Med* **7**, 552–556).

Breast cancer is the most common cancer in women. Men do get breast cancer, but the probability is about 100 times less than for women. There are marked geographical differences in risk (see Figure 4.2). Mortality from breast cancer is decreasing in developed countries due to the introduction of breast screening to detect early cancers and improved treatment regimens.

Colorectal (Figure A.4)

- Adenocarcinoma (90%) or mucinous adenocarcinoma (10%).

- Lifetime risk of getting colorectal cancer: 1 in 20 (men and women).

- Five-year survival rate: c. 60% (but see Table 12.1).

- Risk factors: family history, inflammatory bowel disease, diet (see Table 4.1).

- Metastasis: locally and to liver and lymph nodes.

- Inherited gene changes: *APC*, *MLH1*, *MSH2* (see Tables 8.3–8.5).

- Sporadic gene changes: *APC*, ras, *p53*, *MLH1* (see Figure 2.11 and Table 2.1), *p53* (see Figures 5.11 and 6.12.)

Figure A.4

Colon. Epithelial cells give rise to cancers. The endocrine cells secrete peptides and can form tumours (APUDomas); they are not described in this book. See also Figures 3.2 and 11.2.

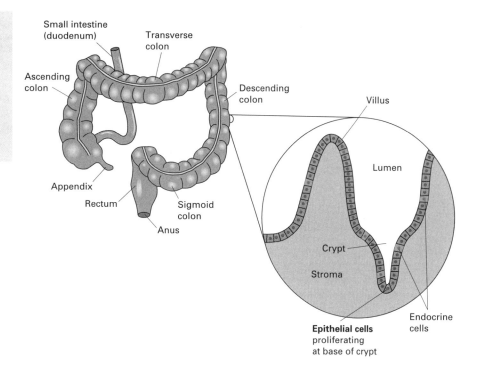

Colorectal cancer is a common cancer in elderly people in developed countries. High-risk families can be screened using colonoscopy and treated using polypectomies. Stool testing is being developed to screen for faecal occult blood and free colonocytes (Davies, R.J., *et al.* (2005). *Nat Rev Cancer* **5**, 199–209). Decreasing meat consumption and increasing intake of fruit and vegetables may reduce the incidence of this cancer.

Leukaemia (Figure A.5)

Leukaemia results from blocked haemopoietic cell differentiation. The type of leukaemia is determined by the stage at which differentiation is blocked (see Figure 9.19 and the accompanying text). Each type of leukaemia has its own characteristics; the information given below contains major generalisations. Leukaemias constitute one-third of childhood cancers. Gene changes in leukaemias vary with the type of leukaemia, but chromosome translocations are common. Chronic myeloid leukaemia (*abl* oncogene) and acute promyelocytic leukaemia (retinoic acid alpha receptor) are described in Figures 10.8 and 5.7, respectively. Inheritance of ataxia telangiectasia and Bloom's syndrome (see Table 8.3) predisposes individuals to a risk of developing leukaemia. The lifetime risk of getting leukaemia is 1 in 400.

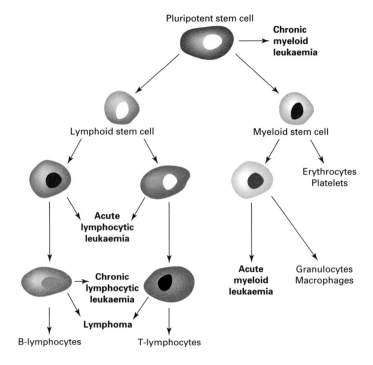

Figure A.5

Leukaemia. Only the major types are shown.

Chronic leukaemia

- Mostly B–cell (95%) but some T–cell (5%) leukaemias. Variants include chronic myeloid leukaemia (see Chapter 2).

- Five-year survival rate: 80%.

- Risk factors: uncertain; not increased by radiation.

- Abnormal cells accumulate in blood, bone marrow and spleen.

- Gene changes: the hallmark of chronic myeloid leukaemia is the Philadelphia chromosome, t(9;22), and formation of the chimeric gene *BCR-ABL* (see Figure 10.8).

Chronic leukaemia is the most common type of leukaemia; it is twice as common in men as in women. The use of imatinib and autologous bone-marrow transplantation has greatly improved survival rates.

Acute leukaemia

- Acute myeloid leukaemia (acute non-lymphocytic leukaemia) is five times more common than acute lymphocytic leukaemia. Variants include acute promyelocytic leukaemia (see Figure 5.7).

- Aggressive condition with 90% mortality within 1 year of diagnosis.

- Risk factors: Down's syndrome, Bloom's syndrome (see Chapter 8), radiation (see Figure 4.4), T-cell leukaemia virus, previous chemotherapy for other cancers.

- Accumulation of abnormal cells in bone marrow and other organs.

- Gene changes: in acute lymphocytic leukaemia *TEL-AML* fusion gene, translocations involving the *MLL* gene.

Men are marginally more susceptible than women. Acute leukaemia is ten times more common in adults than in children, but it accounts for 75% of childhood leukaemias (see Figure 1.1). Chemotherapy has improved survival of people with childhood acute leukaemias.

Lung (Figure A.6)

- Non-small-cell (90%) and small-cell (10%) variants of bronchial epithelial cancers exist. Small-cell carcinomas are derived from epithelial cells, with features of neuro-endocrine origin, as they secrete neuropeptides such as vasopressin and ACTH. Non-small-cell carcinomas have squamous (35%), glandular (adenocarcinoma, 40%) or large (10%) cell features. They may all derive from a common stem cell. Cancers of the mesothelial lining of the lungs (mesothelioma) are associated closely with asbestos exposure. There are epithelial and sarcomatous variants.

- Lifetime risk of getting lung cancer: men, 1 in 12; women, 1 in 23.

- Five-year survival rate: c. 15%.

Figure A.6

Lung. Respiratory epithelium and mesothelial lining give rise to cancers.

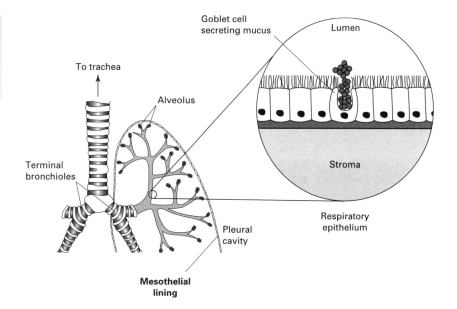

- Risk factors: smoking and passive smoking (see Chapter 4), asbestos (mesothelioma), radon from geological seepage (see Chapters 6 and 13).

- Metastasis: lung, bone, liver.

- Gene changes:

  - Small-cell variant: *Bcl2, Rb, myc, telomerase, p53.*

  - Non-small-cell variant: *ras, Bcl2, p53, Rb, p16^{INK}*, telomerase.

  - Mesothelioma: *p16^{INK}.*

  - *p53* changes in lung cancers are described in Figures 4.6, 5.11 and 6.12 and Table 6.9.

Lung cancer is the most common cancer worldwide and is the leading cause of death from cancer. Smoking is the cause of 80% of lung cancers in men and 70% in women. Lung cancer has a poor response to chemotherapy.

Lymphoma (Figure A.7)

- Two categories: Hodgkin's lymphoma and non-Hodgkin's (lymphocytic or malignant) lymphoma. Non-Hodgkin's lymphomas are mainly of B-cell origin,

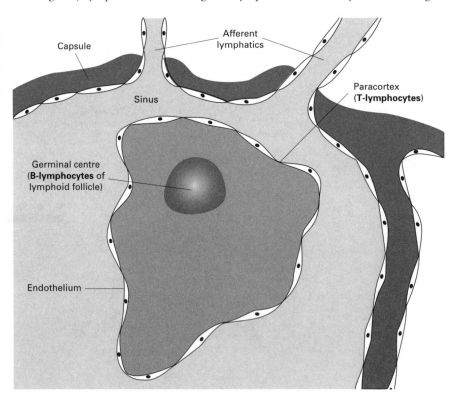

Figure A.7

Lymph node. T-lymphocytes and B-lymphocytes give rise to cancers.

including Burkitt's lymphoma (see Figure 5.5). Hodgkin's lymphoma possibly has a multi-lineage aetiology. The nodular form of Hodgkin's lymphoma is a B-cell tumour.

- Lifetime risk of getting lymphoma: Hodgkin's, 1 in 300; non-Hodgkin's, 1 in 40.

- Five-year survival rate: Hodgkin's, 79%; non-Hodgkin's, 52%.

The following items refer to non-Hodgkin's lymphoma, which is much more common than Hodgkin's lymphoma:

- This is the seventh most common cancer in men and the sixth most common in women.

- There are many risk factors, the main ones being age, sex (more men than women are affected), radiation, chemicals and disorders of the immune system.

- Symptoms include swelling of lymph nodes in the neck, armpit and groin. Further tests involve blood tests, scans and lymphangiograms.

- Gene changes: in Burkitt's lymphoma, there is a characteristic translocation of the oncogene *C-MYC* from chromosome 8 to chromosome 14, 2 or 22. Gene-expression profiling is aiding prognosis.

Early stages are non-aggressive, and so there is a wait-and-see policy. Thereafter, radiotherapy and chemotherapy are used. Five-year survival: 60–70%.

Ovary (Figure A.8)

- Over 90% arise in the epithelial layer surrounding the ovary. The cancers appear as mucinous cystadenocarcinoma (12%), serous cystadenocarcinoma (42%) or endometrioid carcinoma (15%), with a further fraction being undifferentiated carcinomas (17%).

- Lifetime risk of getting ovarian cancer: 1 in 56 (women).

- Five-year survival: c. 50% (see Table 12.1).

- Risk factors: family history, ovulation, fertility treatment, pregnancy (decreased risk), combined oral contraceptive use (decreased risk; see Chapter 13).

- Metastasis: surface shedding into the peritoneum; regrowth on viscera, including the other ovary.

- Inherited gene changes: *BRCA1* and *BRCA2* (see Table 8.5).

- Sporadic gene changes: *p53* (50% of all cases), *ERBB2* (overexpressed in 30% of cases).

Poor prognosis is due to late initial detection.

Figure A.8

Ovary. Coelomic epithelial cells give rise to cancers. Granulosa cells can also give rise to cancers, but they are not described in this book.

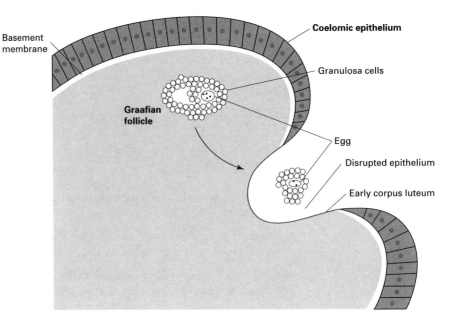

Pancreas (Figure A.9)

- Mostly (80%) ductal adenocarcinoma of the exocrine pancreas.

- Lifetime risk of getting pancreatic cancer: 1 in 60 (men and women).

- Five-year survival: c. 4% (see Table 12.1).

- Risk factors: smoking, pancreatitis.

- Metastasis: intraperitoneal spread to viscera, lung, bone.

- Inherited gene changes: *BRCA2*, *p16^{INK4A}*.

- Sporadic gene changes: many, e.g. *p53*, *KRAS*, *p16^{INK4A}*, *DCC*, *DPC4/SMAD4*.

Treatments ineffective.

Prostate (Figure A.10)

- Adenocarcinomas of luminal epithelium.

- Lifetime risk of getting prostate cancer: 1 in 14 (men).

- Five-year survival rate: c. 95% (see Table 12.1).

- Risk factors: age, high-fat diet (see Chapter 4), low physical activity, family history, race (black people > white people > Asian people) (see Table 4.1 and Figure 4.2).

Figure A.9

Exocrine pancreas. Glandular epithelial cells give rise to cancers.

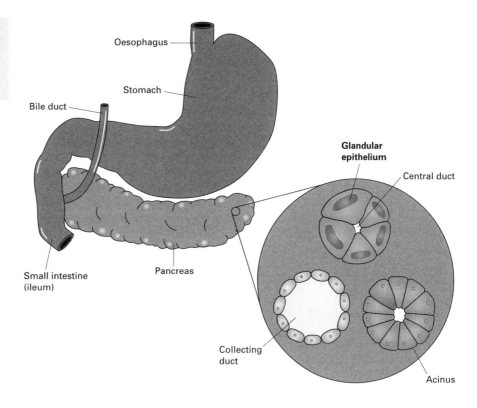

Figure A.10

Prostate gland. Glandular epithelial cells give rise to cancers.

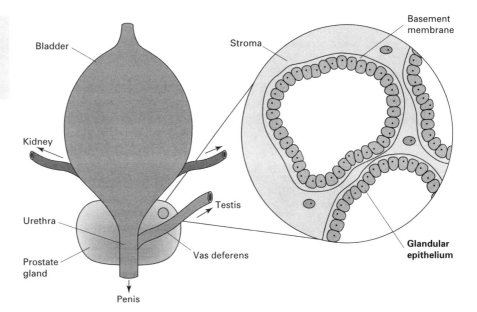

- Metastasis: lymph nodes and bone.

- Inherited gene changes: *BRCA2* (see Table 8.5), *HPC1*. Sporadic gene changes: many − prostate cancer is genetically unstable.

Prostate cancer is the most common cancer in men. Its incidence is increasing. The reasons for this are unclear, but they include improved diagnostic efficiency. Autopsy analysis indicates that most men have occult cancers of the prostate. There are marked geographical variations (see Table 4.1 and Figure 4.2).

Skin (Figure A.11)

- Three cell types can develop into cancers. Basal cell carcinoma (basal epithelium) accounts for 75% of all skin cancers, with squamous cell carcinoma (keratinocytes) contributing another 20%. Malignant melanoma (melanocytes) contributes only 5% of the total. Melanoma can also occur in the eye and vulva.

- Lifetime risk of getting skin cancer: 1 in 60 (melanoma), 1 in 3 (other).

- Basal cell cancers are curable as they rarely metastasise; squamous cell carcinomas are curable if detected early. Five-year survival rate for malignant melanoma: 85%.

- Risk factors for all types of skin cancer: ultraviolet light, fair skin (white people are ten times more likely than black people to get melanoma).

- Melanoma metastasises to lymph nodes, skin and lung.

- Gene changes: individuals who have inherited one of the xeroderma pigmentosum gene defects (see Table 8.3) are at increased risk of getting skin cancers. $p16^{INK}$

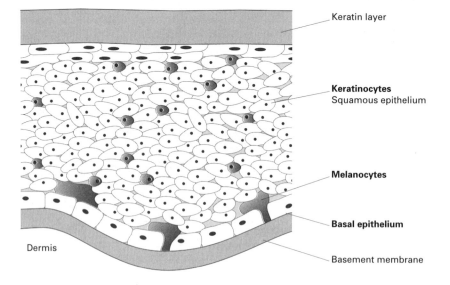

Figure A.11

Skin. Melanocytes, keratinocytes and basal epithelium give rise to cancers.

Keratin layer

Keratinocytes
Squamous epithelium

Melanocytes

Basal epithelium

Basement membrane

Dermis

is involved in the formation of familial and sporadic melanoma (see Table 8.3). *p53* is connected with basal cell carcinoma.

Incidence of skin cancer is the same for men and women. Incidence figures for melanoma are increasing at a rate of 4% per year; this is probably due to an increased ultraviolet component in sunlight.

Uterus (Figure A.12)

Cervix

- Most occur as squamous carcinomas (95%); the rest occur in the endocervical columnar cells as adenosquamous carcinoma (5%).

- Lifetime risk of getting cancer: 1 in 100 (cervical), 1 in 77 (all uterine).

- Five-year survival: 67%.

- Risk factors: Exposure to strains of human papilloma virus (predominantly HPV16 and HPV18), age of first intercourse, number of partners, smoking (see Figure 5.4).

- Metastasis: lymph nodes, distant metastases are rare.

- Gene changes: human papilloma virus contributing the *E6* and *E7* genes (see Table 5.2).

Figure A.12

Uterus. Glandular and squamous epithelia give rise to cancers.

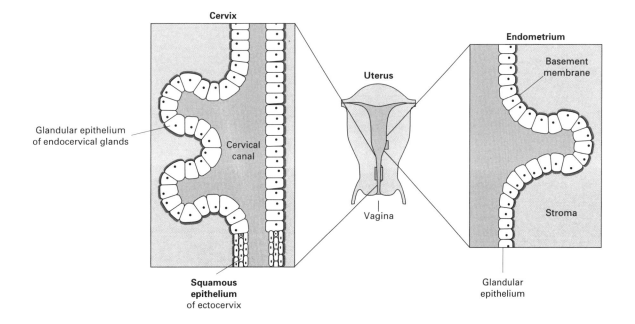

The major cause of cervical cancer is infection with HPV16 and HPV18 (see Table 4.2), which is transmitted by intercourse. Vaccines against the causal agents have been very successful in reducing the incidence of this cancer. It is likely that vaccination will greatly reduce the occurrence of this cancer in the future.

Endometrium

- Mostly adenocarcinomas (95%) of the epithelial cells, sarcomas (5%).

- Lifetime risk of getting endometrial cancer: 1 in 120.

- Five-year survival: 83%.

- Risk factors: oestrogen unopposed by progestins (oestrogen-replacement therapy), obesity, history of infertility, early menarche, late menopause, combined oral contraceptive pill (reduces risk; see Figure 13.2).

- Metastasis: myometrial and cervical invasion.

Good prognosis, as endometrial cancer is detected early because of associated menstrual problems.

Glossary

Acquired resistance: drug resistance resulting from previous drug exposure.

Adjuvant chemotherapy: chemotherapy given at the time of surgery or radiotherapy.

Adjuvant therapy: treatment given in addition to the major type of therapy.

Alkylating agent: electrophilic chemical that alkylates nucleic acids; carcinogenic and used in chemotherapy.

Allele: gene on one chromosome that has a homologue on the other chromosome of a diploid cell.

Anaplasia: lack of differentiated features.

Anchorage dependence: property of cells that require a substrate on which to grow. Cells are described as anchorage independent if substrate is not necessary (suspension growth).

Aneuploid: inexact multiple of normal DNA (chromosome) content.

Angiogenesis: growth of new blood vessels.

Angiogenic factors: peptides that favour the development of new blood vessels.

Anti-angiogenic factors: substances that favour the destruction of new blood vessels.

Antigen: molecule capable of generating an immune response.

Antimetabolite: chemotherapeutic drug that blocks metabolic pathways.

Anti-oncogene: poor alternative term for a tumour suppressor gene (see Chapter 5).

Apoptosis: active cell death (suicide) that requires new gene expression for its initiation.

Apoptosome: protein complex containing protease responsible for final stage of apoptosis.

Ascitic fluid: peritoneal fluid; can contain cells.

Athymic mouse: *see* Nude mouse.

Autocrine: secretion of regulatory molecules that function on the producing cell.

Autosome: chromosome that is not one of the sex chromosomes.

B-cell: lymphocyte capable of being activated to produce antibodies (see Chapter 4).

Benign: a tumour that is not malignant (see Table 3.2).

Biological response modifiers: heterogeneous group of chemicals that influence cells of the immune system and affect other cells. Include interferons, interleukins and tumour necrosis factor.

Cachexia: body wasting associated with advanced cancer.

Cadherins: family of calcium-dependent molecules concerned with cell–cell adhesion.

Cancer: unregulated growth that is invasive and capable of spreading elsewhere (metastasis).

Carcinogen: agent capable of causing cancer.

Carcinogenesis: processes involved in the production of a cancer.

Carcinoma: epithelial cell cancer (see Table 3.3).

Carcinoma *in situ*: early stage of cancer that has not invaded its surroundings.

Case–control study: epidemiological method in which people with one characteristic are compared retrospectively with people without that feature.

cDNA: DNA sequence complementary to an mRNA.

Cell cycle: cycle of events required for cell multiplication.

Chimera: mixed function/cell type.

Chromatin: nuclear DNA plus its attached proteins.

Chromosome: structural unit that contains genetic material.

Clone: group of cells derived from a single ancestor.

Coding region: part of a gene that is transcribed into mRNA and codes for amino acids.

Codon: three-base sequence in DNA that codes for one amino acid.

Cohort study: prospective epidemiological study in which the characteristics of a group of people are followed over a period of time.

Colony-stimulating factors (CSFs): growth factors concerned specifically with haemopoiesis.

Contact inhibition: *see* Density regulation.

Cyclins: proteins expressed transiently at specific points in the cell cycle.

Cytokines: peptides concerned with communications between cells.

Cytostatic: agent that stops the growth of cells.

Cytotoxic: agent that kills cells.

Density regulation: process in which cells stop proliferating when they contact adjacent cells (contact inhibition).

Differentiation: development of specialist function by a cell.

Diploid: describes normal DNA content of cells with a double complement of each chromosome.

Disseminated: a cancer consisting of dispersed cells, e.g. leukaemia.

Domain: region of a protein serving one specific function.

Dominant: a mutation that overcomes the influence of the other allele in a diploid cell. Change that results in a gain of function (see Table 5.1).

Dominant-negative: a dominant mutation that has a negative effect on function (see Table 5.1).

Endocrine: chemical signals carried to the target cells by the bloodstream.

Enhancer: DNA sequence in regulatory region of a gene that is activated by appropriate DNA-binding proteins (transcription factors) (see Figure 5.1).

Epigenetic: regulation of gene activity by means other than altering gene structure.

Epitope: region of an antigen that is recognised by an antibody.

Exons: transcribed regions of a gene that are translated into protein (see Chapter 5).

Extravasation: escape of cancer cells from blood vessels and lymphatics during metastasis.

G_0, G_1, G_2: phases of the cell cycle (see Chapter 9).

Gatekeeper gene: gene in which a functional change is essential for carcinogenesis.

Gene: DNA containing regulatory and coding sequences for one protein (see Chapter 5).

Genotoxic: an agent that damages DNA.

Genotype: genetic (DNA) make-up of a cell.

Germ cell: sperm or egg whose genetic complement can be passed to children.

Grade: histological classification of a cancer based on mitoses, nuclear shape and differentiation (see Chapter 12).

Growth factor: secreted polypeptide that regulates growth. Usually stimulatory but can be inhibitory.

Haemopoietic cells: cells that will form blood cells.

Haploid: half the normal DNA content. Single complement of chromosomes.

Heterodimer: dimer (protein) composed of dissimilar subunits (see Chapter 5).

Heterozygous: having different alleles of one gene.

Homodimer: dimer (protein) composed of similar subunits (see Chapter 5).

Homologous recombination: recombination between similar regions of DNA base sequence on each allele.

Homozygous: having the same alleles of one gene.

Hyperplasia: increased cell number.

Hypertrophy: increased cell size.

Hypoxia: low oxygen level.

Immune surveillance: processes by which the immune system monitors the body for foreign antigens such as cancer cells.

Incidence: number of new cancers developing in a defined population over a defined time.

Initiation: initial stage of carcinogenesis.

Interferons: protective factors secreted by cells in response to viral or fungal infection.

Interleukins: cytokines concerned with haemopoiesis and other functions.

Interphase: period between mitoses.

Intravasation: entry of cancer cells into the bloodstream and lymphatics.

Intrinsic resistance: basic level of drug resistance of a cell.

Intron: gene sequences that are transcribed into RNA but removed before translation.

Invasion: spread into adjacent tissue.

Karyotype: chromosome complement analysed by size, shape and banding pattern of each chromosome.

Knock-out mice: mice in which both alleles of a gene have been deleted. Also called null or $^{-/-}$ mice (see Box 2.1)

Ligand: agent that binds to a receptor.

Linkage: proximity of two genes on a chromosome.

Loss of heterozygosity: loss of the second allele of a gene (see Table 5.1).

M phase (M): mitosis phase of the cell cycle.

Malignant: tumour cancer cells that invade adjacent tissues and metastasise (see Table 3.2).

Mesenchyme: bone, fat, connective tissue and blood vessels derived from embryonic mesoderm.

Metaplasia: reversible replacement of one normal cell type with another.

Metastasis: process by which cancers escape to other parts of the body.

Mitosis: phase of the cell cycle when chromosomes are visible under a microscope.

Mitotic index: percentage of cells in mitosis.

Mutation: a heritable change in the genetic material.

Necrosis: cell death due to membrane disruption and release of lytic enzymes. Does not require RNA or protein synthesis.

Neoadjuvant therapy: chemotherapy given as a primary treatment.

Neoplasia: new growth of any type; includes cancers and benign growths.

Non-genotoxic carcinogen: carcinogen that does not damage DNA.

Nude mouse: genetically athymic mouse that has no cell-mediated immunity. Used experimentally as a host for human tumours.

Oligomers: multiple subunits.

Oncogene: a gene whose protein product contributes to carcinogenesis. Mutations relevant to carcinogenesis are dominant. Normal cellular oncogene is abbreviated to *c-onc* and viral oncogene to *v-onc* (see Chapter 5).

Overall survival: period from first diagnosis to death.

Paracrine: secretion of growth factors by one cell type that influences a nearby cell of a different type.

Phenotype: the combination of characteristics expressed by a cell (organism).

Pleural effusion: liquid plus cells in the space between the pleural membranes of the lung.

Ploidy: DNA (chromosome) content of a cell.

Primary cancer: site of first formation of a cancer.

Prognosis: future outlook for a patient.

Prognostic factor: factor that helps define prognosis.

Progression: changes that result in increased aggressiveness (dedifferentiation) of a cancer.

Promotion: stage of carcinogenesis after initiation.

Promotor: (1) agent that promotes carcinogenesis; (2) regulatory region of a gene that initiates transcription.

Proteasome: ubiquitin-containing complex responsible for selective degradation of individual proteins.

Proto-oncogene: gene that, as a result of mutation, can become an oncogene (see Chapter 5).

Provirus: viral DNA in host genome that can be transcribed into an RNA virus.

Purine: adenine or guanine base, or derivative thereof.

Pyrimidine: cytosine, uracil or thymine base, or derivative thereof.

Recessive: describes a gene whose function is lost as a result of mutation (see Table 5.1).

Relapse: reappearance of a cancer.

Relapse-free survival: period between first diagnosis and appearance of secondary growths.

Relative risk: risk of developing a cancer in one group compared with that in a control group.

Remission: decline in cancer size as a result of treatment.

Replisome: complex responsible for DNA synthesis.

Repressor gene: *see* Tumour suppressor gene.

Restriction fragment length polymorphism (RFLP): DNA sequences cut with restriction nucleases that are different lengths in different individuals.

Retrovirus: RNA virus.

S phase: phase of the cell cycle in which DNA is synthesised.

Sarcoma: mesenchymal cell cancer.

Screening: the testing of a normal population to detect preclinical/clinical disease.

Secondary growth: a metastasis or local recurrence.

Selectins: molecules concerned with cell–substrate and cell–cell adhesion.

Silencer: regulatory DNA sequences that bind appropriate proteins to produce gene inactivation (see Chapter 5).

Somatic cell: a non-germ cell, so genetic complement cannot be passed to children.

Stage: tumour classification based on size, nodal status and metastasis (see Chapter 12).

Stem cell: cell capable of an unlimited number of divisions.

Suppressor gene: *see* Tumour suppressor gene.

T-cell: class of lymphocyte with various subtypes (see Chapter 4).

Telomerase: enzyme that extends telomere length (see Chapter 9).

Telomere: repeated DNA sequences at the end of a chromosome (see Chapter 8).

Therapeutic index: ratio of maximal tolerated dose to minimal effective anticancer dose.

Totipotent cell: cell that has not differentiated and is capable of developing along several alternative pathways.

Transcription: RNA synthesis from DNA (see Figure 5.1).

Transcription factor: protein that regulates transcription (see Chapter 5).

Transfection: transfer of foreign DNA into cells by experimental techniques such as micro-injection.

Transformation: change of cell characteristics from normal to more like those of a cancer.

Transgenic mouse: mouse carrying experimentally introduced genes in every cell of the body.

Transition: mutation that changes a purine to another purine (adenine/guanine) or a pyrimidine to another pyrimidine (cytidine/thymine).

Translation: protein synthesis from RNA (see Figure 5.1).

Transversion: mutation that changes a purine to a pyrimidine, or vice versa.

Tumour: growth that can be benign or malignant.

Tumour antigen: tumour cell antigen capable of eliciting an immune response.

Tumour marker: antigen that provides prognostic information about a cancer.

Tumour suppressor gene: gene that inhibits malignant changes in a cell.

Index

Notes: When the cited pages contain relevant figures or tables, an asterisk (★) is included. Where necessary, individual cancers or genes have been classified into clinical, gene or other subcategories. Clinical includes natural history, epidemiology and pathology details. Gene contains references to familial cancers. The sections designated 'other' contain functional (cellular) details.